Uncommon Ulcers of the Extremities

Ajay K. Khanna • Satyendra Kumar Tiwary
Editors

Uncommon Ulcers of the Extremities

Springer

Editors
Ajay K. Khanna
Institute of Medical Sciences
Department of Surgery
Banaras Hindu University
Varanasi, India

Satyendra Kumar Tiwary
Institute of Medical Sciences
Department of General Surgery
Banaras Hindu University
Varanasi, India

ISBN 978-981-99-1784-6 ISBN 978-981-99-1782-2 (eBook)
https://doi.org/10.1007/978-981-99-1782-2

This Springer imprint is published by the registered company Springer Nature Singapore Pte Ltd.
The registered company address is: 152 Beach Road, #21-01/04 Gateway East, Singapore 189721, Singapore

Paper in this product is recyclable.

Preface

Surgical care has been part of human history as conflicts, battles, injuries and trauma have been associated with its evolution. Ulcers or wounds are the most ancient surgical components, which is evident in their manifestation, but chronic wounds have been the tendo-achilles due to complexity and undefined multi-aetiological association with some of the rare causes missing in the workup, sometimes leading to high morbidity and longer healing time. Nearly 6 years ago, we published the book *Ulcers of the Lower Extremity* (2016) by Springer (Eds. AK Khanna & SK Tiwary), which was a milestone in the scientific literature on wound management. After decades of clinical practice in surgical patient care in a tropical country where a large number of patients present with wounds, there was a need for a book on uncommon ulcers, considering the abundance of academic resources in our surgical journey thus far covered. Considering the focussed and targeted approach for diseases in the twenty-first century, this idea of a book about uncommon ulcers is the next part of our previous publication and it was in mind, vision, observations, and discussions leading to final shape after years of work by us.

The last century witnessed radical changes in approach, understanding and outcomes in many fields, including surgical science . Following wound care protocols after understanding the aetiology and implementing targeted therapies to enhance healing and minimise morbidity are essential and recent developments. Various components and diversified aspects of diseases have seen new fields of developments, with molecular, genetic, immunological, inflammatory, degenerative and neoplastic aspects becoming more defined than ever before and uncommon ulcers have also seen more lucid information. Less prevalent conditions of uncommon ulcers may be missed during aetiological assessment, leading to improper treatment sometimes. Patients with uncommon ulcers are frequently referred from one department to another such as plastic surgery, general surgery, vascular surgery, rheumatology, haematology, oncology, orthopaedics, neurology, physical medicine and rehabilitation, considering the complex clinical condition and inadequate assessment of the condition within a single speciality. The book on uncommon ulcers will serve as a bridge to fill the gaps in information, which will facilitate a better understanding of the disease and management subsequently.

This book has been compiled with contents that aim to address the queries regarding *Uncommon Ulcers of the Extremities*. It fills the gap in scientific knowledge and serves as a valuable source of information for General Surgeons, Plastic

Surgeons, Vascular surgeons, Oncologists, Orthopaedicians, Family Physicians, trainees and fellows across different disciplines when they encounter cases of Uncommon Ulcers. Our earnest desire is that this book becomes a valuable source for understanding and managing the complex clinical condition of Uncommon Ulcers of the Extremities to students, trainees, fellows, nurses and clinicians who may face challenges in wound management at times.

We acknowledge the help of Dr. Naren Agarwal, Ms. Jagjit Kaur Saini, Ms. Vijaya Shuruthi Chandran and Mr. Ejaz Ahmad from Springer Nature to bring out the book in the present form with their assistance and valuable inputs. We are indebted to our family members Anuradha, Divya and Soumya, Rishi, and Hema, Apoorva and Advaita for providing us all moral support and encouragement.

We dedicate this book to all the patients with chronic wounds managed during our entire career, as they have been our resource and inspiration in managing this complex clinical condition.

We conclude our words with the commitment that *Uncommon Ulcers of the Extremities* is a part of our endeavour to search the truth about uncommon wounds. The pursuit of truth has always been an integral part of the journey of human civilization, serving as the cornerstone of science, medicine and religion, which has been said almost 3500 years back by Aadikavi Valmiki, First Great Poet of Ancient Language Sanskrit in his Epic "Valmiki Ramayana".

सत्यमेवेश्वरो लोके सत्यं पद्माश्रिता सदा।
सत्यमूलानिसर्वाणिसत्यान्नास्तिपरंपदम्।।(वाल्मीकि रामायण2.109.13।।)

(Truth is God. The goddess of wealth always takes refuge in truth. Truth is the root of everything. It is supreme and there is nothing above it)

Varanasi, Uttar Pradesh, India Ajay K. Khanna
Varanasi, Uttar Pradesh, India Satyendra Kumar Tiwary

Contents

Editors and Contributors

About the Editors

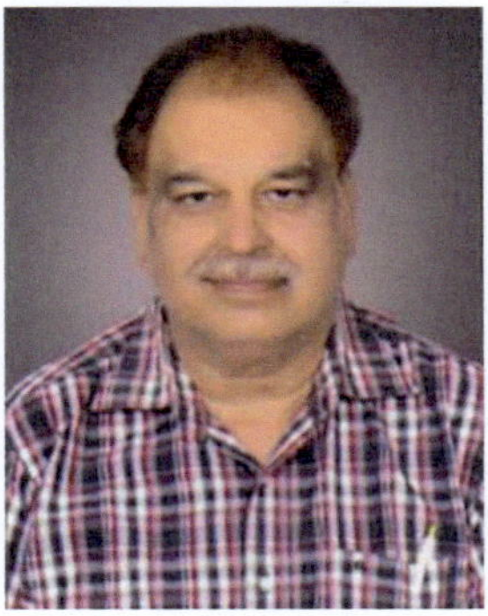

Ajay K. Khanna MS, FRCS, FAMS, FACS, FICS, FACRSI, MNAMS, MBA, DSc, FRSTMH, FAIS, FUICC, FUWAI, FFIM, FMAS, PDCR, is Professor of Surgery and Ex Head of the Department of General Surgery at the Institute of Medical Sciences, Banaras Hindu University (BHU), Varanasi, India. Prof. Khanna has a teaching experience of more than 42 years and has been awarded with Young Outstanding Teacher and Eminent Surgical Teacher. He is the examiner for MBBS, MS, BDS, DNB and FNB in minimal access surgery and M.Ch in endocrine surgery. He has guided more than 50 theses for MS course. He is fellow/member of 33 societies. He regularly started vascular surgery in the Department of Surgery at BHU. Prof. Khanna has delivered more than 100 CME lectures, more than 200 guest lectures in various national and international conference in India, UK, USA, Japan, Poland, Egypt, etc., and presented more than 350 presentations in various national and international conferences. He has more than 370 publications in various national and international journals and 70 chapters in various books to his credit. He is the editor of five books on various subjects. He served as President of Varanasi Surgical Society, President of Uttar Pradesh chapter of the Association of Surgeons of India (ASI), Governing Council Member of ASI, Vice President of ACRSI and Executive Member of UP chapter of ASI, AMASI, VAI, ATVSI and IASO. He has delivered more than 16 orations. He has received various fellowship awards, viz. Clinical Research Fellowship and Registrar at the Department of Surgery, University of Wales College of Medicine, Cardiff, Wales, UK; Metrogyl Travelling Fellowship by Gastrointestinal Research Society; Commonwealth Scholarship; and Indo-Czechoslovakian Cultural Exchange Program, among others. Prof. Khanna's name appears in Asia's Who's Who reference book, Marquis Who's Who in the World, Five Hundred Leaders of Influence, International Directory of Distinguished Leadership, Man of the Year and American Biographical Institute, and he received several other awards. He is fellow of the Royal College of Surgeons of England, fellow of United Writers' Association, fellow of the Indian National Science Academy, fellow of the American College of Surgeons, fellow of the International College of Surgeons, fellow of the Association of Colorectal Society of India, fellow of the Royal Society of Tropical Medicine, fellow of the Association of Surgeons of India, fellow of Union Internationale Cancer controlle and fellow of Minimal Access Surgeons of India. Prof. Khanna was the joint editor of *Indian Journal of Surgery*. He has organised more than 30 conferences and workshops. He was the Chief Inspector for quality assurance review of the Department of Clinical Surgical Sciences, the University of the West Indies, St Augustine Campus, Trinidad and Tobago, and is in the Expert Selection Committee of UPSC, Uttar Pradesh; BPKIMS, Dharan, Nepal; Aligarh Muslim University, Aligarh; KGMU Lucknow; Public Service Commission, J&K; MCI Inspector; DNB Inspector; IGIMS, Patna; PGIMER, Chandigarh; and the Indian Institute of Information Technology, Allahabad.

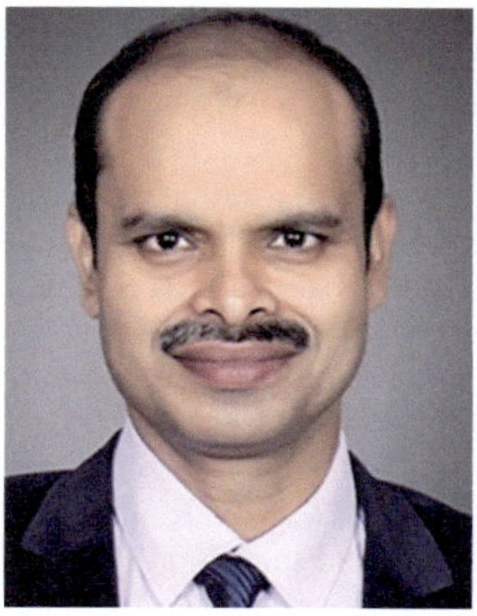

Satyendra Kumar Tiwary MBBS (Hons), MS (Surgery), FMAS, FICS, FCLS, is Professor of General Surgery at the Institute of Medical Sciences, Banaras Hindu University, Varanasi, India. He graduated and postgraduated from Patna Medical College, Patna, India. Dr. Tiwary has around 130 publications in various national and international journals and has delivered numerous oral, poster presentations and invited lectures. He has edited five books (three international books from Springer ***Ulcers of the Lower Extremity*** **(Springer 2016),** ***Vascular Malformations*** **(Springer 2021),** ***Approach to Lower Limb Oedema*** **(Springer 2022)** and another book ***COVID-19: Challenges Ahead*** published by CBS in 2020 and one book ***Annual Updates in Surgery*** in 2020). He has published 15 chapters in different books. He has keen interest in academics and research with special interest in phlebology, vascular medicine, wound management and lower limb pathology.

Contributors

Sandeep Agarwal Institute of Vascular and Endovascular Sciences, Sir Ganga Ram Hospital, New Delhi, India

Teresa Alonso-León Division of Dermatology, Hospital General "Dr. Manuel Gea González", Mexico City, Mexico

Disha Arora Department of Medicine, IMS, BHU, Varanasi, India

Tuhina Banerjee Department of Microbiology, Institute of Medical Sciences, Banaras Hindu University, Varanasi, India

Sankha Shubhra Chakrabarti Department of Geriatric Medicine, Institute of Medical Sciences, Banaras Hindu University, Varanasi, Uttar Pradesh, India

Jaya Chakravarty Department of Medicine, Institute of Medical sciences, Banaras Hindu University, Varanasi, India

Paulo Ricardo Criado Dermatology Department, Hospital das Clinicas da Faculdade de Medicina da, Universidade de Sao Paulo, Sao Paulo, Brazil

Faculdade de Ciências Médicas de Santos (Fundação Lusíada—UNILUS), Santos, SP, Brazil

Valentina Dini Department of Dermatology, University of Pisa, Pisa, Italy

Shantonu Kumar Ghosh Department of Vascular Surgery, National Institute of Cardiovascular Diseases and Hospital, Dhaka, Bangladesh

Madhuri Gore Former Chief of Surgery, LTMMC and LTMGH, Consultant Surgeon, Dr. Gores' Clinic, Mumbai, India

Sanjeev Kumar Gupta Department of General Surgery, Institute of Medical Sciences, Banaras Hindu University, Varanasi, India

D. Harnanan Department of Clinical Surgical Sciences, University of the West Indies, St. Augustine, Trinidad and Tobago, West Indies, Trinidad

P. Harnarayan Department of Clinical Surgical Sciences, University of the West Indies, St. Augustine, Trinidad and Tobago, West Indies, Trinidad

Jai Prakash Jaiswal Norvic Int'l Hospital, Kathmandu, Nepal

Abhinay Jayanthi Department of Anaesthesiology, Institute of Medical Sciences, Banaras Hindu University, Varanasi, India

Upinder Kaur Department of Pharmacology, Institute of Medical Sciences, Banaras Hindu University, Varanasi, Uttar Pradesh, India

Ayman Khalil AMC Hospital, Hurghada, Red Sea, Egypt

Ajay K. Khanna Department of Surgery, Institute of Medical Sciences, Banaras Hindu University, Varanasi, India

Divya Khanna Department of Preventive Oncology, Mahamana Pandit Madan Mohan Malviya Cancer Centre, Tata Memorial Centre, Varanasi, India

Rahul Khanna Department of Surgery, Institute of Medical Sciences, Banaras Hindu University, Varanasi, India

Ritika Khanna Department of Dermatology, Institute of Medical Sciences, Banaras Hindu University, Varanasi, UP, India

Seema Khanna Department of Surgery, Institute of Medical Sciences, Banaras Hindu University, Varanasi, India

Soumya Khanna Department of Surgery, Institute of Medical Sciences, Banaras Hindu University, Varanasi, India

Puneet Kumar Department of Surgery, Institute of Medical Sciences, Banaras Hindu University, Varanasi, India

Rohit Kumar Singh Department of Surgery, Institute of Medical Sciences, Banaras Hindu University, Varanasi, India

Adriana Lozano-Platonoff Division of Dermatology, Wound and Ostomy Care Center, Hospital General "Dr. Manuel Gea González", Mexico City, Mexico

Shomita S. Mathew-Steiner McGowan Institute for Regenerative Medicine, Department of Surgery, University of Pittsburgh School of Medicine, Pittsburgh, PA, USA

Alessandra Michelucci Department of Dermatology, University of Pisa, Pisa, Italy

Himanshu Mishra Department of Radiotherapy and Radiation Medicine, Institute of Medical Sciences, Banaras Hindu University, Varanasi, India

Ritusha Mishra Department of Radiotherapy and Radiation Medicine, Institute of Medical Sciences, Banaras Hindu University, Varanasi, India

Harikrishna K. R. Nair Wound Care Unit, Kuala Lumpur Hospital, Kuala Lumpur, Malaysia

Anisha Najeeb Department of Dermatology and Venereology, Institute of Medical Sciences, Banaras Hindu University, Varanasi, India

V. Naraynsingh Department of Clinical Surgical Sciences, University of the West Indies, St. Augustine, Trinidad and Tobago, West Indies

Varadraj V. Pai Department of Dermatology, Goa Medical College, Bambolim, Goa, India

Abhishek Pandey Department of Medicine, IMS, BHU, Varanasi, India

Meenakshi Pandey Department of Paediatrics, Institute of Medical Sciences, Banaras Hindu University, Varanasi, India

Sandeep Raj Pandey Norvic Int'l Hospital, Kathmandu, Nepal

Rajniti Prasad Department of Paediatrics, Institute of Medical Sciences, Banaras Hindu University, Varanasi, India

Tulika Rai Department of Dermatology, Institute of Medical Sciences, Banaras Hindu University, Varanasi, India

Angampally Rajeev Heart and Vascular Care of Georgia, Newnan, GA, USA

Amrita Rath Department of Anesthesiology, Institute of Medical Sciences, Banaras Hindu University, Varanasi, India

Marco Romanelli Department of Dermatology, University of Pisa, Pisa, Italy

Paolo Romanelli Department of Dermatology and Cutaneous Surgery, University of Miami Miller School of Medicine, Miami, FL, USA

D. Saadoun Department of Internal Medicine and Clinical Immunology, Sorbonne Universités, AP-HP, Groupe Hospitalier Pitié-Salpêtrière, Paris, France

Chandan K. Sen McGowan Institute for Regenerative Medicine, Department of Surgery, University of Pittsburgh School of Medicine, Pittsburgh, PA, USA

Swati Sharma Department of Microbiology, Institute of Medical Sciences, Banaras Hindu University, Varanasi, India

Kanhaiya Singh McGowan Institute for Regenerative Medicine, Department of Surgery, University of Pittsburgh School of Medicine, Pittsburgh, PA, USA

Priyanka Singh Department of Microbiology, Institute of Medical Sciences, Banaras Hindu University, Varanasi, India

Sanjay Singh Department of Dermatology and Venereology, Institute of Medical Sciences, Banaras Hindu University, Varanasi, India

Satyendra Kumar Tiwary Department of General Surgery, Institute of Medical Sciences, Banaras Hindu University, Varanasi, India

M. Vautier Department of Internal Medicine and Clinical Immunology, Sorbonne Universités, AP-HP, Groupe Hospitalier Pitié-Salpêtrière, Paris, France

Chandraprakash Verma Department of Radiotherapy and Radiation Medicine, Institute of Medical Sciences, Banaras Hindu University, Varanasi, India

Vandana Yadav Department of Dermatology and Venereology, Institute of Medical Sciences, Banaras Hindu University, Varanasi, India

Approach to a Case of Ulcer of Extremity

1

Ajay K. Khanna and Soumya Khanna

An ulcer is a break in the skin or mucus membrane caused by the microscopic death of tissues. Ulcers can occur in any portion of the body, at any age, and in either gender. Ulcers can be either acute or persistent. Acute ulcers normally heal quickly, but chronic ulceration occurs when the ulcer lasts longer than 6 weeks and shows no signs of healing after three or more months. Ulcers are lesions that have a "full thickness depth", and chronic ulcers heal slowly. Skin ulceration may be extremely painful and even fatal in severe cases. Chronic ulcers are frequently difficult to heal and may be related with a variety of psychological issues. It has a negative impact on one's quality of life since it is connected with discomfort, swelling, and discharge that can be foul-smelling or bleeding. They may be linked with local infection, systemic infection, bacteraemia, or even septicaemia, and need powerful antibiotics, repeated debridement, and even amputation to preserve the patient's life since it may cause death. Wound care and therapy are extremely difficult for the patient, society, and the treating team, and can be quite costly. The patient may experience psychological stress, helplessness, and sadness. Because the patient's movement is limited, social contacts and the difficulties in carrying out day-to-day activities exacerbate the disease.

There are several reasons of persistent ulceration in the extremities, particularly the lower extremities. Traumatic, venous, arterial, neurogenic, tropical, diabetic, blood dyscrasia, and other non-specific ulcerations exist, as do particular ulcers such as TB, syphilis, actinomycosis, and others, as well as malignant ulcers such as squamous cell carcinoma, basal cell carcinoma, and melanoma. Most cutaneous ulcers of the lower extremities are caused by venous insufficiency, arterial insufficiency, or neuropathy (particularly of diabetic origin), and they are often easy to

A. K. Khanna (✉) · S. Khanna
Department of Surgery, Institute of Medical Sciences, Banaras Hindu University, Varanasi, India

A. K. Khanna, S. K. Tiwary (eds.), *Uncommon Ulcers of the Extremities*,
https://doi.org/10.1007/978-981-99-1782-2_1

detect. Ulcers linked with or caused by systemic inflammatory diseases, on the other hand, are frequently a major diagnostic and therapeutic problem.

1.1 Prevalence

Ulceration is becoming more common as the population grows, as are risk factors like as atherosclerosis, smoking, obesity, and diabetes. Chronic ulceration of the lower limbs is a somewhat common ailment in adults, and ulcers are often characterised by discomfort, friable granulation tissue, bad odour, and wound degradation despite healing. As a result, there is psychological suffering, social distress, and significant financial commitment. Because leg ulcers are caused by a variety of reasons, a multidisciplinary approach is necessary to determine the aetiology, a definite diagnosis, and the best therapy. An accurate diagnosis is required to avoid incorrect therapy, which may induce wound worsening or injury to the patient. Chronic leg ulcer (CLU) is said to affect nearly every part of everyday life: pain is common, sleep is frequently disrupted, mobility and work ability are limited, and it is a costly business. It eventually restricts social activities owing to fear of damage and a bad body image. Chronic leg ulcers (CLU) is typically linked with severe morbidity, high healthcare costs, lost productivity, and decreased quality of life [1]. CLUs afflict 0.6–3% of people over the age of 60, rising to more than 5% of those over the age of 80. CLU is a prevalent cause of morbidity, with a population frequency ranging from 1.9% to 13.1% [2]. While there have been few research on the epidemiology of chronic wounds in India, one study estimated the incidence to be 4.5 per 1000 people. The rate of acute wounds was more than doubled, reaching 10.5 per 1000 people [3].

1.2 Relevant Points of Interest

A thorough history is required to establish a conclusive diagnosis of the condition. The crucial details are where the disease began, how far the lesion progressed, if it was associated with pain or fever, any therapy used, and the outcome. Any systemic condition, such as hypertension or diabetes, must be investigated. A medical history of connective tissue illnesses, heart disease, renal disease, inflammatory bowel disease, hepatitis, coagulopathies, past pregnancy, and cancer may point to a specific diagnosis. It is critical to have a smoking and drinking history.

Physical examination: The patient should be evaluated as a whole, not only the hole (ulcer). It is critical to pay close attention to the surrounding skin as well as other regions of the integument such as the oral mucosa and nails. Cutaneous signs such as livedo reticularis (a netlike violaceous staining encircling a paler core region), palpable purpura, petechiae, nail splinter haemorrhages, and/or mouth ulcers support an inflammatory origin of the ulceration. Lipodermatosclerosis, which often manifests as redness, induration, and darkening of the lower extremity skin, aids in the diagnosis of venous insufficiency. Pulse, blood pressure, and neurological tests are required to rule out arterial insufficiency, venous illness, and/or neuropathy as reasons of the ulceration. The ulcer's edge and floor are crucial indicators of the ulcer's healing potential. Necrosis and the presence of an eschar, for example, indicate a thrombotic disease. Violaceous margins signify pyoderma gangrenosum; a reddish yellow plaque encircling the ulcer indicates necrobiosis lipoidica diabeticorum (NLD), which is commonly linked with diabetes. Swelling, infection, irritating contact dermatitis from wound drainage or dressings, and allergic contact dermatitis from topical treatments and dressings are all common complications of ulcers. A foul-smelling ulcer with purulent discharge is most likely secondary infected or highly colonised and will benefit from systemic/topical antibiotics or topical antiseptic therapy. Necrosis and eschar development in a patient with normal pulses might benefit from surgical debridement, especially in diabetics. Leg oedema should be treated with compression when blood flow is not jeopardised. In addition to ulcer size, using a score system may be a helpful objective approach to track progress. As always, the wound bed must be adjusted in accordance with known wound bed preparation principles in order to promote healing and make available therapies more effective. Pain management is essential for ensuring treatment adherence; referral to a pain management provider may be required at times.

It is equally necessary to provide wound care with the aim of maximising wound healing by reducing oedema, managing the bacterial load, and minimising irritating or allergic contact dermatitis. Treatment of the underlying condition will frequently improve the ulceration. Because these disorders are rare, no particular recommendations have been produced. Treatment should be carefully considered, with an emphasis on reducing potential problems. To handle these patients, a multidisciplinary approach is required, and consults with diverse specialists should be the norm. If the ulcers do not respond to therapy, the diagnosis and management should be reconsidered [4]. The time principle (T: Tissue Debridement, I: Inflammation/ Infection, M: Moisture Balance, E: Edge) is critical for wound healing in order to prepare the wound bed for future grafting or flap repair.

1.3 Common Ulcerations Causes (Table 1.1)

Chronic venous insufficiency (70%): Stasis ulcers in the Gaiters region surrounding the medial or lateral malleolus are common in primary or secondary varicose veins. These ulcers are typically superficial, never penetrate deep fascia, and are often painless unless infected. Brown haemosiderin staining of the lower thigh is rather prevalent. It is also possible to have prominent veins, venous eczema, oedema, and lipodermatosclerosis. Ulcers will not heal unless sufficient care is taken, particularly four-layer bandaging and attention to the refluxing section [5].

Chronic vascular insufficiency (10%): Arterial ulcers can occur on the foot, heel, or toe. It can arise in adults with Buerger's disease or in the elderly with atherosclerosis. These ulcers are quite painful, especially when they are raised. Punctured ulcer and penetrated deep fascia skin that is cold, white, glossy and hairless, indicating persistent Ischaemia. 0.9 is the ankle-brachial pressure index is usually less than 0.9. Pulses are weak or non-existent.

Table 1.1 Causes of extremity ulcers

Vascular	Venous, arterial, lymphatic, vasculitis
Metabolic	Diabetes mellitus, gout, necrobiosis lipoidica, porphyria, Hemocystinuria, Prolidase deficiency, hyperoxaluria, ulcerative colitis, avitaminosis, calcinosis
Infection	Pyogenic, osteomyelitis, tuberculosis, syphilis, tropical diseases fungal diseases, leishmaniasis, histoplasmosis, herpes, lupus vulgaris, amoebiasis, chromoblastomycosis, coccidiomycosis, viral, Corona
Traumatic	Pressure ulcers, radiation damage, thermal burns, decubitus ulcers, iatrogenic
Neoplastic	Basal cell carcinoma, squamous cell carcinoma, melanoma, lymphoma, Marjolin's ulcer, Kaposi sarcoma, sarcoma, Bowen disease
Hypertensive	Martorell
Connective tissue disorders	Inflammatory bowel disorders, pyoderma gangrenosum, rheumatoid arthritis, scleroderma, systemic lupus erythematous, pemphigoid, dermatomyositis, Sjogren's syndrome, polyarteritis nodosa
Haematological	Sickle cell anaemia, Leukaemia, thrombocytosis, thalassemia, spherocytosis, G-6 PD deficiency, thrombocytopenia, granulocytopenia, Polycythaemia
Neuropathic	Diabetes, spinal abnormalities, leprosy, nerve damage
Other causes	Drugs, cryofibrinogenaemia, antiphospholipid syndrome, coagulopathies, calciphylaxis, cholesterol embolisation, necrobiosis Lipoidica, erythema nodosum

Neuropathic ulceration (neurogenic/trophic ulcer): A neuropathic ulcer develops on the anaesthetised skin. Diabetes, spinal abnormalities, leprosy, nerve damage, and other conditions can all produce neuropathy. Ulcers form on pressure sites such as the heel, first and fifth metatarsals, and the gluteal area. Unnoticed damage might result in a painless ulceration. Because they penetrate deep into the bones, they are also known as Perforating Ulcers.

Tropical ulcer: It occurs in tropical nations and is caused by malnutrition, a lack of immunity, humid environments, trauma, or insect bite. Bacteroides induce the infection, which begins as a pustule and progresses to ulceration, which spreads swiftly and kills surrounding tissue (Phagedenic Ulcer).

Diabetic foot ulcers are generally caused by a combination of factors. They might be caused by neuropathy, bacterial infection, or atherosclerosis-related ischaemia. Diabetes risk factors include males above the age of 50, diabetes for more than 10 years, uncontrolled diabetes, peripheral neuropathy, aberrant foot architecture, peripheral vascular disorders, smoking, hypertension, and dyslipidaemia.

Ulcers caused by pressure: Pressure ulcers, often known as bed sores, are produced by unrelieved pressure. Occur on bony prominences, sacrum, and heel, especially in paralysed, debilitated, or bedridden individuals. Frequently infected, resulting in septicaemia and osteomyelitis.

Hypertensive ulceration, commonly known as Martorell ulcer, is caused by uncontrolled hypertension. Typically appear on the back of the lower thigh. More prevalent in females between the ages of 50 and 60. They are excruciatingly painful. A biopsy reveals thicker arteriolar walls.

Skin cancer manifests as a slow-growing plaque or nodule. The majority of skin cancers occur in sun-exposed areas. Skin malignancies that appear as ulceration in the extremities include basal cell carcinoma, squamous cell carcinoma, and melanomas. In HIV patients, sarcomatous lesions may show as ulceration as Kaposi sarcomas. Biopsy is used for diagnosis.

Inflammatory causes: Leg ulcers can be caused by inflammatory process. Inflammatory causes of leg ulcers can be difficult to identify and treat. If an inflammatory cause of leg ulceration is suspected, diagnostic tests may include a deep skin biopsy of the ulcer edge for histology, fungal/mycobacterial culture, direct immunofluorescence, CBC, CRP/ESR, c/p-ANCA, metabolic panel, protein electrophoresis and immunoglobulins, coagulation studies, antiphospholipid antibody, cryoglobulins, cryofibrinogen, ANA, complement, and hepatitis B/C serology.

Pyoderma gangrenosum: Pyoderma gangrenosum is an autoinflammatory condition that has been linked to IBD, rheumatoid arthritis, myeloid dysplasia, and gammopathy. A wide and deep ulcer expansion is typical. Ulcers are extremely painful, with a weakened necrotic edge, pustules, and a necrotic foundation. A non-specific or neutrophilic infiltration is seen on biopsy.

Small vessel vasculitis manifests as palpable purpura with haemorrhage, ischaemia, and infarction. Ulcers can form in vascular lesions. Ulcers are more common on the lower legs and ankles. A biopsy may reveal leukocytoclastic vasculitis.

Medium vessel vasculitis (e.g. polyarthritis, granulomatosis with polyangiitis) causes livedo reticularis, arterial nodules, and gangrene. Lower leg ulcers are often painful, punched-out, and irregular. A biopsy reveals vasculitis in medium-sized vessels.

Rheumatoid ulceration is caused by a combination of factors, including venous and arterial disease, diabetes, vasculitis, and unknown cause. They are excruciatingly painful. It usually results in an ulcer near the ankle. Other vasculitis symptoms include minor nail fold infarcts, digital ischaemia, scleritis, mononeuritis multiplex, pericarditis, pleuritis, fever, and weight loss. A biopsy taken from the ulcer's margin may reveal medium vessel vasculitis.

Necrobiosis lipoidica: In 50% of instances, necrobiosis lipoidica is related with type 1 diabetes. Plaques are yellow-red, atrophic, and telangiectatic. Plaques are most commonly encountered on the shins. Ulceration is extremely difficult to cure. Atrophic epidermis and dermal necrobiotic collagen are seen in the biopsy.

Systemic sclerosis. Fibrin-occlusive vasculopathy is caused by systemic sclerosis. Antiphospholipid antibodies are related with 50% of the cases. This frequently leads in bilateral, painful lower leg ulcers. Raynaud's phenomenon causes painful ischemic digital ulcerations.

Livedoid vasculopathy: Coagulation problems are related with livedoid vasculopathy. Ankles develop little painful superficial sores. Atrophie blanche may be present.

Skin necrosis caused by warfarin: Warfarin-induced skin necrosis occurs 3–10 days after starting warfarin medication. Ecchymosis develops suddenly and leads to a necrotic ulcer. A biopsy reveals intravascular thrombi but no vasculitis.

Heparin-induced necrosis: Heparin-induced necrosis occurs 4–12 days after the start of heparin treatment. Most, but not all, patients may experience heparin-induced thrombocytopenia. Platelet aggregates are seen intravascularly in biopsies.

Other types of coagulopathy: Ulceration can also be caused by antiphospholipid syndrome, protein S and protein C deficiency, and other factors. A necrotic ulcer develops from acute thrombosis. A biopsy reveals intravascular thrombi but no vasculitis.

Cholesterol emboli: Cholesterol emboli are frequently the result of an endovascular surgical operation or the start of anticoagulant medication (days to months later). Purpura, cyanosis, blue toes, digital gangrene, and painful subcutaneous lumps are among symptoms of Livedo reticularis. Fever, weight loss, myalgia, anaemia, and renal failure are examples of systemic symptoms. On histopathology, a biopsy reveals a biconvex needle-like gap in arteries.

Septic emboli are caused by endocarditis or septicaemia. It might be caused by a variety of species. Purpuric patches, pustules, haemorrhagic bullae, and splinter haemorrhages in the nails are all possible. Ulcers are often tiny and irregular, and they are most commonly found on the foot. A biopsy reveals minor blood vessel blockage and vasculitis.

Calciphylaxis is linked to chronic renal failure, secondary hyperparathyroidism, obesity, liver disease, systemic corticosteroids, diabetes, and coagulation abnormalities. It can be seen on the lower limbs, breasts, belly, and buttocks. Ulcers are deep, painful ulcerations that are preceded by tender, retiform purpura. A biopsy reveals vascular wall calcification, thrombosis, and infarction.

Cryofibrinogenaemia: Cryofibrinogenaemia has been linked to cancer, diabetes, connective tissue disease, and infection, although it is more commonly idiopathic. They might manifest itself as Livedo reticularis, purpura, ecchymosis, malaise, and fever. Typically, the condition manifests as a rapid onset of severe ischemic ulceration. Plasma cryofibrinogen levels are high. A biopsy revealed small and medium vessel vasculitis.

Cryoglobulinaemia is linked to connective tissue disorders, haematological malignancies, and hepatitis. Arthralgia and weakness are examples of systemic symptoms. Cold exposure or extended standing causes purpura. Cryoglobulins have been found in serum. A biopsy revealed small and medium vessel vasculitis.

Cocaine vasculopathy caused by levamisole: Occlusive vasculopathy can arise from cocaine laced with levamisole. It is similar to small vessel vasculitis.

It has been observed that ulcers caused by venous insufficiency account for 70% of leg ulcer presentations, arterial disease 10%, and ulcers of mixed origin 15%. The remaining 5% of leg ulcers are caused by less prevalent pathophysiological reasons, and this category of Unusual ulcers requires a lot of diagnostic and treatment Challenges [6, 7].

1.4 Step-Wise Approach

The first step in diagnosing a leg ulcer is to get a thorough history and evaluation of the patient. This should include general health status, social and occupational circumstances, past and current medical history of relevant diseases (such as deep vein thrombosis, diabetes, autoimmune disorders, inflammatory bowel disease, and connective tissue disease), skin condition, current vascular status, limb size and shape, and the history and status of the ulcer to be seen. Lower extremity discomfort, paraesthesia, anaesthesia, and claudication should all be discussed with the patient. It is critical to assess the length of the ulceration and if it is a new or recurring occurrence. Unless there is a neuropathic component, pain is a substantial issue for people with leg ulcers. As a result, the absence of pain implies a neuropathic origin. Patients should be questioned about their mobility as well. The clinical history of the ulcer may indicate its cause. Diabetes, hypertension, hyperlipidaemia, coronary artery disease, alcohol and cigarette use, thyroid, pulmonary, renal, neurologic, and rheumatic illnesses, peripheral vascular disease, deep vein thrombosis, and cutaneous variables such as cellulitis, trauma, and recent surgery are all things to rule out [8].

Pulse palpation and a search for symptoms of venous hypertension, such as varicose veins, haemosiderin pigmentation, varicose eczema, atrophie blanche, and lipodermatosclerosis, should be included for the leg examination. To rule out peripheral neuropathy, the range of hip, knee, and ankle mobility should be measured and sensation evaluated. The ulcer location, size, look, wound base, exudates level, and surrounding skin should all be examined. Pain, oedema, erythema, warmth, induration, discoloration, maceration, dryness, scarring from prior wounds, hair pattern, gangrenous digits, clubbing, cyanosis, capillary refill, and varicose veins should all be looked for in the surrounding area. It is critical to remember that venous and arterial illness can coexist in the same patient [9]. The Leg Ulcer Measurement Method (LUMT) is a validated tool for quantifying leg ulcer evaluation and tracking changes in wound condition over time [10]. Doppler tests detect arterial insufficiency; arterial duplex ultrasonography provides reliable anatomic and haemodynamic information on the location and extent of vascular disease (non-invasively). When required, magnetic resonance angiography, computer tomographic angiography, or digital subtraction angiography can provide more comprehensive anatomic information for treatment planning.

In patients with ulcers, blood tests such as a complete blood count, erythrocyte sedimentation rate, blood sugar, lipid profile, renal function tests, and liver function tests are required. To rule out osteomyelitis and malignancy, plain radiography of the foot, as well as CT and MRI, should be performed. Urine analysis for proteinuria, haematuria, and cylindruria, routine and immunohistopathology of skin biopsies, antinuclear antibodies, rheumatoid factor, complement C4, circulating immune complexes, paraproteins, immunoglobulin fractions, antineutrophil cytoplasmic antibodies, serological tests, and cultures for underlying infections are all laboratory screening tests for vasculitis. Activated partial thromboplastin time, prothrombin time, thrombin time, factor V (Leiden) mutation (506R fi 506Q), factor II (prothrombin) mutation (20210G fi 20210A), antithrombin III, protein C and protein S, and lupus anticoagulant anticardiolipin are all laboratory screening tests for clotting disorders [11].

When a wound infection is suspected, a quantitative bacterial culture should be done. This is accomplished by curetting or biopsying the ulcer bed. The quantitative biopsy is the current gold standard for determining the amount and quality of microbial pathogens in a wound. The presence of more than 10 X 5 organisms per gramme of tissue in quantitative biopsies is regarded serious, and systemic antibiotic treatment should be explored. If osteomyelitis is suspected, representative cultures from the bone or deepest tissue layers must be acquired [12]. Because these ulcers are prone to malignant transformation, a biopsy is required to make a proper diagnosis and rule out malignancy. This necessitates removing a deep wedge of tissue from the ulcer's margin and is typically performed under local anaesthetic for final diagnosis [13].

1.5 Conclusion

Few common ulcers, such as venous ulcers, arterial ulcers, and neuropathic ulcers, are straightforward to diagnose; however, to detect atypical ulcers, a battery of tests is necessary, and the diagnosis may remain ambiguous. Treatment of uncommon ulcers is extremely tough, and a variety of therapies are necessary to heal the ulcers.

References

1. Agale SV. Chronic leg ulcers: epidemiology, aetiopathogenesis, and management. Ulcers. 2013;2013:9.
2. Rayner R, Carville K, Keaton J, Prentice J, Santamaria XN. Leg ulcers: atypical presentations and associated comorbidities. Wound Pract Res. 2009;17(4):168–85.
3. Shukla VK, Ansari MA, Gupta SK. Wound healing research: a perspective from India. Int J Low Extrem Wounds. 2005;4(1):7–8.
4. Panuncialman J, Falanga V. Unusual causes of cutaneous ulceration. Surg Clin North Am. 2010;90(6):1161–80.
5. Raffetto JD, Ligi D, Maniscalco R, Khalil RA, Mannello F. Why venous leg ulcers have difficulty healing: overview on pathophysiology, clinical consequences, and treatment. J Clin Med. 2021;10:29. https://doi.org/10.3390/jcm10010029.
6. Casey G. Causes and management of leg and foot ulcers. Nurs Stand. 2004;18(45):57–8.
7. Gottrup F, Karlsmark T. Leg ulcers: uncommon presentations. Clin Dermatol. 2005;23(6):601–11.
8. Dean S. Leg ulcers and management. Aust Fam Physician. 2006;35(7):480–5.
9. London NJM, Donnelly R. ABC of arterial and venous disease. Ulcerated lower limb. BMJ. 2000;320(7249):1589–91.
10. Burrows C. Leg ulcers. Wound Care Can. 2008;8(2):16–8.
11. Mekkes JR, Loots MAM, van der Wal AC, Bos JD. Causes, investigation and treatment of leg ulceration. Br J Dermatol. 2003;148(3):388–401.
12. Siddiqui AR, Bernstein JM. Chronic wound infection: facts and controversies. Clin Dermatol. 2010;28(5):519–26.
13. Panuncialman J, Hammerman S, Carson P, Falanga V. Wound edge biopsy sites in chronic wounds heal rapidly and do not result in delayed overall healing of the wounds. Wound Repair Regen. 2010;18(1):21–5.

Hypertensive/Martorell Ulcer

2

Disha Arora and Abhishek Pandey

2.1 Introduction

Chronic wounds pose a major healthcare problem. Due to various differential diagnosis of leg ulcers, there is a diagnostic challenge. Vascular aetiologies compromise the majority of leg ulcers, out of which venous ulcers arev the common aetiology. The major clues to the diagnosis are the clinical presentation, underlying aetiology and pathological hallmarks of the ulcer. Despite adequate treatment, if the ulcer does not heal in 4–12 weeks, it warrants a search for the rare cause of ulcer apart from vascular insufficiency due to atherosclerosis and venous stasis. Hypertensive ulcers are a potentially undiagnosed cause of leg ulcers.

Fernandes Martorell first described Martorell hypertensive ischaemic leg ulcer (HYTILU) in 1945 in Barcelona, Spain, in four hypertensive obese females. One year later, Hines et al. reported the association of these ulcers with hypertrophic occlusive subcutaneous arterioles and called them "hypertensive ischaemic ulcer". They are characterised by localised subcutaneous atherosclerosis. There is a female preponderance. The extreme pain in these hypertensive ulcers is characteristic, which needs to be differentiated from other painful lower extremity ulcers like sickle cell ulcer, vasculitis ulcer, insect bite, pyoderma gangrenosum, aeroembolism, and large vessel occlusive ulcer. The ulcers are so rapidly progressive, and pain is so severe that it can be the sole reason for the patient seeking medical attention.

D. Arora · A. Pandey (✉)
Department of Medicine, IMS, BHU, Varanasi, India

A. K. Khanna, S. K. Tiwary (eds.), *Uncommon Ulcers of the Extremities*,
https://doi.org/10.1007/978-981-99-1782-2_2

2.2 Pathogenesis

Duncan and Faris in 1985 demonstrated that the patient with Martorell ulcers has small and medium vessel changes with normal ankle-brachial index. There is increased local vascular resistance, which causes vasoconstriction. The differentiating feature of these ulcers from arterial ulcers is that pain is not aggravated by exercise or limb elevation, exacerbating an arterial ulcer. Also, an arterial ulcer is deep punched out ulcers seen on the anterior shin, dorsum of the foot or any bony prominence.

Bell and Clausen first described diffuse arteriolar changes in hypertension in 1928 on 420 autopsies of patients with primary hypertension characterised primarily in skin arterioles but also occur in the brain, kidney and other organs.

The average wall to lumen ratio of arteriole is 1:2.14 in people with normal blood pressure, while it is reduced significantly to 1:1.57 in patients with essential hypertension in a study conducted by Farber and Hines. This occurs due to the thickening of the elastic lamina and hyperplasia of the media. This process is called hyalinosis, which leads to increased luminal stenosis. A study was conducted by Duncan and Farries, in which twelve normotensive individuals were compared with eight patients with peripheral vascular disease and six patients with hypertensive leg ulcers. They found that hypertensive ulcer and peripheral vascular disease patients had low skin perfusion compared to normal individuals. There is a local increase in peripheral resistance in Martorell ulcers while reducing blood inflow in peripheral vascular disease. This leads to inadequate vasodilatory response to arterial narrowing, leading to decreased tissue perfusion and ischaemic ulcers.

Vascular insufficiency ulcer may accompany less severe ischaemia coupled with an additional insult like trauma or macrovascular occlusion. Similar changes in the vessel wall are seen in calcific uremic arteriopathy, where medial calcification leads to obliteration of small arterioles. According to the Angiosome model, a branch of an artery supplying an area of skin is called Angiosome. So, even if foot pulse may be palpable, there is a possibility that non-healing ulcers may have different Angiosome; thus, revascularisation may lead to early healing of an ulcer. There can be triggering factors like trauma, although 50% of cases occur spontaneously.

2.3 Clinical Presentation

The typical location is lower one-third of the leg on a lateral dorsal aspect, often involving the Tendo Achilles in 90% of cases. Medial and anterior locations have also been described. It can present as single or multiple small black eschars-like symmetrical lesions with purplish edges and a necrotic base. It initially began as a painful blister that changes its colour from red to blue and black, then finally ulcerates. There can be preceding history of trauma also. Livedo reticularis, pigmentation, and shin spots often precede the development of ulceration.

Satellite lesions with irregular edges often develop in the areas of livedo reticularis, suggesting additional cutaneous necrosis.

Due to local ischaemia and infarction, there is intractable pain often disturbing the sleep of the patient. Pain is disproportionate to the size of the ulcer; this is a pathognomonic feature of these ulcers. This differentiates it from venous ulcers, which are often painless.

Peripheral pulses are often palpable.

2.4 Differential Diagnosis

The most common mimickers of painful Martorell leg ulcers are pyoderma gangrenosum, calciphylaxis, sickle cell, vasculitis and vasculopathies, which needs to be differentiated.

1. **Pyoderma gangrenosum (PG)** typically starts as a papule or pustule, enlarging rapidly and finally ulcerating. Margins have a characteristic violaceous border and rolled margin with a cribriform base and an undermining edge. They are often associated with inflammatory bowel disease, rheumatoid arthritis, malignancies like AML and CML, etc.; it is a diagnosis of exclusion. Skin biopsy is usually done to rule out other causes like infections and vasculitis. Differentiating it from Martrell ulcer is very important as both present as painful ulcers, but treatment modalities of both conditions are diametrically opposite. *Debridement is the key management in Martrell ulcer, which is contraindicated in PG due to pathergy phenomenon where surgical management often worsens the ulcer. Similarly, misdiagnosing a Martorell ulcer as PG leads to mandatory use of immunosuppressants which exposes the patient to the risk of sepsis.*
2. **Vasculitis ulcers** are often distal and bilaterally symmetrical. They can present as multiple, palpable purpuric lesions or as urticarial necrotic ulceration. They are seen in the background of hepatitis C, connective tissue disorders and drugs.
3. **Calciphylaxis** is usually seen in chronic renal insufficiency patients where distal skin necrosis is predominant, although non-uremic calciphylaxis in morbidly obese individuals where proximal skin necrosis is often seen. This is due to eutrophication, where calcification is caused in body water enriched with nutrients or inorganic substances. Martorell HYTILU and non-uremic calciphylaxis both are seen in association with coexisting hypertension and diabetes. Both are characterised by a common hallmark feature, i.e. ischaemic subcutaneous atherosclerosis.

2.5 Diagnosis

Diagnosis of HYTILU is based on the background history of hypertension, clinical presentation and confirmed by *elliptical-shaped biopsy specimen* of size 5 cm × 0.5 cm down to the fascia, including healthy skin at the border of the wound and extending up to the necrotic area. Longitudinal orientation is kept for histological examination. Often the punch biopsies are taken from the base of the ulcer, which is superficial and misses the **subcutaneous occlusive atherosclerosis,** which is the **typical finding for HYTILU**. This finding was confirmed in a series of Martorell ulcers where 50% of such ulcers were erroneously misdiagnosed as pyoderma gangrenosum (due to sheets of neutrophilic granulocytes in the necrotic dermis) and 20% as necrotising vasculitis.

Fifty per cent develop the peripheral arterial disease simultaneously; therefore, vascular assessment should be done at the start of management as revascularisation procedures may be required in case of relevant large vessel arterial occlusions. Vascular assessment involved clinical examination, ankle-brachial pressure index (ABPI) measurement, segmental oscillography, especially for medial calcinosis, and imaging via fine needle angiography.

Interestingly, it can be seen with small and medium vessel atherosclerosis without evident large vessel peripheral arterial disease.

It is essential to rule out end-stage renal disease or identify patients with kidney transplants. Renal function test, parathyroid hormone status and calcium-phosphate product levels are screened in these patients.

2.5.1 Diagnostic Criteria

Martorell described the clinical criteria for the diagnosis of hypertensive ulcer as follows:

1. Location-Inner aspect of lower one-third of lower limb (Figs. 2.1 and 2.2).
2. Diastolic hypertension in lower limbs.

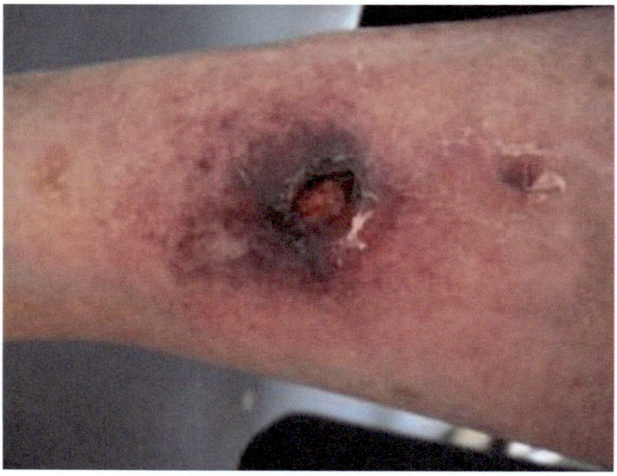

Fig. 2.1 Beginning of Martorell HYTILU at the pretibial lower leg after minor trauma. The wound border is progressively inflamed and necrotic. This wound causes excruciating pain. Source: Jürg Hafner, Stephan Nobbe, Severin Läuchli, Katrin Kerl, Lars E. French, Nedzimin Pelivani, Kornelia Böhler, Dieter Mayer, Patricia Senet, Martorell hypertensive ischemic leg ulcer must not be confounded with pyoderma gangrenosum: Management is totally different, Reviews in Vascular Medicine, Volume 1, Issue 1, 2013, Pages 5–8, ISSN 2212–0211, https://doi.org/10.1016/j.rvm.2012.08.001. (https://www.sciencedirect.com/science/article/pii/S2212021112000033)

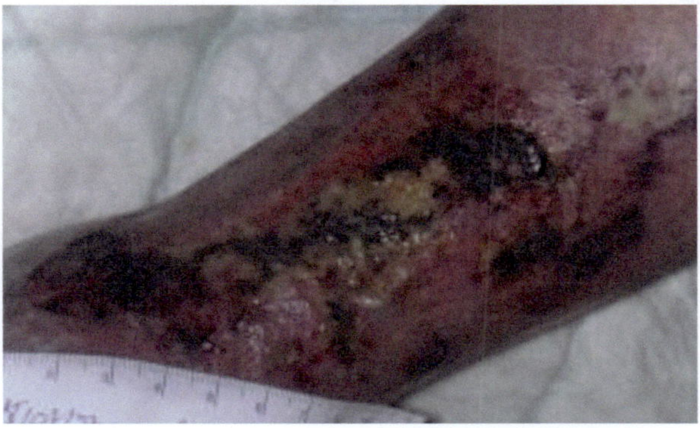

Fig. 2.2 Progressively necrotic livedo at the laterodorsal leg leading to a skin infarction. Source: Jürg Hafner, Stephan Nobbe, Severin Läuchli, Katrin Kerl, Lars E. French, Nedzimin Pelivani, Kornelia Böhler, Dieter Mayer, Patricia Senet, Martorell hypertensive ischemic leg ulcer must not be confounded with pyoderma gangrenosum: Management is totally different, Reviews in Vascular Medicine, Volume 1, Issue 1, 2013, Pages 5–8, ISSN 2212–0211, https://doi.org/10.1016/j.rvm.2012.08.001. (https://www.sciencedirect.com/science/article/pii/S2212021112000033)

3. Arterial calcinosis must be absent, and arteries must be "hyperpulsatile" in bilateral lower limbs.
4. Chronic venous insufficiency must be ruled out.
5. Lesions must be symmetrical or evidence of residual hyperpigmentation of the previous ulcer in the inner aspect of lower limbs.
6. Pain must increase in the horizontal position.
7. More common in women.

2.6 Histopathological Diagnosis

Typical histological findings include necrobiosis of the three skin layers, i.e. epidermis, dermis and subcutis. Out of which, the vascular changes are most evident in the subcutaneous fat layer. The pathological hallmark is thickened vessel wall due to atherosclerotic arterioles leading to narrowing of the vascular lumen as evident by increased wall to lumen ratio. Hyperplasia of the intima, medial wall calcinosis is seen in 70% of the arterioles, along with the partial canalised thrombosed vessel walls. (Fig. 2.3).

2.7 Management

Early diagnosis of this ulcer is of utmost importance to avoid unnecessary pain and to guide appropriate therapy.

Conservative management—based on the size of the ulcer, HYTILU re-categorised as small <3 cm, medium >3 cm and large >6 cm diameter. Conservative

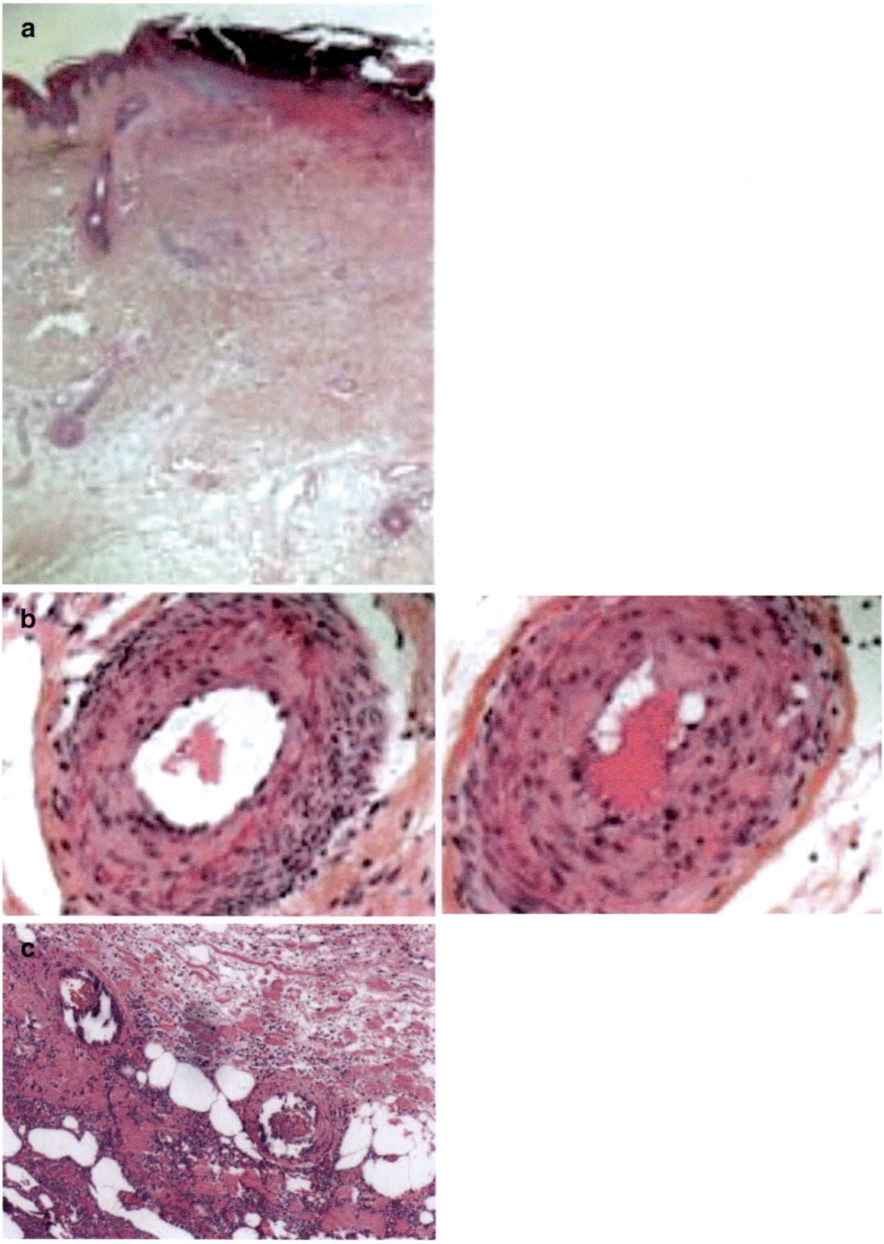

Fig. 2.3 (**a**) Haematoxylin eosin stain: destruction of epidermis and superficial dermis with arteriolosclerosis of vessels at the dermo-hypodermal junction. (**b**) Arteriolosclerosis: hypertrophy of the media and intimal hyperplasia results in a reduced wall-to-lumen ratio. (**c**) Subcutaneous arterioles in Martorell hypertensive ischaemic leg ulcer show in 70% of slides a thickened vessel wall with medial calcification. The lumen is narrowed and in some instances thrombosed. Source: Jürg Hafner, Stephan Nobbe, Severin Läuchli, Katrin Kerl, Lars E. French, Nedzimin Pelivani, Kornelia Böhler, Dieter Mayer, Patricia Senet, Martorell hypertensive ischemic leg ulcer must not be confounded with pyoderma gangrenosum: Management is totally different, Reviews in Vascular Medicine, Volume 1, Issue 1, 2013, Pages 5–8, ISSN 2212–0211, https://doi.org/10.1016/j.rvm.2012.08.001. (https://www.sciencedirect.com/science/article/pii/S2212021112000033)

management may be tried in small-sized ulcers. Also, it can be done in freshly grafted patients with progressive wound borders if the patient is doing well.

Conservative management compromises:

- Local wound care.
- Topical antimicrobial and antiseptic ointments.
- Limited regular debridement.
- Applying non-adherent gauzes.
- Topical negative pressure devices.
- Intravenous sodium thiosulfate should be considered in cases of extensive necrosis. It is an inorganic salt that dissolves calcium phosphate. This is extensively being used in uremic and non-uremic calciphylaxis. For renal compromised patients, it is being used as mixed with dialysis fluid instead of intravenous form.
- Usage of topical occlusive dressings has been associated with critical colonisation of bacteria in the setting of compromised wounds leading to maceration and hence should be discouraged.

2.8 Skin Grafting

1. Surgical debridement and split-thickness skin graft.
2. Mesh split-thickness skin graft.

First, dead necrotic tissue is completely excised, leaving behind a surgical wound extending up to the fascia with a healthy ulcer border; this is called necrosectomy. Following this, there are two approaches split skin graft can be immediately placed, or it can be done after wound conditioning as mentioned in the wound bed preparation paradigm. Selective cases may have local negative pressure management.

This strategy most effectively alleviates the intractable pain from ongoing and progressive skin infarction.

A retrospective case series by Hafner et al. in 2010 showed that in 31 patients, 94% achieved successful complete healing by using split skin grafting.

Dagregorio et al. in 2006 studied 20 patients retrospectively for mesh split-thickness graft which showed 14 of 20 complete healing in 2 weeks after discharge and 100% pain relief.

Extensive curettage under local anaesthesia can be carried out after checking the perfusion.

2.9 Pain Management

Due to chronic persistent pain, the quality of life of suffering patients is affected significantly. The key factor in the wound bed preparation paradigm is controlling pain until the patient is ready for surgical management.

Causes of pain in Martorell ulcer

1. Nociceptive pain is stimulus-dependent, and characteristic features are throbbing, gnawing or aching quality of pain. It is best managed by WHO pain ladder medications like nonsteroidal anti-inflammatory medications, including aspirin and narcotics.
2. Neuropathic pain is a spontaneous pain characterised by stabbing, burning or shooting type of sensation. Such pain responds well to tricyclic antidepressants like nortriptyline, desipramine, gabapentin, and pregabalin.

2.10 General Measures

- Adequate blood pressure control

  Orbach showed the first response to antihypertensive medications in treating hypertensive ulcers.

  Beta-blockers cause local vasoconstriction and thus aggravate ischaemic ulcers and impair the healing of hypertensive leg ulcers. Therefore, they are contraindicated in such a scenario.

  Calcium channel blockers: one randomised controlled trial was done in 1995 by Nikolova in which 30 outpatients received nifedipine 10 mg orally thrice a day for 2 months. Significant reduction in ulcer surface area and symptomatic improvement in pain were observed in the nifedipine group compared to placebo although the mean difference in the systolic blood pressure was only 5 mm Hg at the end of 2 months (165.5 ± 12.2 mm Hg for nifedipine vs 170.8 ± 13.1 mmHg for placebo). This study highlights two important facts:
  - Pathophysiology of hypertensive ischaemic ulcer combines two phenomena: localised atherosclerosis and inappropriate local vasoconstriction. Such a different response of antihypertensive medications can affect ulcer healing.
  - Secondly, drugs reducing local vasoconstriction like calcium channel blockers and angiotensin-converting enzyme promote rapid healing of ulcers.
- **Control of diabetes.**
- **Cessation of smoking.**
- **Compression banding stockings to control oedema (especially when coexistent venous wall disease).**
- **Control obesity.**
- **Avoid trauma.**
- **Role of antibiotics:**

  Infection commonly complicates chronic ulcers with decreased blood supply starting from the contamination; bacteria colonise the wound leading to superficial and deep tissue infection. Increased bacterial burden impairs the natural healing power. This can be managed by applying topical antimicrobials for superficial ulcers and systemic antimicrobial agents for deep infection.
- **Role of antiseptic and dressings:**

  Silver dressings and honey dressings have a topical anti-inflammatory action. These are other novel therapies with limited success.
- ***Role of anticoagulation***

Vitamin K antagonists, apart from anticoagulation action, also inhibit vitamin k-dependent calcification protecting protein. This enhances small and medium vessel circulation leading to better wound healing.

- ***Role of vasodilators.***
- ***Role of nontraumatic moisture balance.***
- ***Negative pressure wound therapy.***
- ***Role of hyperbaric oxygen:***

  By correcting the local superficial ischaemia, hyperbaric oxygen therapy is nowadays being utilised in wound healing. A case report was published by Frada et al. in 1989 in which one patient wound was healed by using HBO.
- ***Role of intravenous infusion of prostaglandin E1:***

  Pacific et al., in 2011, conducted a study in 6 hypertensive patients treated with antihypertensive vs four patients treated with PGE1 infusion revealed that intravenous infusion of prostaglandin improves peripheral perfusion.
- **Becaplermin:**

  It is a recombinant platelet-derived growth factor-BB. However, in a randomised control trial conducted by senet et al. in 2011, 64 patients were compared between topical becaplermin topical gel once daily and topical hydrogel, in which 5 out of 28 healed with becaplermin and 3 out of 31 healed with hydrogel. After 12 weeks, no significant results were seen in both the groups revealing that becaplermin was not superior to hydrogel in the management of Martorell ulcer.
- **Spinal cord stimulation:**

  Apart from treating chronic ischaemic pain, this modality can also be utilised for healing a wound by using device-related stimulation of wound healing. Further prospective studies are required before accepting this electrical stimulation related to wound healing stimulation as a primary modality for wound healing. A case report was done by De Andres et al. in 2011, in which a spinal cord stimulator was used, and it was shown that due to an increase in the blood flow to the ischaemic area, there is both pain relief and a decrease in the size of the ulcer.

2.11 Management of Residual Wounds

Instead of aggressive tissue debridement, non-traumatic gentle removal of slough should be carried out. In this case, the prevention of secondary bacterial infection is prioritised over tissue toxicity by the antiseptic agents, as the infected limb can be life-threatening. Cleansing with normal saline flowed by povidone-iodine or polyhexamethylene biguanide, which are the antiseptic agents, is commonly used nowadays. However, these measures are a bridge to appropriate surgical management, which is reported to be a 100 % healing rate in a case series of Martorellulcers.

2.12 Prognosis

Failure to recognise the diagnosis accurately leads to months of ineffective local therapy and significant morbidity due to extreme pain causing prolonged disability in patients with hypertensive leg ulcers. The antihypertensive drugs inhibiting local arteriolar vasoconstriction are important in successful treatment. This is similar to diabetic microvascular disease, where a more aggressive blood pressure control goal of 140/90 mm hg is kept. Surgery is the mainstay of treatment. Timely diagnosis and treatment lead to rapid healing of ulcer along with symptomatic improvement in pain.

2.13 Clinical Pearls

1. Martorell ulcer clinically presents as a painful ulcer with a necrotic base in the lower one-third of the laterodorsal aspect of the leg or Tendo Achilles.
2. Patients with metabolic syndrome having long-standing hypertension with or without diabetes are particularly prone.
3. Pain is not associated with intermittent claudication, aggravated by exercise or leg elevation, thus differentiating it from arterial ulcer.
4. Deep elliptical skin biopsy is required for confirmation.
5. The most effective treatment modality is surgery in which solid skin grafting is done following necrosectomy.

3 Rheumatoid Ulcers

Sankha Shubhra Chakrabarti

3.1 Introduction

Rheumatoid arthritis is the most common type of autoimmune arthritis characterised by pain, swelling, and tenderness of peripheral joints in a symmetrical pattern. It is also characterised by prominent extra-articular manifestations. These include rheumatoid nodules, pulmonary involvement, vasculitis, and systemic effects [1]. Ulcers of the extremities have been reported in around 10% cases of rheumatoid arthritis, but in contrast, rheumatoid arthritis is a rare cause of ulcers of the extremities [2]. When one thinks of rheumatoid limb ulcers, the general idea that comes to mind is of cutaneous ulcers related to rheumatoid vasculitis. However, there may be other aetiologies of limb ulcers in rheumatoid arthritis, with ulcers due to imbalances in foot pressure resulting from deformities being some of the common ones [3]. Infective and iatrogenic ulcers, ulcers resulting from co-existent diseases such as chronic venous insufficiency, atherosclerotic peripheral vascular disease, ulcers resulting from cutaneous dystrophic calcinosis, and multifactorial ulcers have also been observed in large retrospective studies involving patients of rheumatoid arthritis [4, 5]. A particularly interesting entity is pyoderma gangrenosum, which is responsible for chronic non-healing ulcers in the limbs. Pyoderma gangrenosum is an uncommon inflammatory disorder of the skin characterised by neutrophilic infiltration. The spectrum of skin manifestations ranges from papules or pustules to painful ulcers. Rheumatoid arthritis is one of the major systemic inflammatory conditions associated with pyoderma gangrenosum [6]. In this chapter, we will discuss the epidemiology of rheumatoid

S. S. Chakrabarti (✉)
Department of Geriatric Medicine, Institute of Medical Sciences, Banaras Hindu University, Varanasi, UP, India
e-mail: sankha.chakrabarti1@bhu.ac.in

A. K. Khanna, S. K. Tiwary (eds.), *Uncommon Ulcers of the Extremities*,
https://doi.org/10.1007/978-981-99-1782-2_3

ulcers of the extremities, the pathogenesis of major aetiologies of rheumatoid limb ulcers, their presenting clinical manifestations, diagnostic approach to them, and treatment options for such ulcers.

3.2 Epidemiology of Rheumatoid Limb Ulcers

Rheumatoid arthritis is the most common autoimmune arthritis and affects around 0.5–1% of the world population [7]. Higher prevalence has been reported for some native American populations such as the Pima Indians and Chippewa Indians. On the other hand, Chinese and Japanese populations have reported lower prevalence and some studies on rural populations in South Africa and Nigeria failed to identify any cases of rheumatoid arthritis despite good sample sizes [7]. Like most autoimmune diseases, rheumatoid arthritis has a female preponderance with a two–three-fold higher prevalence [8]. Previously thought to be a disease of younger adults, it is now widely accepted that the elderly are also affected by rheumatoid arthritis. In fact, rheumatoid arthritis is one of the most common inflammatory diseases of the elderly. Elderly onset rheumatoid arthritis is defined as having an onset above 65 years of age, and like rheumatoid arthritis of the young, also has a predilection for females [9].

As far as ulcers of the extremities are concerned, rheumatoid arthritis and other inflammatory conditions are rare aetiologies overall but do account for a considerable proportion of non-healing chronic limb ulcers. Experience from a multidisciplinary wound healing and limb preservation clinic from the University of Pittsburgh revealed that around 7% of leg ulcerations had a reasonably certain collagen vascular aetiology [10]. While the experience from less specialised and more peripheral centres may turn up lower numbers, autoimmune diseases must be suspected as potential causes of non-vascular chronic limb ulcers. Foot ulcer prevalence is around 10% in patients of rheumatoid arthritis in the course of their disease. Prevalence of extremity ulceration may be higher if upper limb vasculitic ulcers are also included. Those developing rheumatoid foot ulcers have a nearly 50% recurrence rate at same and different sites [3]. The major classes of ulcers of the extremities in rheumatoid arthritis patients are ulcers due to co-existent arterial or venous insufficiency, ulcers due to deformities leading to differential load distribution on the limbs, and vasculitic ulcers. Besides contributing to the pathogenesis of ulcers of the extremities, rheumatoid arthritis is also a cause for impaired healing of the ulcers, leading to chronicity.

3.3 Pathogenesis

The pathogenesis of a rheumatoid limb ulcer is complex and multifactorial. It is depicted in Fig. 3.1 and can be discussed under varied sub-headings.

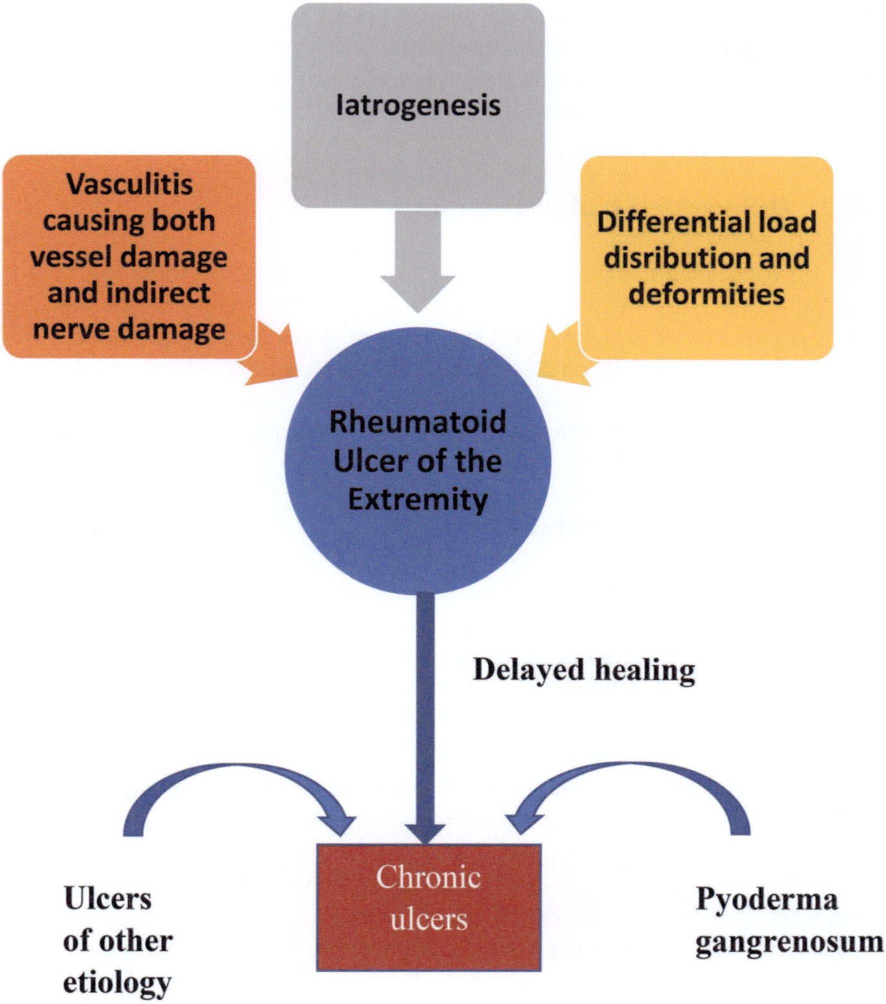

Fig. 3.1 Pathogenesis of rheumatoid limb ulcer

3.3.1 Vasculitis and Inflammation

The hallmark of a non-healing rheumatoid limb ulcer is inflammation and vasculitis, albeit as a subtype these ulcers are rarer. Rheumatoid vasculitis is undifferentiable from other causes of vasculitis. It is classified as a "vasculitis associated with systemic disease" as per the 2012 revised Chapel Hill consensus conference nomenclature criteria [11]. Rheumatoid vasculitis affects vessels of any calibre but more frequently small and medium-sized vessels and is characterised by infiltration of vessel walls by mononuclear cells or neutrophils [12]. An association with specific genotypes of the *HLA-DRB1* shared epitope has been reported, and markers of immune involvement such as high titres of rheumatoid factor and anti-cyclic citrullinated polypeptide (anti-CCP) and decreased complement levels are also observed [12, 13]. Mononeuritis multiplex is another typical feature of rheumatoid vasculitis. This may result in sensory loss in the extremities, leading to both development of new neuropathic ulcers and non-healing of existing ones [13].

3.3.2 Differential Load Distribution

Foot deformities are a common feature of rheumatoid arthritis. These lead to differential load bearing on the feet, predisposing some parts to undergo damage due to higher pressures. The concomitant sensory neuropathy also aggravates the problem. A unique British study on determinants of foot ulceration in rheumatoid arthritis patients determined loss of protective sensations, abnormal ankle brachial pressure index, and forefoot deformities to be strongest risk factors [3].

3.3.3 Associated Conditions

Even in patients of rheumatoid arthritis, the majority of limb ulcers are not attributable to disease-related vasculitis and inflammation but rather to presence of comorbidities. A 7-year retrospective case review of all patients with leg ulcers seen at the National Skin Centre at Singapore identified venous disease as the most common aetiology of leg ulcers in those with rheumatological conditions [4]. Other ulcers identified included multifactorial ones, those due to atypical mycobacterial infection, and ulcers due to pyoderma gangrenosum, ischaemic microangiopathy, and iatrogenic ulcers [4]. Since the burden of comorbidities may be high in rheumatoid arthritis patients, especially in elderly patients, chronic venous ulcers in the setting of varicose veins and ulcers of diabetic foot due to neuropathy and atherosclerotic vascular disease may be quite common.

Pyoderma gangrenosum is a complex neutrophilic dermatosis. It may be often seen in association with cases of rheumatoid arthritis as also other autoimmune and inflammatory disorders. The pathogenesis of this entity is complex, not fully elucidated, and involves not only neutrophils but T cells, inflammasomes, keratinocyte apoptosis, and epigenetic changes [14]. There is an increased migration of neutrophils to the dermis which is the hallmark of this disease. In this it resembles other entities such as Behçet's disease and Sweet's syndrome. Genetic susceptibility plays an important role in pyoderma gangrenosum.

3.3.4 Iatrogenic

While several medications and therapeutic interventions may cause chronic extremity ulcers, two noteworthy agents are methotrexate and leflunomide. These two disease-modifying anti-rheumatic drugs (DMARDs) form the cornerstone of the usual triple drug regimen utilised for rheumatoid arthritis [15]. They are also extensively used as first-line monotherapy. Both methotrexate and leflunomide are known to cause leg ulcers. Methotrexate-induced skin ulcers in patients of rheumatoid arthritis have been reported mostly in the elderly. They often develop after years of therapy, and have a predilection for the lower limbs, hands, and elbows. The pathogenesis is related to the inhibition of the folate biosynthesis pathway, and DNA replication [16, 17]. Other agents such as steroids, biologicals, and non-steroidal anti-inflammatory drugs (NSAIDS) may have an accelerant role if taken simultaneously [16]. Leflunomide induces cutaneous ulcers by inhibiting dihydroorotate dehydrogenase involved in pyrimidine synthesis, as well as by blunting the action of growth factors such as the epidermal derived growth factor (EDGF). Inflammation in the dermis and subcutaneous tissue with necrosis of collagen fibres, presence of granulation tissue, and giant cell granulomas are visualised on histopathological examination [18, 19].

3.3.5 Impaired Healing

Rheumatoid arthritis is a systemic inflammatory disease and results in a state of chronic inflammation which is inevitably characterised by the typical features of anaemia and hypoalbuminemia especially in the elderly, loss of muscle mass, and delayed wound healing [20, 21]. Impaired wound healing adds to the chronicity of limb ulcers which increase prevalence rates. Steroids which are often part of treatment protocols for acute flares of rheumatoid arthritis may also impair healing.

3.4 Clinical Features

In this section, we will primarily discuss the presentation of classical vasculitic ulcers of the extremities which are observed in patients of rheumatoid arthritis. Some salient features of ulcers due to comorbid illness or iatrogenic ulcers are briefly mentioned in Table 3 .1. Pyoderma gangrenosum is discussed separately.

3.4.1 Vasculitic Ulcers of the Extremities

Although the most common extremity ulcers in patients of rheumatoid arthritis are of other aetiology, vasculitic ulcers are the pathognomonic ulcers of any connective tissue disorder. Notably, vasculitic rheumatoid ulcers may affect both the lower and upper extremities, unlike the commoner venous ulcers which have a definite lower limb predilection. However, these ulcers are again commoner on the lower limbs and in the sacral region, sometimes giving a false diagnosis of bedsores (pressure sores/decubitus ulcers) [31]. The spectrum of cutaneous manifestations varies from palpable purpura to nodules to ulcers, and digital necrosis [12]. Deep, painful ulcers may suggest a vasculitic origin, but histopathological evidence is usually needed to make a definitive diagnosis, and even then, it may not be always feasible [32].

Table 3 .1 Salient features of non-vasculitic ulcers in rheumatoid arthritis [3, 5, 16, 19, 22–30]

Ulcers due to differential load distribution	These occur in the setting of foot deformities which are common in rheumatoid arthritis, especially if left untreated. Common deformities of the feet in rheumatoid arthritis include hallux valgus, hallux rigidus, mallet toe, claw toe, splay toe deformities (forefoot), pes planus (mid foot), and calcaneal varus and valgus deformities (hind foot). Raised plantar pressures, and ill-fitting footwear due to deformities may also contribute to these ulcers
Venous ulcers	These are seen mostly in the setting of a long history of varicose veins, especially neglected ones. They are shallow, painful, poorly demarcated ulcers located over bony prominences. The medial malleolus is a common site. Associated skin changes such as itching and scaling may be present
Ulcers due to peripheral arterial disease	These are a common finding in smokers or patients with other risk factors for atherosclerotic peripheral vascular disease. Those with history of coronary or cerebrovascular atherosclerosis or acute events may have such ulcers. A history of limb claudication may also exist. Common sites are the toes, heels, and bony prominences of the foot. These ulcers are usually deep, round or punched out, with a clearly demarcated edge. There may be absent or feeble peripheral arterial pulses or audible bruits. Gangrene of digits or limb may be associated
Diabetic foot ulcers	Diabetic foot ulcers are usually multifactorial. Diabetes is a risk factor for both peripheral arterial diseases leading to arterial ulcers as described above, and neuropathy. Autonomic neuropathy, small fibre sensory neuropathy, and large fibre neuropathy combine with arterial disease to cause the characteristic diabetic foot. There is associated paresthesias, hypoesthesia, and anhidrosis due to autonomic neuropathy. While ulcers due to predominant peripheral arterial disease follow the patterns described above for arterial ulcers, neuropathic ulcers commonly occur over the weight-bearing areas such as the plantar metatarsal head, great toe, and heels
Ulcers due to ischemic microangiopathy	Occlusive microangiopathy due to thrombotic or anatomic occlusion is seen in rheumatoid arthritis if there are associated conditions such as livedo reticularis, calciphylaxis, or antiphospholipid antibodies syndrome. The ulcers may be similar in location and morphology to inflammatory microangiopathic ulcers which are seen in classical vasculitis and in pyoderma gangrenosum. However, minor variations in clinical features may be present depending on the aetiology
Ulcers in the setting of co-existent other connective tissue/ inflammatory disorders	Rheumatoid arthritis may be associated with other connective tissue disorders such as systemic lupus erythematosus, scleroderma, Behçet's disease (as part of overlap syndromes), or other conditions such as calcinosis cutis, inflammatory myositis, or psoriasis. The ulcers specific to these disease types may be seen in such cases. Leukocytoclastic vasculitis is a generally skin-limited vasculitis which may be idiopathic or secondary to rheumatoid arthritis or other systemic diseases. It may lead to skin ulceration on the extremities in patients of rheumatoid arthritis
Iatrogenic ulcers	Methotrexate-induced skin ulcers are commonly located over the lower limbs, hand, and elbows. These resolve well within weeks after drug discontinuation. Cutaneous ulcers on lower limbs and forearms have been reported with leflunomide use, mainly in elderly females after months of therapy. The healing of these ulcers after drug withdrawal is delayed

Suspicion should be strong when the ulcers do not heal with standard vascular interventions and local wound care [33]. Sometimes, an association with vasculitic involvement of other organs may exist, and this portends a poor prognosis [12]. Necrotising vasculitis and associated vasculitic nerve involvement may also be observed in some cases of rheumatoid arthritis with cutaneous ulcers [34].

3.4.2 Pyoderma Gangrenosum

Pyoderma gangrenosum, as described above, is a neutrophilic dermatosis which may be idiopathic but is usually seen associated with immune-inflammatory conditions such as rheumatoid arthritis [35]. In the ulcerative variant of pyoderma gangrenosum, tender inflammatory nodules or pustules are the initial manifestations developing most commonly at sites of trauma, especially on the anterior lower extremities. The pre-tibial region is commonly affected [36]. They rapidly evolve into necrotic ulcers with violaceous undermined borders and surrounding erythema. Pyoderma gangrenosum also has bullous, pustular, vegetative, peristomal, post-operative subtypes [35].

3.5 Diagnosis

The diagnosis of an ulcer of the extremity in a patient of rheumatoid arthritis is clinical. History of pre-existing disease and presence of associated skin lesions and examination findings as described for the individual entities above allows an empirical diagnosis of the cause of the ulcer. A detailed neurological examination may be warranted in cases of co-existing morbidities such as diabetes when ruling out neuropathic ulcers is important. A 10G monofilament test may be performed to identify loss of protective sensation [37]. Histopathological evidence from a biopsy of the lesion may have additive value in pin-pointing the exact diagnosis. The salient feature of a typical vasculitic ulcer of the extremity is mononuclear cell or neutrophilic infiltration of the vessel wall of small and medium vessels. The vessel wall may be destroyed, with necrosis, and disruption of the internal and external elastic lamina [12]. Leukocytoclasis or the presence of debris of neutrophils within the blood vessel walls may be seen. A sensitive and specific finding for vasculitis in rheumatoid arthritis is perivascular infiltrates of mononuclear or polymorphonuclear cells with greater than/equal to three cell layers [38].

In suspected cases of pyoderma gangrenosum, biopsies taken early in the course from the border show an infiltrate of chronic inflammatory cells confined to the dermis. A perivascular lymphocytic infiltrate and fibrinoid necrosis of the vessel wall may be noted. Later in the course of ulceration, a polymorphonuclear cell infiltrate with features of ulceration, infarction, and abscess formation is more common [39]. Histopathological examination also allows the exclusion of chronic mycobacterial infections and malignancies which may develop in the setting of long-standing wounds [33].

Some additional diagnostic tests are often needed to evaluate the status of comorbidities which are a common cause of ulcers of the extremities in rheumatoid arthritis. A doppler ultrasonographic imaging of the arterial and venous systems of the lower limbs is useful to diagnose venous insufficiency, concomitant deep venous thrombosis as well as peripheral arterial atherosclerotic lesions. A routine haematological and biochemical panel including metabolic parameters such as glycosylated haemoglobin and lipid profile may be useful. Serology to rule out overlap connective tissue disorders and systemic vasculitis syndromes may also be needed. Common serological investigations include estimation of anti-nuclear antibody (ANA), anti-double-stranded DNA antibody (anti-ds-DNA), anti-Smith antibody (anti-Sm), anti-centromere antibody, anti-Scl-70 antibody, anti-Ro/La antibodies, cytoplasmic and perinuclear anti-neutrophil cytoplasmic antibodies (c- and p-ANCAs). The details of the connective tissue disorders identified by these tests are not within the domain of this chapter. Pus culture from the wound site with antibiotic sensitivity testing against bacterial and fungal pathogens may also guide the therapeutic protocol.

3.6 Management

The management of rheumatoid ulcers of the extremities is based on three planks—local wound care, coverage for secondary infections, and immunosuppression targeting the underlying disease. Additional therapy may be warranted in case of specific co-existent aetiologies. In venous disease, compression stockings and limb elevation strategies may be useful. In atherosclerotic peripheral arterial disease, use of antiplatelets, statins, dual antiplatelet-vasodilator medications (cilostazol), and hemorheological medications such as pentoxifylline may be beneficial. Anticoagulants may be needed lifelong in case of associated antiphospholipid antibody syndrome resulting in thrombosis and ulcers of vascular origin. A trained podiatrist may be able to design a therapeutic and prophylactic plan for deformity-related ulcers which are caused by differential load distribution. Endovascular therapy for occlusive vascular lesions is being attempted in recent times and may be useful in select cases.

3.6.1 Local Wound Care

The local care of vasculitic ulcers is based on eliminating necrotic tissue, control of infection, maintenance of moistness of the wound, and eliminating pockets from the wound margin. Cadexomer iodine ointment aids in achieving the first two goals whereas silver sulfadiazine cream and povidone iodine ointment are useful for infection control. Occasionally, if the ulcers are extensive and evidence of systemic (blood stream) infection exists, systemic antibiotics may be added. Moistness of the wound may be ensured using Cadexomer or povidone iodine when exudates are excessive and using silver sulfadiazine cream when exudates are lacking.

Occasionally in cases of painful ulcers, white petrolatum or a petrolatum-based ointment may be useful. Debridement may be useful in patients with significant dead and necrotic tissue. Both debridement and use of occlusive dressing must be done with added care, considering the tendency of these ulcers to rapidly deteriorate [40]. Innovative solutions are being developed to enhance healing of vasculitic ulcers. These include the use of bovine collagen glycosaminoglycan matrices, split thickness skin grafting and corrective operations for foot deformities [41–43]. A consultative approach between a surgeon with expertise in chronic non-healing wounds, a physician with expertise in rheumatology, and a dermatologist may provide the best outcomes.

3.6.2 Coverage for Secondary Infections

Local site infections are usually bacterial but may rarely be caused by fungi, mycobacteria, and also viruses or leishmania in exceptional cases. Systemic antibiotic coverage usually is targeted against locally prevalent organisms [44]. A broad-spectrum beta lactam covering both gram positive and negative organisms may be the standard of care. Anti-pseudomonal coverage with fluoroquinolones (levofloxacin) or anti-pseudomonal beta lactams (piperacillin-tazobactam, ceftazidime, or meropenem) for hospitalised patients may be needed, especially in patients with co-existent diabetes. Piperacillin-tazobactam, meropenem, amoxycillin-clavulanate, metronidazole, and clindamycin provide good coverage against anaerobic organisms. Coverage for methicillin-resistant *Staphylococcus aureus* (MRSA) is needed if culture reports suggest MRSA or if there is a history of prolonged hospitalisation or surgical interventions. Linezolid may be a good oral option in such cases [44]. Guidelines recommend the use of dapsone, an anti-mycobacterial antibiotic useful in the treatment of leprosy, in the management of rheumatoid vasculitis. However, it plays a mainly immunomodulatory role [40].

3.6.3 Systemic Immunosuppression

Systemic immunosuppression is the cornerstone of the treatment of rheumatoid arthritis. Since the vasculitic process is intricately linked with the core pathogenesis of rheumatoid arthritis, treatment of rheumatoid vasculitic ulcers also utilises immunosuppressants. These include both standard disease-modifying anti-rheumatic drugs (DMARDs) as well as biological DMARDs, and other immune-suppressants. The first-line management for rheumatoid vasculitis is high-dose steroids, such as prednisolone 0.5–1 mg/kg/day. Methotrexate is the DMARD of first choice for management of rheumatoid arthritis and may be used similarly in management of skin ulcers due to rheumatoid vasculitis. If non-responsive to these therapy, cyclophosphamide and azathioprine have been suggested as additional therapeutic options [12, 40]. Newer biological DMARDs such as anti-TNFα therapies (infliximab, adalimumab, etanercept, etc) may also be useful sometimes, though concerns have been raised regarding ulcers and vasculitis developing or worsening occasionally while on anti-TNF therapy. Stoppage of these agents or switching to safer options has been recommended in guidelines for such cases [40, 45]. The guidelines of the Japanese Dermatological Association also advice the use of cyclosporine, cyclophosphamide, and intravenous immunoglobulin (IVIg) in non-responsive cases [40].

3.6.4 Management of Pyoderma Gangrenosum

The management of this condition is non-specific and mostly focused on treating the underlying systemic disease and local wound care. Topical steroids, topical tacrolimus and pimecrolimus are sometimes used. Systemic immunosuppression with high-dose prednisolone (1–2 mg/kg/day) and high-dose cyclosporine either alone or with steroids may be utilised. Dapsone, sulfasalazine, and the other immunosuppressants discussed above in the management of rheumatoid vasculitis may also be effective in certain cases [36].

3.7 Conclusion

Ulcers of the extremities are common in patients of rheumatoid arthritis. Chronic non-healing limb ulcers are a major source of morbidity in these patients and adversely affect the quality of life. Although vasculitic ulcers are pathognomonic, the more common ulcers are venous and arterial ulcers, and also those related to deformities. Histopathological examination usually provides support to what is commonly a clinical diagnosis. The management of rheumatoid ulcers of the extremities rests on local wound care, coverage of secondary infections, and adequate use of disease-modifying anti-rheumatic drugs and other systemic immunosuppressants.

References

1. Smolen JS, Aletaha D, McInnes IB. Rheumatoid arthritis. Lancet. 2016;388(10055):2023–38. https://linkinghub.elsevier.com/retrieve/pii/S0140673616301738.
2. Thurtle OA, Cawley MI. The frequency of leg ulceration in rheumatoid arthritis: a survey. J Rheumatol. 1983;10(3):507–9.
3. Firth J, Waxman R, Law G, Nelson EA, Helliwell P, Siddle H, et al. The predictors of foot ulceration in patients with rheumatoid arthritis. Clin Rheumatol. 2014;33(5):615–21.
4. Chia HY, Tang MB. Chronic leg ulcers in adult patients with rheumatological diseases—a 7-year retrospective review. Int Wound J. 2014;11(6):601–4.
5. Hida T, Minami M, Kubo Y. Bilateral leg ulcers secondary to dystrophic calcinosis in a patient with rheumatoid arthritis. J Med Invest. 2017;64(3.4):308–10. http://www.ncbi.nlm.nih.gov/pubmed/28955003.
6. Ibrahim I, Shereef H, Hashim A, Habbal H, Mahmood R, Mohamed MA. Winning the battle after three years of suffering: a case of a refractory pyoderma Gangrenosum treat-

ment challenge. Case Rep Rheumatol. 2021;2021:8869914. http://www.ncbi.nlm.nih.gov/pubmed/33777473.
7. Silman AJ, Pearson JE. Epidemiology and genetics of rheumatoid arthritis. Arthritis Res. 2002;4(Suppl 3):S265–72. http://www.ncbi.nlm.nih.gov/pubmed/12110146.
8. Gerosa M, De Angelis V, Riboldi P, Meroni P. Rheumatoid arthritis: a female challenge. Women's Health. 2008;4(2):195–201. https://doi.org/10.2217/17455057.4.2.195.
9. Kobak S, Bes C. An autumn tale: geriatric rheumatoid arthritis. Ther Adv Musculoskelet Dis. 2018;10(1):3–11. https://doi.org/10.1177/1759720X17740075.
10. Goslen JB. Autoimmune ulceration of the leg. Clin Dermatol. 1990;8(3–4):92–117. https://linkinghub.elsevier.com/retrieve/pii/0738081X9090050B.
11. Jennette JC, Falk RJ, Bacon PA, Basu N, Cid MC, Ferrario F, et al. 2012 revised international Chapel Hill consensus conference nomenclature of vasculitides. Arthritis Rheum. 2013;65(1):1–11. https://doi.org/10.1002/art.37715.
12. Bartels CM, Bridges AJ. Rheumatoid vasculitis: vanishing menace or target for new treatments? Curr Rheumatol Rep. 2010;12(6):414–9. https://doi.org/10.1007/s11926-010-0130-1.
13. Ghosh SK, Bandyopadhyay D, Biswas SK, Darung I. Mucocutaneous manifestations in patients with rheumatoid arthritis: a cross-sectional study from eastern India. Indian J Dermatol. 2017;62(4):411–7. http://www.ncbi.nlm.nih.gov/pubmed/28794554
14. Ahn C, Negus D, Huang W. Pyoderma gangrenosum: a review of pathogenesis and treatment. Expert Rev Clin Immunol. 2018;14(3):225–33. https://doi.org/10.1080/1744666X.2018.1438269.
15. Fraenkel L, Bathon JM, England BR, St.Clair EW, Arayssi T, Carandang K, et al. 2021 American College of Rheumatology Guideline for the treatment of rheumatoid arthritis. Arthritis Care Res (Hoboken). 2021;73(7):924–39. https://doi.org/10.1002/acr.24596.
16. Kurian A, Haber R. Methotrexate-induced cutaneous ulcers in a nonpsoriatic patient: case report and review of the literature. J Cutan Med Surg. 2011;15(5):275–9. https://doi.org/10.2310/7750.2011.10078.
17. Tekur V. Methotrexate-induced nonhealing cutaneous ulcers in a nonpsoriatic patient without pancytopenia. Indian Dermatol Online J. 2016;7(5):418. http://www.idoj.in/text.asp?2016/7/5/418/190509.
18. Jakob A, Porstmann R, Rompel R. Skin ulceration after leflunomide treatment in two patients with rheumatoid arthritis. JDDG. 2006;4(4):324–7. https://doi.org/10.1111/j.1610-0387.2006.05934.x.
19. McCoy CM. Leflunomide-associated skin ulceration. Ann Pharmacother. 2002;36(6):1009–11. https://doi.org/10.1345/aph.1A347.
20. Kurnick JE. Mechanism of the Anemia of chronic disorders. Arch Intern Med. 1972;130(3):323. https://doi.org/10.1001/archinte.1972.03650030011003.
21. Avishai E, Yeghiazaryan K, Golubnitschaja O. Impaired wound healing: facts and hypotheses for multi-professional considerations in predictive, preventive and personalised medicine. EPMA J. 2017;8(1):23–33. https://doi.org/10.1007/s13167-017-0081-y.
22. Roy Choudhury A, Roy CA. Leukocytoclastic Vasculitis in a patient with rheumatoid arthritis. Cureus. 2021;13:e17124. https://www.cureus.com/articles/67403-leukocytoclastic-vasculitis-in-a-patient-with-rheumatoid-arthritis.
23. Borman P. Foot problems in a group of patients with rheumatoid arthritis: an unmet need for foot care. Open Rheumatol J. 2012;6(1):290–5. http://benthamopen.com/ABSTRACT/TORJ-6-290.
24. Papi M, Papi C. Biologics in Microangiopathic wounds. Int J Low Extrem Wounds. 2018;17(4):205–13. https://doi.org/10.1177/1534734618813767.
25. Werchek S. Diagnosis and treatment of venous leg ulcers. Nurse Pract. 2010;35(12):46–53.
26. Grey JE, Harding KG, Enoch S. Venous and arterial leg ulcers. BMJ. 2006;332(7537):347–50. https://doi.org/10.1136/bmj.332.7537.347.
27. Alexiadou K, Doupis J. Management of diabetic foot ulcers. Diabetes Ther. 2012;3(1):4. https://doi.org/10.1007/s13300-012-0004-9.

28. Oliver TI, Mutluoglu M. Diabetic foot ulcer. In: StatPearls. Treasure Island, FL: StatPearls Publishing; 2021. http://www.ncbi.nlm.nih.gov/pubmed/30726013.
29. Mazzucchelli R, Yebra M, Barbadillo C, Berrocal E, Gea JC, Andreu-Sanchez JL. Double disease in rheumatology: coexistence of rheumatoid arthritis and psoriatic arthritis. Clin Exp Rheumatol. 1992;10(1):83–5. http://www.ncbi.nlm.nih.gov/pubmed/1551285.
30. Iaccarino L, Gatto M, Bettio S, Caso F, Rampudda M, Zen M, et al. Overlap connective tissue disease syndromes. Autoimmun Rev. 2013;12(3):363–73. https://linkinghub.elsevier.com/retrieve/pii/S1568997212001218.
31. Seitz CS, Berens N, Bröcker E-B, Trautmann A. Leg ulceration in rheumatoid arthritis–an underreported multicausal complication with considerable morbidity: analysis of thirty-six patients and review of the literature. Dermatology. 2010;220(3):268–73. https://www.karger.com/Article/FullText/284583.
32. Öien RF, Håkansson A, Hansen BU. Leg ulcers in patients with rheumatoid arthritis—a prospective study of aetiology, wound healing and pain reduction after pinch grafting. Rheumatology. 2001;40(7):816–20. https://doi.org/10.1093/rheumatology/40.7.816.
33. Shanmugam VK, Angra D, Rahimi H, McNish S. Vasculitic and autoimmune wounds. J Vasc Surg Venous Lymphat Disord. 2017;5(2):280–92. https://linkinghub.elsevier.com/retrieve/pii/S2213333X16301809.
34. Puéchal X, Said G, Hilliquin P, Coste J, Job-Deslandre C, Lacroix C, et al. Peripheral neuropathy with necrotizing vasculitis in rheumatoid arthritis. Arthritis Rheum. 1995;38(11):1618–29. https://doi.org/10.1002/art.1780381114.
35. Maverakis E, Marzano AV, Le ST, Callen JP, Brüggen M-C, Guenova E, et al. Pyoderma gangrenosum. Nat Rev Dis Prim. 2020;6(1):81. https://www.nature.com/articles/s41572-020-0213-x.
36. Teagle A, Hargest R. Management of pyoderma gangrenosum. J R Soc Med. 2014;107(6):228–36. https://doi.org/10.1177/0141076814534407.
37. Armstrong DG. The 10-g monofilament: the diagnostic divining rod for the diabetic foot? Diabetes Care. 2000;23(7):887–7. https://diabetesjournals.org/care/article/23/7/887/23931/The-10-g-monofilament-the-diagnostic-divining-rod.
38. Voskuyl AE, van Duinen SG, Zwinderman AH, Breedveld FC, Hazes JMW. The diagnostic value of perivascular infiltrates in muscle biopsy specimens for the assessment of rheumatoid vasculitis. Ann Rheum Dis. 1998;57(2):114–7. https://doi.org/10.1136/ard.57.2.114.
39. Brooklyn T, Dunnill G, Probert C. Diagnosis and treatment of pyoderma gangrenosum. BMJ. 2006;333(7560):181–4. https://doi.org/10.1136/bmj.333.7560.181.
40. Fujimoto M, Asai J, Asano Y, Ishii T, Iwata Y, Kawakami T, et al. Wound, pressure ulcer and burn guidelines—4: guidelines for the management of connective tissue disease/vasculitis-associated skin ulcers. J Dermatol. 2020;47(10):1071–109. https://doi.org/10.1111/1346-8138.15186.
41. Imai M, Kondo N, Kumazaki R, Endo N. Treatment of an intractable forefoot ulcer using realignment osteotomy in a patient with rheumatoid arthritis. Case Rep Orthop. 2020;2020:8817456. http://www.ncbi.nlm.nih.gov/pubmed/32802537.
42. Serra R, Rizzuto A, Rossi A, Perri P, Barbetta A, Abdalla K, et al. Skin grafting for the treatment of chronic leg ulcers—a systematic review in evidence-based medicine. Int Wound J. 2017;14(1):149–57. http://www.ncbi.nlm.nih.gov/pubmed/26940940.
43. Garwood CS, Kim PJ, Matai V, Steinberg JS, Evans KK, Mitnick CDB, et al. The use of bovine collagen-glycosaminoglycan matrix for atypical lower extremity ulcers. Wounds. 2016;28(9):298–305. http://www.ncbi.nlm.nih.gov/pubmed/27701125.
44. Hernandez R. The use of systemic antibiotics in the treatment of chronic wounds. Dermatol Ther. 2006;19(6):326–37. https://doi.org/10.1111/j.1529-8019.2006.00091.x.
45. Ashida A, Murata H, Mikoshiba Y, Ohashi A, Kobayashi A, Koga H, et al. Successful treatment of rheumatoid vasculitis-associated skin ulcer with a TNF-α antagonist. Int J Dermatol. 2014;53(2):e154–6. http://www.ncbi.nlm.nih.gov/pubmed/23557520.

Ulcers in Systemic Sclerosis

4

Anisha Najeeb, Vandana Yadav, and Sanjay Singh

4.1 Introduction

4.1.1 Systemic Sclerosis: Definition and Prevalence

Systemic sclerosis (SSc) is a connective tissue disease characterized by progressive fibrosis of the skin and internal organs and it has important clinical sequelae. The pooled prevalence is 17.6 per 100,000 and the pooled incidence rate is 1.4 per 100,000 person-years [1]. The pooled prevalence and incidence in women is almost five times higher than the pooled estimates in men [1].

4.2 Diagnostic Criteria of Systemic Sclerosis

Diagnostic criteria of systemic sclerosis are as follows (Tables 4.1 and 4.2).

The total score is determined by adding the maximum weight (score) in each category. Patients with a total score of 9 or more are classified as having definite systemic sclerosis.

Anisha Najeeb, Vandana Yadav and Sanjay Singh contributed equally.

A. Najeeb · V. Yadav · S. Singh (✉)
Department of Dermatology and Venereology, Institute of Medical Sciences, Banaras Hindu University, Varanasi, India

A. K. Khanna, S. K. Tiwary (eds.), *Uncommon Ulcers of the Extremities*,
https://doi.org/10.1007/978-981-99-1782-2_4

Table 4.1 The American College of Rheumatology/European League Against Rheumatism (ACR/EULAR) criteria for the classification of systemic sclerosis [2]

I Item	S Sub-items	W Weight/ score
Skin thickening of the fingers of both hands extending proximal to the metacarpophalangeal joints *(sufficient criterion)*		9
Skin thickening of the fingers *(only count the higher score)*	• Puffy fingers • Sclerodactyly of the fingers (distal to the metacarpophalangeal joints but proximal to the proximal interphalangeal joints)	2 4
Fingertip lesions *(only count the higher score)*	• Digital tip ulcers • Fingertip pitting scars	2 3
Telangiectasia	–	2
Abnormal nailfold capillaries	–	2
Pulmonary arterial hypertension and/or interstitial lung disease *(maximum score is 2)*	• Pulmonary arterial hypertension • Interstitial lung disease	2 2
Raynaud phenomenon	–	3
SSc-related autoantibodies (anticentromere, anti-topoisomerase I [anti-Scl-70], anti-RNA polymerase III) *(maximum score is 3)*	Anticentromere Anti-topoisomerase I Anti-RNA polymerase III	3

Table 4.2 Definitions of items/sub-items in the American College of Rheumatology/European League Against Rheumatism (ACR/EULAR) criteria for the classification of systemic sclerosis [2]

I Item	Definition
Skin thickening	Skin thickening or hardening not due to scarring after injury, trauma, etc.
Puffy fingers	Wollen digits—a diffuse, usually nonpitting increase in soft tissue mass of the digits extending beyond the Normal confines of the joint capsule. Normal digits are tapered distally with the tissues following the contours of the digital bone and joint structures. Swelling of the digits obliterates these contours. Not due to other causes such as inflammatory dactylitis
Fingertip ulcers or pitting scars	Ulcers or scars distal to or at the proximal interphalangeal joint not thought to be due to trauma. Digital pitting scars are depressed areas at digital tips as a result of ischaemia, rather than trauma or exogenous causes
Telangiectasia	Telangiectasiae are visible macular dilated superficial blood vessels, which collapse upon pressure and fill slowly when pressure is released. Telangiectasiae in a scleroderma-like pattern are round and well-demarcated and found on hands, lips, inside of the mouth, and/or are large mat-like telangiectasiae. Distinguishable from rapidly filling spider angiomas with central arteriole and from dilated superficial vessels

Table 4.2 (continued)

I Item	Definition
Abnormal nailfold capillary pattern consistent with systemic sclerosis	Enlarged capillaries and/or capillary loss with or without pericapillary haemorrhages at the nailfold. May also be seen on the cuticle
Pulmonary arterial hypertension	Pulmonary arterial hypertension diagnosed by right-sided heart catheterisation according to standard definitions
Interstitial lung disease	Pulmonary fibrosis seen on high-resolution CT or chest radiography, most pronounced in the basilar portions of the lungs, or occurrence of 'Velcro' crackles on auscultation, not due to another cause such as congestive heart failure
Raynaud phenomenon	Self-reported or reported by a physician, with at least a 2-phase colour change in the finger(s) and often toe(s) consisting of pallor, cyanosis, and/or reactive hyperaemia in response to cold exposure or emotion; usually one phase is pallor
SSc-related autoantibodies	Anticentromere antibody or centromere pattern seen on antinuclear antibody testing, anti-topoisomerase I antibody (also known as anti-Scl-70 antibody), or anti-RNA polymerase III antibody. Positive according to local laboratory standards

4.2.1 Ulcers in Systemic Sclerosis

Skin ulcers are one of the most frequent manifestations of systemic sclerosis (SSc). The ulcers may be very painful, often persistent, and recurrent; they may lead to marked impairment of the patient's activities and quality of life.

Systemic sclerosis skin ulcers are defined as loss of substance involving epidermis, basement membrane, and dermis, and frequently deeper skin structures; lesions may be multiple, recurrent, and/or relapsing; they are localized at one or more skin areas, often acral zones of the hands and feet. The ulcers are classified as follows [3]:

1. Digital ulcers.
2. Skin ulcers of the bony prominence.
3. Skin ulcers of calcinosis.
4. Skin ulcers of lower limbs.
5. Skin ulcers or digital ulcers with gangrene.

According to a recent study by Pinto et al., 57.5% of patients with systemic sclerosis had at least one episode of digital ulcer anytime during their illness. The prevalence of skin ulcers on bony prominences was 13%, on calcinosis was 4.8%, on lower limbs was 15.8%, and the ulcer was associated with gangrene in 13% of cases [4].

4.3 Pathogenesis of Vascular Disease in Systemic Sclerosis

The three major pathological events in systemic sclerosis are vasculopathy, inflammation, and fibrosis. Initially, microvascular injury occurs which is followed by infiltration of inflammatory cells of the innate and the adaptive immune systems. Various cytokines like interleukin (IL) 4, 6, 8, 10, 13, and 17, transforming growth factor β (TGF-β), platelet-derived growth factor, and endothelin-1 are overexpressed in the skin which then activate the fibroblasts, eventually causing fibrosis [5].

4.3.1 Pathogenesis of Ulcers

The underlying vasculopathy in systemic sclerosis and the recurrent vasospasm due to Raynaud phenomena contribute to the ischaemic damage leading to the formation of the fingertip digital ulcers. Platelet activation is a prominent feature of scleroderma-associated vasculopathy, which, in turn, leads to intraluminal thrombosis which plays a crucial role in the development of these ulcers [6].

Development of ulcers over bony prominences like the phalangeal joints and elbows is due to the repetitive trauma at the sites of chronic contractures. The tissue overlying these sites is usually atrophic and avascular which leads to poor healing. As their pathogenesis is different from the ulcers located at distal digits, vasodilators are generally less effective in treating them [6].

4.3.2 Ulcers over the Sites of Calcinosis

Patients with systemic sclerosis are also prone to develop ulceration at the sites of underlying calcinosis. Repetitive trauma is thought to contribute to calcinosis, as it is preferentially located in the dominant hand and other acral sites. Due to the underlying proliferative obliterative vasculopathy in systemic sclerosis, there is impairment in the compensatory angiogenesis at the sites of trauma which makes them more susceptible to ulcerations [7].

4.4 Clinical Features

Digital ulcers on the tips of fingers or toes, which may result in tender and painful pitting scars, are the most common types of ulcers in systemic sclerosis (Fig. 4.1). The ulcers may occur over the extensor surfaces of bony prominences as a result of microtrauma. The other common sites of ulcers on the upper limbs are elbows followed by metacarpophalangeal joints, proximal interphalangeal joints, and the wrist [4]. Skin ulcers may also develop over the pre-existing calcinosis cutis. Calcinosis cutis occurs most frequently in the hands, followed by proximal upper extremities, knees, or proximal lower extremities and hip, in that order [7]. Skin ulcers presenting on lower limbs are most common over the malleoli, followed by the plantar

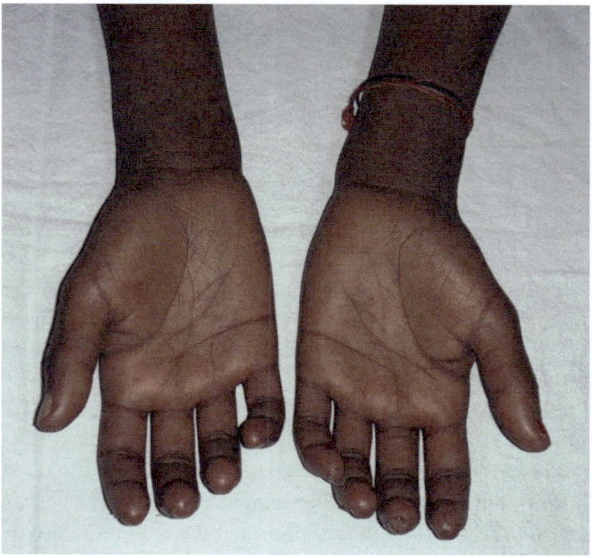

Fig. 4.1 Digital ulcers in an 11-year-old girl with systemic sclerosis. She had skin thickening extending proximal to the metacarpophalangeal (MCP) joints, digital tip scarring, dilated nailfold capillaries, and the Raynaud phenomenon

aspect of the feet [4]. Digital ulcers may be associated with severe local pain and a major impact on the quality of life. Other complications which are associated with skin ulcers in systemic sclerosis include critical digital ischaemia, paronychia, infections, gangrene, osteomyelitis, and finger pulp loss or amputation [8].

4.5 Investigations

Investigations for skin ulcers are performed mainly to assess the microvascular abnormalities and macrovascular damage, to know the extent of ulcers, and to evaluate the presence of secondary infection.

Structural microvascular abnormalities can be easily detected noninvasively with nailfold video capillaroscopy (NVC). NVC is a reliable tool for early diagnosis of SSc and assessment of disease progression. NVC scleroderma patterns have been reported to predict clinical complications of the disease, including the development of future DUs [9].

Colour Doppler ultrasonography is a useful technique to identify morphological and functional digital arteries abnormalities. Narrowed arteries, or chronically or acutely occluded arteries, are typical ultrasonographic findings [10]. Colour Doppler ultrasonography can also be used to detect changes in blood flow and vascular resistance parameters.

X-ray and magnetic resonance imaging (MRI) should be performed in deep ulcers to see the extent of the ulcer. MRI is a useful tool for the early detection of osteomyelitis.

Pus culture and antibiotic susceptibility test may be done in large and chronic non-healing ulcers if the secondary bacterial infection is suspected.

4.6 Management

Digital ulcers require a multidisciplinary approach with cooperation between physicians and specialist nursing and other allied health professionals to ensure appropriate treatment and provide patient education.

4.6.1 Lifestyle Changes

A correct education of patients with SSc for an appropriate lifestyle is advisable with specific instructions for individuals with severe Raynaud phenomenon and complicating digital ulcers. Therefore, all patients should be advised to wear a hat, gloves, scarf, coat, and warm socks and shoes during winter weather. Considering that some drugs can trigger episodes of Raynaud phenomenon, it is necessary to avoid medicines that contain ergotamine, appetite suppressants, beta-blockers, and hormonal contraceptives; in addition, all patients are strongly advised to stop smoking, avoid emotional stress, and to take adequate measures to avoid physical trauma to the extremities.

4.6.2 Drug Treatment

Current local management of digital ulcers includes a combination of nonpharmacologic care, antibiotics (in case of infection), analgesia, and wound dressing, if necessary. Meticulous attention should be directed towards wound care, including keeping the digital ulcer clean and using a suitable dressing; if the digital ulcer is dry then an attempt should be made to wet it (alginates and antimicrobials) and vice versa for wet digital ulcers (hydrogel and hydrocolloids) [11].

4.6.3 Prostanoids (Level of Evidence: Meta-Analysis)

Prostanoids are potent vasodilators and also inhibit platelet aggregation and vascular smooth muscle cell proliferation. Prostanoids can be administered by various routes: oral, intravenous (i.v.), and subcutaneous; however, side effects are common to all, including systemic hypotension, dizziness, flushing, gastrointestinal disturbance, jaw pain, and myalgia.

Intravenous iloprost is efficacious in healing DUs in patients with SSc. One meta-analysis published in 2013 included four randomized controlled trials (RCT), two with intravenous iloprost (0.5–2 ng/kg/min for 3–5 consecutive days), one with oral iloprost (100 or 200 μg/day vs placebo for 6 weeks), and one with oral treprostinil (slow release up to 16 mg two times a day for 20 weeks) [12–16]. This analysis showed a trend towards a beneficial effect of prostanoids over placebo for healing of digital ulcers with the greatest effect seen with intravenous iloprost, but it did not show significant effects of prostanoids for the prevention of new DUs in SSc. The greatest effect was seen with intravenous iloprost. Because of the risk of side effects and route of administration usually requiring hospitalization, intravenous iloprost may be considered in particular in patients with SSc with DUs not responding to oral therapy.

4.6.4 Endothelin Receptor-1 Antagonists (Level of Evidence: Meta-Analysis)

Bosentan, a dual receptor antagonist, was found to be effective in reducing the number of new DUs in patients with SSc in two high-quality RCTs [17, 18]. A meta-analysis [14] showed that bosentan was successful in ulcer prevention, with a statistically significant reduction in the mean number of new ulcers per patient. Bosentan should be considered for reduction of the number of new DUs in SSc, especially in patients with multiple DUs despite the use of calcium channel blockers, phosphodiesterase type-5 (PDE-5) inhibitors, or iloprost therapy. There are two major concerns related to the use of bosentan and other endothelin receptor antagonists (ERA), potential liver injury and teratogenicity. Hormonal contraceptives may not be reliable if co-administered with bosentan, because bosentan may reduce their efficacy by interference with the cytochrome P450 system.

4.6.5 Phosphodiesterase Type-5 Inhibitors (Level of Evidence: Meta-Analysis)

Phosphodiesterase type-5 inhibitors inhibit the degradation (and therefore increase the bioavailability) of cyclic GMP, with subsequent vasodilatation. A meta-analysis of RCTs [14] investigating various selective PDE-5 inhibitors (sildenafil 50 mg twice daily, modified-release sildenafil 100 mg/day increased up to 200 mg/day or tadalafil 20 mg on alternate days) indicates that PDE-5 inhibitors improve healing of DUs in patients with SSc. Moreover, the results of one small RCT [19] indicate that PDE-5 inhibitors may prevent the development of new DUs in SSc. Side effects associated with the usage of PDE-5 inhibitors were common and included different forms of vasomotor reactions, myalgias, allergic reactions, chest pain, dyspepsia, nasal stuffiness, and visual abnormalities.

4.6.6 Calcium Channel Blockers (Level of Evidence: Randomized Controlled Trial)

There are not many studies on calcium channel blockers to examine their efficacy in healing or prevention of digital ulcers, although many clinicians prescribe calcium channel blockers in this context (often for concomitant severe Raynaud phenomenon). In a randomized, double-blind study comparing oral nifedipine (30 mg daily for 4 weeks and then 60 mg daily for 12 weeks) and i.v. iloprost for Raynaud phenomenon (both with concomitant placebo infusions and capsules, respectively), the mean number of DUs was reduced from 4.3 to 1.4 after 16 weeks of treatment with nifedipine [20].

4.6.7 Combination Therapy (Level of Evidence: Case Report)

No randomized controlled trials are addressing vasoactive therapies used in combination for DUs. Two case reports have suggested that the combination of PDE-5 inhibitors and endothelin receptor antagonist (ERA) therapies (either both at low dose or initial PDE5 inhibitor with subsequent ERA) is efficacious in refractory DU disease [21, 22].

4.6.8 Other Drug Therapies that Have Been Explored

4.6.8.1 Statins (Level of Evidence: Randomized Controlled Trial)

In a randomized trial, which included 84 patients with SSc, 4 months of treatment with atorvastatin (40 mg; compared with placebo) was associated with a reduction in the number of new DUs (1.6 vs 2.5) during the treatment period [23].

4.6.8.2 Anticoagulant and Antiplatelet Agents (Level of Evidence: Randomized Controlled Trial)

In a randomized controlled trial, 24 weeks of open-label treatment with s.c. low-molecular-weight heparin was not associated with a significant difference in new DUs [24].

4.6.9 Surgical Strategies

4.6.9.1 General Approach

Surgical intervention is required only in a minority of patients with DU, usually in those who have failed medical management. The main aim of debridement is to relieve pain by removing necrotic tissue and/or pus. Despite the therapeutic intervention, amputation of the affected digit may be necessary [25, 26]. Indications for surgical intervention include failure of DU healing, severe pain, osteomyelitis, and underlying calcinosis.

4.6.9.2 Sympathectomy and Injection of Botulinum Toxin (Level of Evidence: Retrospective Case Series and Case Series)

There is increasing experience worldwide with these techniques for the treatment of DUs, although the evidence base in SSc-related digital vasculopathy is limited. In a retrospective analysis of 26 patients with DUs, improvement in pain was reported in 92.3% post-sympathectomy, with DU healing in the majority, and with only two patients later requiring surgical intervention (at 6 months and 4.5 years) [27].

Botulinum toxin has also been reported to be associated with the healing and prevention of DUs in SSc. In a case series of botulinum toxin, in five patients with refractory DU disease, all DUs had healed by 12 weeks (and one within 2 weeks) [28].

Treatment	Level of evidence
Prostanoids	Meta-analysis
Endothelin receptor-1 antagonists	Meta-analysis
Phosphodiesterase type-5 inhibitors	Meta-analysis
Calcium channel blockers	Randomized, double-blind study
Combination therapy	Case report
Statins	Randomized trial
Anticoagulant and antiplatelet agents	Prospective parallel-group, randomized study

4.6.10 Prognosis

Skin ulcers in SSc are often recurrent and difficult to heal because of local complications, mainly infections; the latter were observed in over two-thirds of individuals and were often responsible for more severe complications, namely osteomyelitis, gangrene, and/or amputation [3]. The development of SSc-skin ulcer was significantly associated with lower patients' mean age at the disease onset, male gender, diffuse cutaneous subset, calcinosis, telangiectasia, melanodermia, abnormal pulmonary arterial pressure, and/or altered inflammation reactant (CRP) [3]. Recurrent and slow to heal DUs are significantly associated with severe pain, hand disability, and reduced quality of life [29].

References

1. Bairkdar M, Rossides M, Westerlind H, Hesselstrand R, Arkema EV, Holmqvist M. Incidence and prevalence of systemic sclerosis globally: a comprehensive systematic review and meta-analysis. Rheumatology (Oxford). 2021;60:3121–33.
2. van den Hoogen F, Khanna D, Fransen J, Johnson SR, Baron M, Tyndall A, et al. 2013 classification criteria for systemic sclerosis: an American college of rheumatology/European league against rheumatism collaborative initiative. Ann Rheum Dis. 2013;72:1747–55.
3. Giuggioli D, Manfredi A, Lumetti F, Colaci M, Ferri C. Scleroderma skin ulcers definition, classification and treatment strategies our experience and review of the literature. Autoimmun Rev. 2018;17:155–64.
4. Pinto B, Janardana R, Kaimal S, Charles BS, Sangeeta KN, Mathew J, et al. Nondigital skin ulcers in systemic sclerosis: a neglected entity. Indian J Rheumatol. 2021;16:139–44.
5. Orteu CH, Denton CP. In: Griffiths CEM, Barker J, Bleiker T, Chalmers R, Creamer D, editors. Systemic sclerosis. Rook's textbook of dermatology. 9th ed. West Sussex: Wiley Blackwell; 2016. p. 56.1–56.23.
6. Chung L, Fiorentino D. Digital ulcers in patients with systemic sclerosis. Autoimmun Rev. 2006;5:125–8.
7. Valenzuela A, Song P, Chung L. Calcinosis in scleroderma. Curr Opin Rheumatol. 2018;30:554–61.

8. Moinzadeh P, Denton CP, Black CM, Krieg T. Systemic sclerosis. In: Kang S, Amagai M, Bruckner AL, Enk AH, Margolis DJ, McMichael AJ, Orringer JS, editors. Fitzpatrick's dermatology. 9th ed. New York: McGraw-Hill; 2019. p. 1086–105.
9. Cutolo M, Pizzorni C, Sulli A, Smith V. Early diagnostic and predictive value of capillaroscopy in systemic sclerosis. Curr Rheumatol Rev. 2013;9:249–53.
10. Schmidt WA, Krause A, Schicke B, Wernicke D. Color Doppler ultrasonography of hand and finger arteries to differentiate primary from secondary forms of Raynaud's phenomenon. J Rheumatol. 2018;35:1591–8.
11. Hughes M, Ong VH, Anderson ME, Hall F, Moinzadeh P, Griffiths B, et al. Consensus best practice pathway of the UK scleroderma study group: digital vasculopathy in systemic sclerosis. Rheumatology. 2015;54:2015–24.
12. Black CM, Halkier-Sørensen L, Belch JJ, Ullman S, Madhok R, Smit AJ, et al. Oral iloprost in Raynaud's phenomenon secondary to systemic sclerosis: a multicentre, placebo-controlled, dose-comparison study. Br J Rheumatol. 1998;37:952–60.
13. Seibold JR, Wigley FM, Schiopu E, Denton CD, Silver RM, Steen VD, et al. Digital ischemic ulcers in scleroderma treated with oral treprostinil diethanolamine: a randomized, double-blind, placebo-controlled, multicenter study [abstract]. Arthritis Rheum. 2011;63:968–9.
14. Tingey T, Shu J, Smuczek J, Pope J. Meta-analysis of healing and prevention of digital ulcers in systemic sclerosis. Arthritis Care Res (Hoboken). 2013;65:1460–71.
15. Wigley FM, Seibold JR, Wise RA, McCloskey DA, Dole WP. Intravenous iloprost treatment of Raynaud's phenomenon and ischemic ulcers secondary to systemic sclerosis. J Rheumatol. 1992;19:1407–14.
16. Wigley FM, Wise RA, Seibold JR, McCloskey DA, Kujala G, Medsger TA Jr, et al. Intravenous iloprost infusion in patients with Raynaud phenomenon secondary to systemic sclerosis. A multicenter, placebo-controlled, double-blind study. Ann Intern Med. 1994;120:199–206.
17. Korn JH, Mayes M, Matucci-Cerinic M, Rainisio M, Pope J, Hachulla E, et al. Digital ulcers in systemic sclerosis: prevention by treatment with bosentan, an oral endothelin receptor antagonist. Arthritis Rheum. 2004;50:3985–93.
18. Matucci-Cerinic M, Denton CP, Furst DE, Mayes MD, Hsu VM, Carpentier P, et al. Bosentan treatment of digital ulcers related to systemic sclerosis: results from the RAPIDS-2 randomised, double-blind, placebo-controlled trial. Ann Rheum Dis. 2011;70:32–8.
19. Agarwal V, Ghosh P, Sharma A, Bhakuni DS, Kumar S, Singh UN. Efficacy of tadalafil in Raynaud's phenomenon secondary to systemic sclerosis: a double-blind randomized placebo-controlled parallel group multicentric study. Arthritis Rheum. 2010;62:S872.
20. Rademaker M, Cooke ED, Almond NE, Beacham JA, Smith RE, Mantet TG, et al. Comparison of intravenous infusions of iloprost and oral nifedipine in treatment of Raynaud's phenomenon in patients with systemic sclerosis: a double-blind randomised study. BMJ. 1989;298:561–4.
21. Ambach A, Seo W, Bonnekoh B, Gollnick H. Low-dose combination therapy of severe digital ulcers in diffuse progressive systemic sclerosis with the endothelin-1 receptor antagonist bosentan and the phosphodiesterase V inhibitor sildenafil. J Dtsch Dermatol Ges. 2009;7:888–91.
22. Moinzadeh P, Hunzelmann N, Krieg T. Combination therapy with an endothelin-1 receptor antagonist (bosentan) and a phosphodiesterase V inhibitor (sildenafil) for the management of severe digital ulcerations in systemic sclerosis. J Am Acad Dermatol. 2011;65:102–4.
23. Abou-Raya A, Abou-Raya S, Helmii M. Statins: potentially useful in therapy of systemic sclerosis-related Raynaud's phenomenon and digital ulcers. J Rheumatol. 2008;3:1801–8.
24. Denton CP, Howell K, Stratton RJ, Black CM. Long-term low molecular weight heparin therapy for severe Raynaud's phenomenon: a pilot study. Clin Exp Rheumatol. 2000;18:499–502.
25. Denton CP, Krieg T, Guillevin L, Schwierin B, Rosenberg D, Silkey M, et al. Demographic, clinical and antibody characteristics of patients with digital ulcers in systemic sclerosis: data from the DUO registry. Ann Rheum Dis. 2012;71:718–21.
26. Hachulla E, Clerson P, Launay D, Lambert M, Morell-Dubois S, Queyrel V, et al. Natural history of ischemic digital ulcers in systemic sclerosis: single-center retrospective longitudinal study. J Rheumatol. 2007;34:2423–30.

27. Momeni A, Sorice SC, Valenzuela A, Fiorentino DF, Chung L, Chang J. Surgical treatment of systemic sclerosis-is it justified to offer peripheral sympathectomy earlier in the disease process? Microsurgery. 2015;35:441–6.
28. Motegi S-I, Yamada K, Toki S, Uchiyama A, Kubota Y, Nakamura T, et al. Beneficial effect of botulinum toxin a on Raynaud's phenomenon in Japanese patients with systemic sclerosis: a prospective, case series study. J Dermatol. 2016;43:56–62.
29. Morrisroe K, Stevens W, Sahhar J, Ngian G, Ferdowsi N, Hill CL, et al. Digital ulcers in systemic sclerosis: their epidemiology, clinical characteristics, and associated clinical and economic burden. Arthritis Res Ther. 2019;21:299.

Livedoid Vasculopathy: Clinical, Histopathological, and Therapy Evaluation

5

Paulo Ricardo Criado

What's known?
- Atrophie blanche and painful ulcers were the most frequent cutaneous manifestation.
- Livedoid vasculopathy (LV) treatment is a challenge and relapses are frequent.

What's new?
- Our Brazilian retrospective review of 75 cases diagnosed as VL over the last 15 years was made, the largest study in Latin America.
- The Caucasian ethnic group was the most prevalent even in a country with significant racial miscegenation.
- Associated thrombophilic factors are common in LV, mainly high levels of lipoprotein (a), followed by antiphospholipid antibodies and elevated serum levels of coagulation factors VIII/IX.

5.1 Introduction

Livedoid vasculopathy (LV), livedo vasculopathy is classified as a rare disease [1], with an estimated prevalence in general North American population is around 1 case per 100,000 inhabitants [2], and this disease is an orphan-condition (Orphanet classification for rare diseases ORPHA:542643) [3]. It is a chronic disorder that usually presents as recurrent reticulated purpura and/or livedo racemosa on the lower limbs, with recurrent, painful purpuric and/or necrotic macules that may lead to often

P. R. Criado (✉)
Dermatology Department, Hospital das Clinicas da Faculdade de Medicina da, Universidade de Sao Paulo, Sao Paulo, Brazil

Faculdade de Ciências Médicas de Santos (Fundação Lusíada—UNILUS), Santos, SP, Brazil

A. K. Khanna, S. K. Tiwary (eds.), *Uncommon Ulcers of the Extremities*,
https://doi.org/10.1007/978-981-99-1782-2_5

ulcerative lesions, especially the ankles and dorsum of the feet [4]. The pain, functional disability, and cosmetic defects in these patients lead to severe impairment in quality of life [5].

The ulcers often are multiple in distinct stages of healing and subsequently over weeks or months, resulting in atrophic and reticulated porcelain-like white scars, named *Atrophie Blanche*, surrounded by punctate telangiectasias with livedoid brownish pigmentation [1]. The main pathogenic mechanism is a vaso-occlusive phenomenon due to intraluminal thrombosis of the dermal blood vessels and occasionally in the subcutis [1].

5.2 Our Casuistic

We performed a retrospective and transversal study in a Brazilian tertiary centre reviewing the epidemiological and clinical data, the histopathological findings on the haematoxylin-eosin stain and direct immunofluorescence, as well as the therapy of our patients with LV. We aimed to assess the comorbidities, the age of disease's onset, dermatological and laboratory findings, therapies applied, and time of follow-up of our patients. There are few articles in the Latin America reviewing clinical and epidemiological data of the patients with LV.

5.3 Methods

This retrospective study identified patients with LV from our database from January 1, 2005, to December 31, 2019. Patients included in the study presented with typical LV based on both clinical symptoms and signs (painful recurrent ulcers on legs or feet, livedo racemosa or livedo-like hyperpigmentation, and atrophie blanche), histopathology findings (intraluminal thrombosis of dermal and/or subcutis), and other criteria as (1) the absence of polymorphonuclear neutrophils and nuclear fragmentation in the vicinity of the dermal vessels early in the process, (2) the absence of permeation vascular wall by leukocytes, (3) fibrin deposition and hyalinization of the vascular wall, and (4) normal serum complement levels in most patients and the absence of detectable circulating immune complexes [1, 6]. The exclusion criteria were vasculitis with leukocytoclasis in skin biopsies or another cause for the leg ulceration had been elucidated as pyoderma gangrenosum, sarcoidosis, factitial dermatitis, conditions induced by drugs, and ulcers due to infectious-parasitic diseases. This study was approved by local Ethical Committee under the number 2.371.020.

On the first visit, patient's history was taken as age, sex, race, and the patient was asked about their age at first symptoms, treatment, occurrence of the previous thrombosis, pain during flare of the LV, paraesthesia on limbs, pruritus during healing of ulcers, concomitant diseases, familiar history of LV and thrombosis. The history or practice of smoking and other comorbidities: thyroid diseases, diabetes mellitus, systemic arterial hypertension, kidney diseases, autoimmune, infectious, neurological, heart diseases, and obesity (body mass index, BMI >30) was registered. The patients underwent a general and dermatological physical exam. All data from patients, including details on epidemiology, clinical characteristics, histopathology, treatment, and follow-up were collected from their physical or electronic records of our institution and registered in chart reviews and transferred for a table of Excel® for Windows®.

On dermatological exam, we registered the presence of active ulcers, their location, the presence of livedo racemosa on lower and/or upper limbs, presence of scars (*atrophie blanche*, AB), presence of venous stasis signs (varices, lower limb oedema), lower limbs arterial pulses, presence of tinea pedis and/or onychomycosis on feet.

All histopathological findings of cutaneous biopsies underwent for LV diagnosis purposes were registered, including presence or not of: fibrinoid necrosis of blood wall vessels, intraluminal fibrinoid thrombi and/or intraluminal fibrin-platelets thrombi in upper dermis and/or lower dermis and/or subcutis, perivascular lymphomononuclear infiltrate, perivascular neutrophil infiltrate, presence or not of leukocytoclasis, and collagen fibres augmentation in dermis.

Direct immunofluorescence (DIF) was performed as previously reported by Aoki et al. [7] and the data were collected.

Laboratory testing for diagnosing the established abnormalities associated with LV were recommended for all patients with LV, including hypercoagulable states (factor V G1691A gene mutation [Leiden], prothrombin G20210A gene mutation, methylenetetrahydrofolate reductase mutation and homocysteine serum levels, protein C and/or protein S deficiency, antithrombin deficiency, lipoprotein(a) serum levels, elevation of activity of Factor VIII and Factor IX, lupus anticoagulant, and anticardiolipin antibodies (ACA) IgM and IgG (2 distinct exams >20 MPL and > 20 GPL, at least), hepatitis B and C infection and autoimmune diseases (antinuclear antibodies, antineutrophil cytoplasmic antibody, rheumatoid factor). Serum levels of Lp(a) were measured by immunoturbidimetry (DiaSorin®, Sallugia, Italy). Values higher than 30 mg/dL (international cut-off for cardiovascular risk) were classified as "elevated levels".

The results of electromyographic exams were registered as mononeuritis multiplex or axonal sensitive and/or motor polyneuropathy on lower and/or upper limbs and analysed by the same neurology group.

All patients were submitted to arterial and venous Doppler ultrasound studies in our institution and the abnormal results were registered.

All drugs or procedures applied on the treatment of patients with LV, neuropathy, and relief of pain were registered.

5.4 Results

Seventy-five patients were included, 59 women (78.66%) and 16 men (21.34%), in the distribution of 3.68 ♀: ♂. During the study period, we observed that 5 women became pregnant, having normal newborns and not showed new lesions of LV through the pregnancy. Nine (12%) patients were smokers.

The median age of the patients at the first consultation in our Institution was 39.97 years (SD 16.54, range 13–78 years). The median age noticed by patients at the onset of the LV symptoms was 34.65 years (SD 17.41, range 8–77 years). The age group between 20 and 48 years of age (42 patients, 56%) was the most frequent. Fourteen (18.66%) patients noticed the onset of the disease until 18 years of age. Among 75 patients with LV, the racial/ethnic distribution was 61 (81.33%) white, 9 (12%) mulatto, 4 (5.33%) black, and 1 (1.33%) Asian.

The pain was referred by 70 patients (93.33%) and pruritus during ulcers healing in 35 (46.66%) of 75 patients. Hypoesthesia symptoms were noticed in 33 patients (44%) (15 patients on right lower limb, 15 patients on the left lower limb, and 3 patients on hands). Electroneuromyography studies were obtained in 11 (33.33%) of 33 symptomatic patients and showed: 8 (72.72%) peripheral axonal sensitive-motor polyneuropathy in LL, 2 (18.18%) patients with sensitive mononeuritis multiplex in LL, and 1 (9.09%) with peripheral axonal sensitive-motor polyneuropathy in upper limbs.

Flares of LV (new ulcers) related to seasonality were reported by 29 patients (38.66%) of 75 patients. Most of them occurred during spring/summer in 23 patients (79.92%) and during autumn/winter in 6 patients (20.68%). Unfortunately, 36 patients did not relate their LV flares in any season.

LV lesions observed during the first consultation in our institution in 75 patients were distributed as active ulcers in 62 patients (82.66%), AB in 75 patients (100%), hyperpigmented scars in 30 patients (40%), purpuric lesions in 45 patients (60%), telangiectasis on scars in 70 patients (93.33%), hemosiderosis on legs in 35 patients (46.66%), bilateral lesions on lower limbs (LL) in 71 patients (94.66%), unilateral lesions on LL in 4 patients (5.33%), bilateral livedo racemosa (LR) on LL in 48 patients (64%), bilateral LR on upper limbs in 7 patients (9.33%), LR on trunk in 1 patient (1.33%).

The interval of time recovered in 65 patients (86.66%), since the first symptoms of LV until a physician diagnosis, based on dermatological signs and histopathology findings range 1–20 years (median 6.65, SD 4.50).

Symptoms of chronic venous stasis or positive findings of venous insufficiency on legs were observed in 19 patients (25.33%) and lipodermatosclerosis in 5 (1.33%). Peripheral arterial diseases in lower limbs occurred ultrasound Doppler studies in 6 patients (8%), Raynaud phenomenon in 3 (4%), dyslipidaemia in 8 patients (10.66%) (7 hypercholesterolemia and 1 hypertriglyceridemia).

Systemic arterial hypertension (SAH) was present in 16 patients (21.33%), obesity in 29 patients (38.66%), diabetes mellitus in 7 (9.33%), hypothyroidism in 2 (2.8%), asthma in 1 (1.33%), chronic C hepatitis in 1 patient (1.33%), and congestive heart insufficiency in 1 (1.33%). Autoimmune conditions: primary antiphospholipid syndrome (APS) in 4 patients (5.33%), secondary APS due to systemic lupus erythematosus (SLE) in 1 (1.33%), SLE in 2 patients (2.66%), rheumatoid arthritis in 1 (1.33%), and chronic spontaneous urticaria in 1 (1.33%). History of thromboembolic conditions: previous venous thrombosis in lower limbs in 6 patients (8%), and one case (1.33%) of each follow conditions in distinct patients:

thrombosis in retinal arteria, deep venous thrombosis plus lung emboli plus sagittal thrombosis sinus, and another patient with retroperitoneal venous thrombosis.

Dermatological comorbidities found were tinea pedis in 11 patients (14.66%) and onychomycosis on feet in 10 (13.33%), regressive congenital cutaneous haemangioma in the same site of unilateral LV lesions in 1 (1.33%), and cutaneous primary malignant melanoma in 1 (1.33%).

Extracutaneous cancer was registered in 3 patients (4%): kidney cancer (1.33%) and 2 breast cancer (2.66%) (one of them before LV diagnosis and another after LV diagnosis).

All thrombophilia exams described in the methods section were completed or partially performed by 72 patients (96%) and not in 3 patients. Thrombophilic factors were found in 48 patients (66.66%) and absent in 24 (33.33%). Two or more concomitant thrombophilic factors were retrieved in 26/71 patients (36.61%) with our complete screening. Heterozygous Factor V (Leiden) mutation in 3/71 (4.22%), heterozygous Prothrombin gene mutations in 2/71 (2.81%), reduction of serum Protein C activity in 2/72 (2.77%), reduction of serum Protein S activity in 3/72 (4.16%), reduction of serum Antithrombin activity in 3/72 (4.16%), increase of serum Factor VIII activity in 9/72 (12.5%), increase of serum Factor IX activity in 9/72 (6.94%), hyperhomocystenemia in 5/2 (12.5%) (3 heterozygous and 2 homozygous for methylenetetrahydrofolate reductase, MTHFR, Lupus anticoagulant in 7/72 (9.72%), IgG ACA in 10/72 (13.88%), IgM ACA in 10/72 (13.88%), IgG ACA plus IgM ACA in 8/72 (11.11%), and Lupus anticoagulant plus ACA (IgG and /or IgM) in 5/72 (6.94%).

Serum levels of Lipoprotein (a) [Lp(a)] were the most common thrombophilic factor found in 30 patients (41.66%) (20–216 mg/dL, normal range < 9 mg/dL for women and < 11 mg/dL for men), medium value 78.5 mg/dL, SD 49.42 mg/dL, among 72 patients. Among these 30 patients, 24 (80%) showed levels of cardiovascular risk (> 30 mg/dL), medium value 92.63 mg/dL, SD 45.63 mg/dL. Taken these data from thrombophilic states together Lp(a), antiphospholipid antibodies, and elevated serum of Factors VIII and IX were the more relevant factors involved in pathogenesis of LV in our patients.

Eight (13.33%) in 60 patients showed elevated plasma levels of fibrinogen. Unspecific antinuclear antibodies (ANA) were increased (title ≥1:320) in 14/72 (19.44%), and one patient with rheumatoid factor (RF) positive. The antineutrophil cytoplasmic antibody (ANCA) test was negative in 72 patients. Reactive-C-protein (CRP) was elevated in only 2/72 (2.77%) and complement levels were reduced only in 4 patients, 3 with SLE diagnosis and 1 with RA of 72 patients. Only 1/72 (1.38%) demonstrated IgG monoclonal gammopathy of uncertain significance.

The biopsies obtained by punch 5 mm of diameter from 75 LV patients, often on lesions as purpuric macules or surrounding the AB, under haematoxylin-eosin stain, the follow findings were observed: fibrinoid necrosis of the dermal vessels in 36 patients (48%); segmental hyalinization of the wall vessels in the dermis in 60 patients (80%); intraluminal hyaline thrombi in the dermal vessels in 67 patients (89.33%) found in upper dermis in 60 patients (69.33%), lower dermis in 52 (69.33%) and subcutis in 9 (9.33%); intraluminal fibrin-platelet thrombi in 7 patients

(9.33%); erythrocytes extravasation in 65 patients (86.66%); perivascular lymphomononuclear infiltrate in 68 patients (90.66%); mild perivascular lymphomononuclear infiltrate with few neutrophils without leukocytoclasis in 10 patients (13.33%), and collagen fibres augmented in dermis in 24 patients (32%) (Fig. 5.1). Twenty-four (32%) of our 75 patients need more than at least two different skin biopsies to meet the histopathological criteria for LV diagnosis. Fifteen patients (20%) obtained a positive histopathological feature of LV when the biopsies were taken from plantar cavum, where livedo-like macules and/or purpura were present.

DIF was performed in 37 patients (49.33%) of 75 patients and at least one positive immunoreactant was observed in 27 patients (72.97%). Immunoreactants positive in both upper and lower dermis were found in 23 patients (62.16%). Distinct immunofluorescence patterns were retrieved: granular C3 in the wall vessels in 18/37 (48.64%); granular C3 in the BZM in 6/37 (16.21%); homogeneous C3 in the wall vessels in 7 (18.42%); homogeneous C3 in the BZM in 2/37 (5.4%); granular IgM in the wall vessels in 15/37 (40.54%); granular IgM in the BZM in 3/37 (8.1%); homogeneous IgM in the wall vessels in 2 (5.4%); homogeneous IgM in the BZM in 1/37 (2.7%); granular IgG in the wall vessels in 2/37 (5.4%); homogeneous IgG in the BZM in 1/37 (2.7%); granular IgA in the wall vessels in 4/37 (10.81%); and homogeneous IgA in the BZM in 1/37 (2.7%) (Fig. 5.1).

Several drugs were used for the treatment of our 75 patients. Some medications were disposable in our Institution, and it was accessible for distribution for our patients and other drugs, or procedures were not (cilostazol, hyperbaric oxygen therapy, pentoxifylline, rivaroxaban). The following drugs or treatments were applied for our 75 patients to treat LV: acetylsalicylic acid (ASA) (100–200 mg/day) for 57 patients (76%), pentoxifylline (800–1200 mg/day) for 54 (72%), diosmin/hesperidin (450/50 mg, t.i.d) for 36 (48%), cilostazol (100–200 mg/day) for 18 (24%), hyperbaric oxygen therapy (median of 20 sessions, per LV flare) for 18 (24%), danazol (100–200 mg/day) for 12 (16%), enoxaparin (40–80 mg/day) for 15 (20%), rivaroxaban (20–30 mg/day) for 11 (14.66%), warfarin (INR $1.5 \leq 2$) for 7

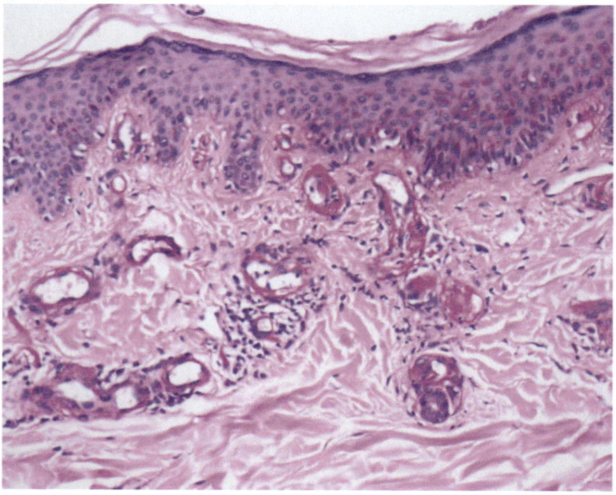

Fig. 5.1 Classical findings on chronic lesions of livedoid vasculopathy. Fibrin deposition into upper dermal blood vessels (HE, 200x)

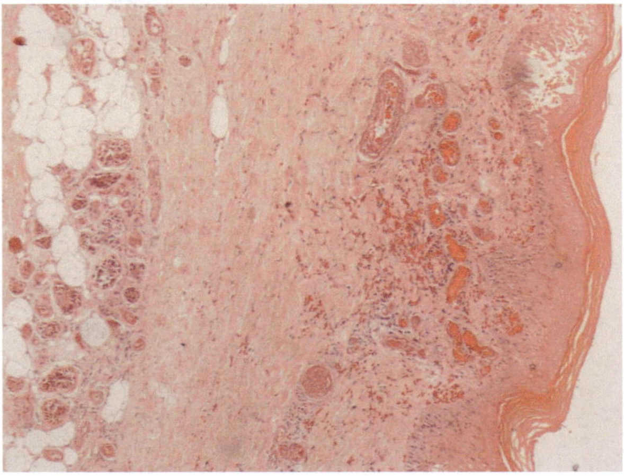

Fig. 5.2 Histopathological findings on acute lesions of livedoid vasculopathy. Multiple thrombi into upper dermal blood vessels (HE, 100x)

(9.33%), nicotinic acid (1.500 mg/day) for 5 (6.66%), unfractionated heparin (UFH) (Heparin sodium 5000 I.U./mL, 5000 I.U subcutaneous each 12 h/day) for 4 (5.33%), folic acid plus B vitamin complex for 4 (5.33%), colchicine (0.5 mg t.i.d/day) for 4 (5.33%), and dipyridamole (300 mg/day) for 1 (1.33%) (Fig. 5.2). Only one patient who received danazol developed amenorrhoea due to hormonal disbalance, but 50% of patients who received pentoxifylline and/or ASA noticed dyspeptic symptoms or headache. Any patient noticed episodes of bleeding during the use of anticoagulant drugs as warfarin, UFH, enoxaparin, or rivaroxaban.

Patients received these drugs for peripheral neuropathy treatment symptoms and/or signs: prednisone (40–60 mg/day) for 16 (21.33%), methotrexate (15–20 mg/week) for 5 (6.66%), azathioprine (150–300 mg/day) for 4 (5.33%), hydroxychloroquine (400 mg/day) for 4 (5.33%), cyclophosphamide pulse for 1 patient (91.33%), and methylprednisolone pulse for 1 (1.33%). For pain control, the patients were treated with paracetamol plus codeine (500/10 mg t.i.d) for 30 (40%), gabapentin (300–1800 mg/day) for 5 (6.66%), and tramadol (200–400 mg/day) for 10 (13.33%).

The time of follow-up in our institution varied between 1 and 168 months (median 58.07; SD 38.5). Ten patients lost the follow-up in our hospital. Among the other 65 patients, 11 (16.92%) were discharged after at least 2 years without new flares of LV (probable remission), and 54 patients were under treatment until December 2019.

5.5 Discussion

In this single-institution retrospective study, we analysed the data of 75 patients, the larger number of LV patients in Brazil and Latin American until 2019, in the literature indexed in PubMed.

In Table 5.1, we reviewed our findings and other 10 other published studies indexed in PubMed, in the last 17 years, enrolled more than 20 patients [10–18]. All

Table 5.1 Data from our findings and other 9 studies published in PubMed in the last 14 years that enrolled findings concerning livedoid vasculopathy. *AB* atrophie blanche, *ACA* anticardiolipin antibodies, *ANA* anti-nuclear antibodies, *Anti-MPO* anti-myeloperoxidase antibodies, *BC* breast carcinoma, *B-cell Ly* B-cell lymphoproliferative disease, *CHD* coronary heart disease, *DIF* direct immunofluorescence, *DM* diabetes mellitus, *HIV* human immunodeficiency virus infection, *IBS* irritable bowel disease, *MTHFR* methylenetetrahydrofolate reductase, *MCTD* mixed connective tissue disease, *NR* rot reported, *PV* polycythemia vera, *RA* rheumatoid arthritis, *Scl* scleroderma, *SD* standard deviation, *SAH* systemic arterial hypertension, *SLE* systemic lupus erythematous, *UCTD* undifferentiated connective tissue disease, *VS* venous stasis

Author (single centre/multicentre) (prospective/ retrospective study design)	Year of publication	Country	Number of patients	Time (years) for disease diagnosis	Mean age (years) at disease onset	Thrombophilia findings	Dermatological findings	More frequent histopathological findings	DIF positive	Comorbidities	Peripheral neuropathy
Gao and Jin [8]	2023	China	55	11.5 (8–15) (for 7 patients whose developed neurological symptoms). No data provided for time to LV diagnosis	22.52 (8–54)	In 7 patients with peripheral neurological symptoms, 2 had protein C deficiency, 2 had elevated serum levels of Lp(a), 1 had lupus anticoagulant positive, 3 not displayed any thrombophilia among of them investigated	Not reported	Not reported	Not reported	Not reported	7 patients: 3 had numbness and hypoesthesia and other 4 only numbness
Criado et al. [9] **(present study)** (single centre) (retrospective)	Our study. Published (2021)	**Brazil**	**75**	**6.65 (1–20) (SD 4.50)**	**34.65 (8–77) (SD ± 17.41)**	**Thrombophilic factors in 48 (66.66%) two or more in 26/71 patients (36.6)**	**AB scars 100%, followed by telangiectasias 93.33% and active ulcers in 82.66%. Bilateral lesions on lower limbs were present in 94.66% and bilateral livedo racemosa on lower limbs in 64%**	**Intraluminal hyaline thrombi in the dermal vessels (89.33%)**	**Positive in 72.95% (27/37). Granular C3 in the wall vessels (48.64%), homogeneous C3 in the wall vessels (18.42%)**	**SAH (21.33%), obesity (38.66%), DM II (9.33%), and symptoms or signs of VS (25.33%). SLE in 2 and RA in 1 patient**	**Hypoesthesia symptoms (44%)**

Gardette et al. [10] (multicentre) (prospective)	2019	France	26	3.4 (range 2.2 months–29.5 years)	35.5 (6–67)	20 (77%) had at least one thrombophilia	Purpura and necrotic ulcers (100%), livedo reticularis (85%), hyperpigmentation and AB (80–100%), peripheral telangiectasia (62%)	Intraluminal thrombosis (100%)	(NR)	SLE in one patient, familial hypertriglyceridemia in one patient, renal transplant In 3 patients (2 of whom were HIV positive)	10/20 patients (50%) had a peripheral neuropathy (median time of 11.4 years)
Weishaupt el al [11]**.** (multicentre) (prospective)	2019	Germany	27	(NR)	53.0 (40.5–68)	11/25 (44%) had at least one thrombophilia factor	Livedo racemosa 23/27 (85%), AB in 27/27 (100%) and ulcers	(NR)	(NR)	B-cell Ly, esophagitis, migraine, hyperlipidaemia, IBS, lumbago, glaucoma, DM type II, CHD, BC, monoclonal gammopathy, pollinosis, AR, asthma, hyperthyroidism	Peripheral polyneuropathy in one
Lee and Cho [12] (single centre) (retrospective)	2019	Korea	40	(NR)	33 (12–65)	17/40 (42.5%), but none specified	Erythema, ulcers	(NR)	(NR)	VS 3 (7.5%) PV 1 (2.5%)	(NR)
Feng et al. [13] **(single centre) (retrospective)**	2014	China	24	17.0 years old (5: 9–13 years, 17:14–20 years, one: 21–35 years, and one >35 years)	17 (9–37)	ACA in 11/24 patients, β2GP1 antibodies in 6/24 patients	Small ulcers, stellate scars, and variable degree of hyperpigmentation	Vessels showed fibrin deposition both within the wall and inside the lumen	Positive in 7/12 with C3 and immunoglobulin within blood vessels walls	SAH in 1, DM in 3 patients had mild SV on the Lower extremities	(NR)

(continued)

Table 5.1 (continued)

Author (single centre/multicentre) (prospective/ retrospective study design)	Year of publication	Country	Number of patients	Time (years) for disease diagnosis	Mean age (years) at disease onset	Thrombophilia findings	Dermatological findings	More frequent histopathological findings	DIF positive	Comorbidities	Peripheral neuropathy
Gan et al. [14] **(single centre) (retrospective)**	2012	Singapore	70	Median of 39	(NR)	ACA positive (3/45), LAC positive (1/45)	Ulcers, atrophie blanche	63 patients (90%): Dermal vessel thrombosis (57%)	DIF positive 54/55 patients	SLE in one patient and another with RA	Peripheral neuropathy in 6 patients
Feng et al. [15] **(multicentre) (prospective)**	2011	China	30	(NR)	21.02	ACA in 13 (43.33%), and β2 GP I in 9 patients (30%)	3 patients with livedo reticularis in whole leg	(NR)	(NR)	Two patients with SLE	(NR)
Tsai et al. [16] **(multicentre) (prospective)**	2009	Taiwan	56	29.79 ± 12.274	–	Only genotypes CC of the MTHFR mutation C677T	(NR)	(NR)	(NR)	(NR)	(NR)
Hairston et al. [17] **(single centre) (retrospective)**	2006	United States of America	47	1–45 (mean, 6.3)	10–85	Factor V (Leiden) mutation, MTHFR mutation, hyperhomocysteinemia, protein C and protein S deficiency, ACA, LA	Atrophie blanche in 71.1%, ulcers in 68.9%	Dermal blood vessel thrombosis was noted in 44/45 (97.8%)	DIF positive in 31/36 patients (86.1%)	RA in 3, Scl in 1, MCTD in 1, UCTD in 1 patient. VS in 4, solid organ carcinoma in 3, hematologic malignancy in 2 patients	Mononeuritis multiplex in 1 patient

these data included 450 LV patients, 326 women and 134 men (median rate, 2.43♀:1♂). Table 5.1 described some aspects as the country of these studies, prospective, retrospective, single or multicentre study design, age at disease onset, sex distribution, thrombophilic factors retrieved, dermatological lesions, histopathology aspects, treatments, and follow-up [8, 10–18].

Our data were similar to previous publications in single or multicentre studies in countries of Asia, Europe, and North America [8, 10–18].

The sex distribution of 3.68 ♀: ♂ in our patients was more elevated than other previous studies conducted in French [10] and in Germany [11], but almost similar to the data from 70 patients in Singapore [14].

The age group between 20 and 48 years (42 patients, 56%) was the most frequent in our study, with a mean age of 34.65 years (SD 17.41, range 8–77 years). These findings were comparable to the data found of Gan et al. [14] in Singapore (mean age of 39 years, 15–75), among 70 patients, and Gardette et al. [10] in France, (mean age of 35.5 years, 6–67), among 26 patients. In our study was remarkable the presence of 14 (18.66%) patients that referred to the onset of diseases before 18 years old. These findings alert the physicians to this often misdiagnosis in children and adolescents, with painful ulcerations in lower legs.

Brazil is the world's fifth largest country and has the seventh largest GDP, while ranking 71st and 85th for GDP per capita and the human development index, respectively [8], and these aspects can explain some demographic and therapeutic data among our 75 patients, as the few cases (11) of rivaroxaban use and none with other Factor Xa inhibitors or intravenous immunoglobulin, a group of expensive drugs in our country, and not available in Public Health System (SUS) for this International Code Diseases classification (ICD: L95). Nowadays, Brazilian population is estimated in 209 million individuals, and it is highly heterogeneous, as a result of five centuries of admixture of Europeans, Africans, and Amerindians (Native Americans), with a more recent component of Asian people immigration, represented mainly by Japanese, Chinese, and Korean people [19]. According to Callegary-Jacques and Salzano [20], 58% of immigrants who arrived in Brazil between 1500 and 1972 were Europeans, 40% were Africans, and 2% were Asians. In this sense, Brazil might be a "meeting point" for the three major historical-geographical components of humanity, namely distinct composition in the ethnic distribution of our patients, where there was a predominance of white patients 81.33%. Other included 12% mulatto, 5.33% black, and 1.33% Asian patients, an unexpected distribution front to Brazilian ethnic composition. Interestingly, there are few data from African patients with LV in the literature until now, excluding our patients [20]. Based on these data, probably African and Afro-descendants' people are less susceptible to develop LV or these ethnic group, unfortunately, has less access to the health system.

Among our patients the most frequent LV lesions present during the first visit were AB scars 100%, followed by telangiectasias 93.33% and active ulcers in 82.66%. Bilateral lesions on LL were present in 94.66% and bilateral LR on LL in 64%. These findings are especially concordant with patients of Hairston et al. [17] and similar to Gildette et al. [10] patients. In Weishaupt et al. [11], AB was found in all patients.

Intraluminal hyaline thrombi in the dermal vessels were found in 89.33% patients, followed by perivascular lymphomononuclear infiltrate in 90.66%, erythrocytes extravasation in 86.66% and, segmental hyalinization of the wall's vessels in the dermis in 80% of our patients. These histopathological findings are according to the majority of the Gildette et al. [10] patients. Pauci-inflammatory intraluminal thrombosis was the hallmark of LV in our patients.

On DIF study was positive in 72.95% (27/37) of our patients. The most frequent immunoreactant was granular C3 in the wall vessels in 48.64% followed by; homogeneous C3 in the wall vessels in 18.42%. Hsiao and Wu [21] studding DIF in 27 LV patients obtained a tissue expression of C3 in 100% and IgM in 96% of their patients. Hairston et al. [17] described a positive DIF in 31 (86.1%) of 36 patients, and the most prevalent immunoreactants were fibrin>C3 > IgM. All these studies in LV showed a variable sensitivity in DIF, with C3 and IgM as immunoreactants more frequent similar to demonstrated by our findings.

To concern thrombophilic factors together, Lp(a), antiphosholipid antibodies and, the elevated serum of Factors VIII and IX were the more relevant factors involved in the pathogenesis of LV in our patients. Few authors have investigated Lp(a) [22, 23] in LV patients and we are unable to find any LV dosing Factor VIII/ Factor IX. In a review, Algahtani and Stuckey [24] reviewed the association between elevated levels of Factor VIII and concluded that high factor VIII levels are a risk factor for thrombosis, with a greater impact on venous than on arterial thrombosis.

Lp (a) is a cholesterol-rich lipoprotein particle, consisting of a low-density lipoprotein (LDL) domain (containing apolipoprotein B-100) covalently bound to the glycoprotein apolipoprotein(a) [apo(a)] [25]. Due to high structural homology with plasminogen, Lp(a) is capable of inhibiting fibrinolysis by means of competing with plasminogen for stabilized fibrin binding [25]. A convincing association has been widely reported between Lp(a) and a kaleidoscope of vascular occlusive disorders [25]. It has been demonstrated that Lp(a) acts as a pro-thrombotic and antifibrinolytic factor, interfering with clot biology at multiple levels [26], such as the following: (1) impairment of plasminogen activation and/or formation of active plasmin due to Lp(a) similarity to plasminogen; (2) overproduction of PAI-1 induced by oxidized Lp(a) [ox-Lp(a)]; (3) promotion of tissue factor (TF) expression in monocytes; and (4) binding and inhibition of tissue factor pathway inhibitor (TFPI) [27].

We found elevated levels of Lp(a) in 30/72 (41.66%) of patients and Weishaupt et al. [11] found in 5/12 (42%), showing percentages very similar in both only large studies published including thrombophilia screening with Lp(a). Previously, our group published a study demonstrated of Lp(a), deposits in the wall vessels, and in perivascular cells in lesions of LV patients, and it was not significative in normal skin controls [4]. This reinforces the probable pathogenic mechanism of Lp(a) as a co-factor for intraluminal thrombosis in LV or its involvement in ulcers healing.

The most frequent comorbidities in our patients were systemic SHA (21.33%), obesity (38.66%), diabetes mellitus type II (9.33%), and symptoms or signs of venous insufficiency in LL (25.33%). Though the prevalence of venous insufficiency was high in our patients, all cases were documented by ultrasound Doppler and histopathological hallmarks of LV, as the presence of segmental hyalinizing vascular changes and intraluminal thrombi occlusion in dermal vessels, as emphasized by Hairston et al [17]. Weishaupt et al. [11] found hypertension in 70% of LV patients, BMI was elevated in 40%, and diabetes mellitus type II in ≤2 patients, concordant findings with our study.

LV flares were reported occurring during spring/summer in 23/29 (79.92%) and during autumn/winter in 6/29 (20.68%). This VL season exacerbation during summer is clinical behaviour similar to previous descriptions by other authors as Lee and Cho [12].

Our therapeutic experience acquired with these 75 LV patients demonstrated that the pain referred to by 93.33% of them during the acute phase of the ulceration process need an approach with drugs for analgesia (tramadol, paracetamol *plus* codeine) and a specific therapy to enhance the arterial blood supply in skin microcirculation on lower limbs. Rivaroxaban, enoxaparin, hyperbaric oxygen therapy, cilostazol and, danazol, this last especially in cases with Lp(a) high levels were the most useful therapeutic approach in severe LV cases, on the clinical setting of consecutive and multiple ulcerations during the flares [28]. Most of our patients were submitted to maintenance treatment with pentoxifylline and/or ASA during ulcerations remission.

As a long interval of 15 years of this retrospective study, our data collection has some limitations, mainly related to the study design, complementary exams performed, and data obtained from patients. Accuracy of data collection also relied on adequate documentation in the medical records. Our data was published in 2021 and until now this case series is the largest from a single centre indexed in PubMed [9].

5.6 Hallmarks of the Literature

LV is a rare disease and it received distinct nomenclatures since it was described in an Occidental literature by Milian (1929), including "livedo vasculitis", "segmental hyalinizing vasculitis" (Bard and Winkelmann, 1967), "livedo reticularis with summer ulceration", "Milian white atrophy", "atrophie blanche en plaque", and "PURPLE" (painful purpuric ulcers with a reticular pattern of lower extremities) [6]. McCalmont et al. [29] used the term "livedoid vasculopathy" in 1992.

Nowadays, the primary physiopathology of LV is one or more hypercoagulable states, while the inflammation interplays as a secondary role. Then, LV is classified as a biological result of coagulating or antifibrinolytic disorder, essentially a vasculopathy, which occurs when a thrombus forms into the dermal or eventually subcutaneous vessels and compromises the blood flow [6].

This condition shows a chronic course with periodic and recurrent exacerbations, often affecting the legs and feet bilaterally [30].

LV is distinct from vasculitis, which refers to primary inflammation of the vessel wall followed by fibrinoid necrosis [31]. Livedoid vasculopathy is usually associated with phenomena that cause hypercoagulability and thrombus formation, including [30]: chronic venous hypertension of the limbs and varicose veins, autoimmune connective tissue diseases (systemic lupus erythematosus, rheumatoid arthritis, scleroderma, mixed connective tissue disease), thrombophilia states (inherited causes factor V Leiden variant, prothrombin gene G20210A mutation, and protein C, protein S, and antithrombin deficiency, elevated levels of FVIII and Factor IX, elevated lipoprotein A serum levels, polymorphism of plasminogen inhibitor activator gene (PAI) (4G/5G) or acquired causes as acquired homocysteinemia, cryoglobulinemia, cryofibrinogenaemia, antiphospholipid antibody syndrome), neoplasms (solid organ neoplasia, myeloproliferative disorders, paraproteinemia, etc.) and idiopathic forms [31].

The associations between LV and genetic abnormalities show geographical or ethnic differences [6]. PAI-1-675 4G/5G was the most common genetic abnormality, accounting for 85.26% of cases ($n = 81$ of 95), followed by PAI-1 A844G, MTHFR C677T, and MTHFR A1298C variants [6]. Prothrombin G20210A and factor V G1691A were mainly present in patients with LV from Europe, North America, and South America [6].

Burning pain is the main prodromal symptom of LV [6]. Physical examination often reveals lesions in distinct stages of evolution: livedo-like hemosiderosis, white atrophic porcelain-like lesions, telangiectasis, palpable and non-palpable purpura (often better visualized on dermoscopy exam), and small ulcers with necrotic debris (Figs. 5.3, 5.4 and 5.5). The small ulcerations progressively evolve to confluent reticulated ulcers. The main locations of the ulcers are the dorsum of the feet, ankles, and the lower extremities, often bilaterally. Exceptionally, upper extremities may be affected in some patients [6]. Ulcers are characterized by the clinical aspect "punched-out" located on perimalleolar area, heals in a period of time between 3 and 4 months and solve as "atrophie blanche", a non-pathognomonic type of scar small round or stellate porcelain white atrophic lesions surrounded by hyperpigmentation and telangiectasis [6, 29, 30].

The main differential diagnosis is the cutaneous polyarteritis nodosa (cPAN) (cutaneous arteritis), which may simulate the clinical aspects of LV. For cPNA exclusion, the skin biopsies should involve dermis and subcutis, to visualize the

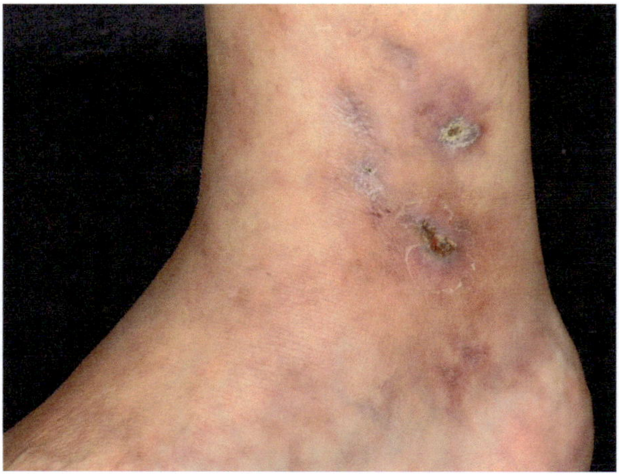

Fig. 5.3 Livedoid vasculopathy. Punched-out and reticulate ulcers on ankle

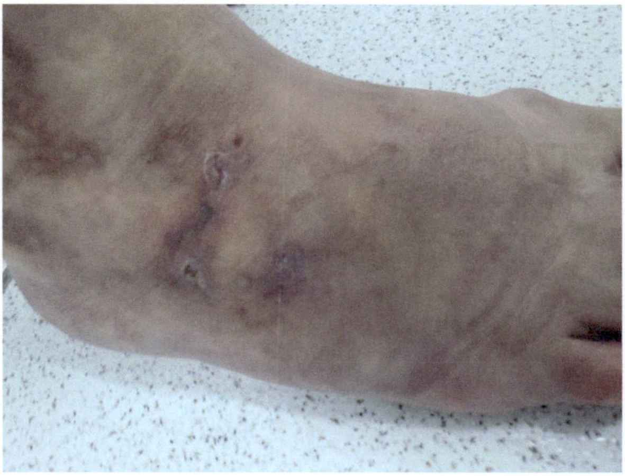

Fig. 5.4 Livedoid vasculopathy. Reticulate purpuric lesions and punched-out ulcers on foot

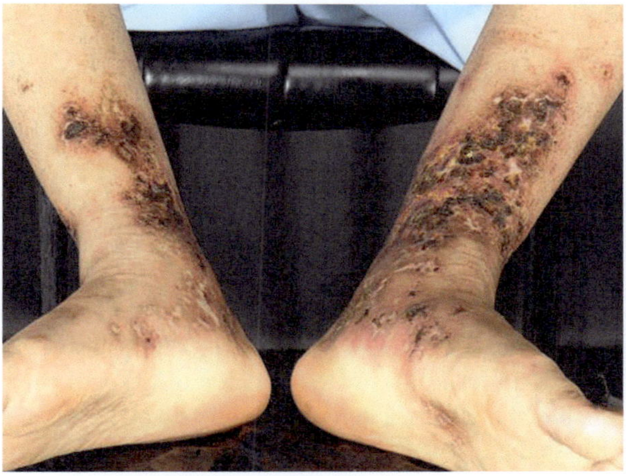

Fig. 5.5 Livedoid vasculopathy. Multiple necrotic and punched-out reticulate ulcers on ankles and feet

histopathology hallmark of cPAN, the leukocytoclastic vasculitis in dermal-hypodermal arteries. The ideal biopsy specimen is a small wedge of tissue that includes adjacent healthy skin and the ulcer margin and is obtained through the dermis and subcutis, or purpura lesion (Figs. 5.1 and 5.2). Other conditions producing reticulated ulcers on legs and feet are differential diagnosis of LV: true leukocytoclastic small vessels vasculitis, peripheral arterial disease, chronic venous insufficiency, cryoglobulinaemic vasculitis or vasculopathy, ANCA-associated vasculitis, sickle cell disease, hydroxyurea ulcers, distinct vasculopathies (cholesterol emboli, atrial myxoma embolization, oxaluria).

The treatment for LV is based on non-drug interventions as smoking cessation without use of nicotine patches or gums, prevention or treatment of venous stasis (flavonoid drugs as diosmin plus hesperidin) and several drug interventions, as [32]: low-dose ASA (acetylsalicylic acid, 100 mg/day), oral pentoxifylline (400 mg t.i.d), oral dipyridamole, folic acid (and possibly vitamin B complex, particularly in patients with methylenetetrahydrofolate reductase mutation), hydroxychloroquine (especially for patients with antiphospholipid antibodies), anabolic steroids (stanazolol or danazol, in patients with cryofibrinogenemia or high serum levels of lipoprotein A), warfarin sodium, heparin, low-dose or low-molecular-weight (enoxiparin), hyperbaric oxygen therapy, tissue plasminogen activator infusion, intravenous immunoglobulin. Recently, there are reports using direct oral anticoagulants (DOACs, as dabigatran, rivaroxaban, apixaban) [33], anti-TNFα agents (etanercept, adalimumab) [34, 35], sulodexide [36], rituximab [37], cilostazol [38].

5.7 Conclusions

Despite the above limitations, we believe that several clinically useful data from Latin America, particularly in Brazil, can be drawn, as predominance in white ethnic group, paraesthesia symptoms (hypoesthesia) on lower limbs in 40% of our patients, the frequency of elevated Lp(a) and Factor VIII/IX serum levels, ACA, symptoms and/or signs of leg venous stasis in 25.33% of our patients. Taking all data together, there are convincing information that multifactorial conditions are related or involved in the LV pathogenesis, as distinct thrombophilic factors and venous stasis, and its association with extracutaneous conditions as peripheral neuropathy, obesity (21.33%), and SAH (38.66%), at least, in a group of these patients. A work-up for lesions with suspicion of livedoid vasculopathy is presented in Fig. 5.6, based on the article review published by Eswaran et al. [39]. In Fig. 5.7 is demonstrated the progessive suggested treatment steps for livedoid vasculopathy.

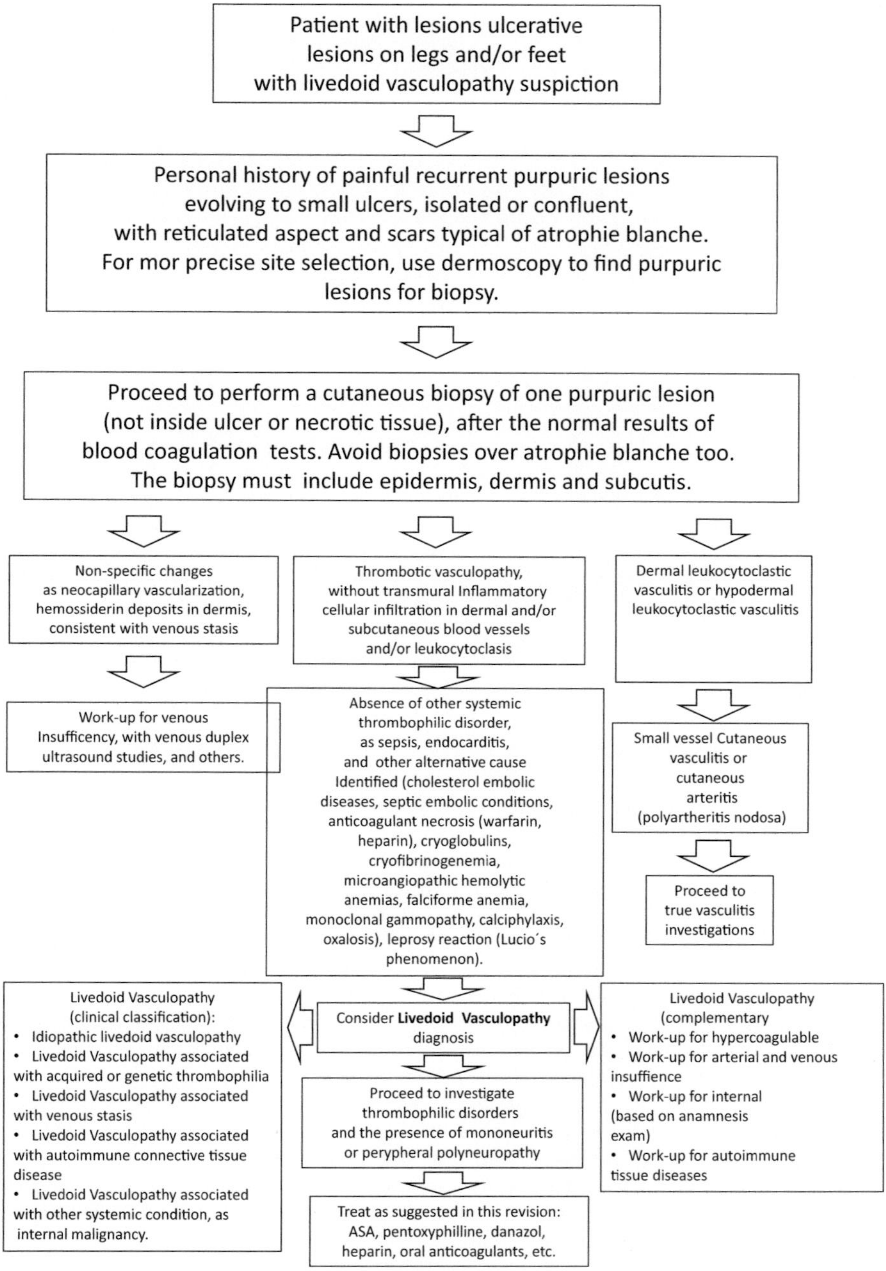

Fig. 5.6 Practical work-up of purpuric and ulcerated lesions on legs and/or feet for diagnosis of livedoid vasculopathy

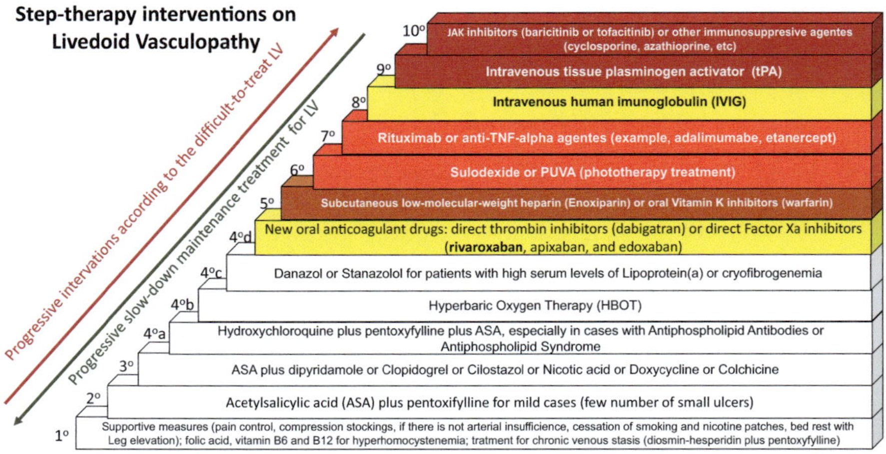

Fig. 5.7 Step-therapy interventions for LV patients are based on disease severity (intensity of pain, number of ulcers, and impact on quality of life). Progression on each step adds economic burden for patients and institutions, potential severe adverse reactions and there is a reduced the number of evidence-based treatments.* In black bold letters are listed the interventions with a greater number of patients allocated in case series published in the literature

References

1. Criado PR, Rivitti EA, Sotto MN, de Carvalho JF. Livedoid vasculopathy as a coagulation disorder. Autoimm Rev. 2011;10:33–60.
2. Stevanovic DV. Atrophie blanche: a sign of dermal blood occlusion. Arch Dermatol. 1974;109:858–62.
3. The portal for rare diseases and orphan drugs. https://www.orpha.net/consor/cgi-bin/Disease_Classif.php?lng=EN&data_id=187&PatId=28055&search=Disease_Classif_Simple&new=1. Accessed 30 Dec 2019.
4. Espinel DPGS, Di Giacomo TB, Pincelli TP, Pereira NV, Sotto MN, Kirsner RS, Criado PR. Analysis of serum levels and cutaneous expression of lipoprotein (a) in 38 patients with livedoid vasculopathy. J Cutan Pathol. 2017;44(12):1033–7.
5. Polo Gascón MR, de Carvalho JF, de Souza Espinel DP, Barros AM, Alavi A, Criado PR. Quality-of-life impairment in patients with livedoid vasculopathy. J Am Acad Dermatol. 2014;71(5):1024–6. https://doi.org/10.1016/j.jaad.2014.06.030.
6. McCalmont CS, McCalmont TH, Jorizzo JL, White WL, Leshin B, Rothberger H. Livedo vasculitis: vasculitis or thrombotic vasculopathy? Clin Exp Dermatol. 1992;17:4–8.
7. Flores G, Culton DA, Prisayanh P, Qaqish BF, James K, Maldonado M, Aoki V, Hans-Filho G, Rivitti EA, Diaz LA. IgG autoantibody response against keratinocyte cadherins in endemic pemphigus foliaceus (Fogo selvagem). J Invest Dermatol. 2012;132(11):2573–80. https://doi.org/10.1038/jid.2012.232; Epub 2012 Jul 19.
8. Suarez-Kurtz G, Paula DP, Struchiner CJ. Pharmacogenomic implications of population admixture: Brazil as a model case. Pharmacogenomics. 2014;15(2):209–19. https://doi.org/10.2217/pgs.13.238.
9. Bilgic A, Ozcobanoglu S, Bozca BC, Alpsoy E. Livedoid vasculopathy: a multidisciplinary clinical approach to diagnosis and management. Int J Womens Dermatol. 2021;7(5Part A):588–99.

10. Weishaupt C, Strölin A, Kahle B, Kreuter A, Schneider SW, Gerss J, Eveslage M, Drabik A, Goerge T. Characteristics, risk factors and treatment reality in livedoid vasculopathy—a multicentre analysis. J Eur Acad Dermatol Venereol. 2019;33(9):1784–91.
11. Gan EY, Tang MB, Tan SH, Chua SH, Tan AW. A ten-year retrospective study on livedo vasculopathy in Asian patients. Ann Acad Med Singap. 2012;41(9):400–6.
12. Feng S, Su W, Jin P, Shao C. Livedoid vasculopathy: clinical features and treatment in 24 Chinese patients. Acta Derm Venereol. 2014;94(5):574–8. https://doi.org/10.2340/00015555-1711.
13. Feng SY, Jin PY, Shao CG. The significance of anticardiolipin antibody and immunologic abnormality in livedoid vasculitis. Int J Dermatol. 2011;50(1):21–3. https://doi.org/10.1111/j.1365-4632.2010.04569.x.
14. Lee JS, Cho S. Livedoid vasculopathy in Koreans: clinical features and response to rivaroxaban treatment. J Eur Acad Dermatol Venereol. 2019;34:e176. https://doi.org/10.1111/jdv.16129; [Epub ahead of print].
15. Tsai TF, Yang CH, Chu CY, Liou YH, Hsiao WC, Lin CT, Wu LS. Polymorphisms of MTHFR gene associated with livedoid vasculopathy in Taiwanese population. J Dermatol Sci. 2009;54(3):214–6. https://doi.org/10.1016/j.jdermsci.2008.
16. Gao Y, Jin H. Livedoid vasculopathy and peripheral neuropathy: a retrospective cohort study of 55 Chinese patients and literature review. Int Wound J. 2023;20(5):1498–505. https://doi.org/10.1111/iwj.14004.
17. Hairston BR, Davis MD, Pittelkow MR, Ahmed I. Livedoid vasculopathy: further evidence for procoagulant pathogenesis. Arch Dermatol. 2006;142(11):1413–8.
18. Gardette E, Moguelet P, Bouaziz JD, Lipsker D, Dereure O, Le Pelletier F, Lok C, Maisonobe T, Bessis D, Conard J, Francès C, Barete S. Livedoid vasculopathy: a French observational study including therapeutic options. Acta Derm Venereol. 2018;98(9):842–7.
19. Callegari-Jacques SM, Salzano FM. Brazilian Indian/non Indian interactions and their effects. Cienc Cult. 1999;51:166–74.
20. Reagin H, Marks E, Weis S, Susa J. Livedoid vasculopathy presenting in a patient with sickle cell disease. Am J Dermatopathol. 2018;40(9):682–5. https://doi.org/10.1097/DAD.0000000000001133.
21. Goerge T, Weishaupt C, Metze D, Nowak-Göttl U, Sunderkötter C, Steinhoff M, Schneider SW. Livedoid vasculopathy in a pediatric patient with elevated lipoprotein(a) levels: prompt response to continuous low-molecular-weight heparin. Arch Dermatol. 2010;146(8):927–8.
22. Weishaupt C, Strölin A, Kahle B, et al. Characteristics, risk factors and treatment reality in livedoid vasculopathy—a multicentre analysis. J Eur Acad Dermatol Venereol. 2019;33(9):1784–91. https://doi.org/10.1111/jdv.15639.
23. Algahtani FH, Stuckey R. High factor VIII levels and arterial thrombosis: illustrative case and literature review. Ther Adv Hematol. 2019;10:2040620719886685. https://doi.org/10.1177/2040620719886685.
24. Salvagno GL, Pavan C, Lippi G. Rare thrombophilic conditions. Ann Transl Med. 2018;6(17):342. https://doi.org/10.21037/atm.2018.08.12.
25. Riches K, Porter KE. Lipoprotein(a): cellular effects and molecular mechanisms. Cholesterol. 2012;2012:923289. https://doi.org/10.1155/2012/923289; Epub 2012 Sep 6. PMID: 22991657.
26. Criado PR, Espinell DP, Barreto P, Di Giacomo TH, Sotto MN. Lipoprotein(a) and livedoid vasculopathy: a new thrombophilic factor? Med Hypotheses. 2015;85(5):670–4. https://doi.org/10.1016/j.mehy.2015.08.009.
27. Criado PR, de Souza Espinell DP, Valente NS, Alavi A, Kirsner RS. Livedoid vasculopathy and high levels of lipoprotein (a): response to danazol. Dermatol Ther. 2015;28(4):248–53. https://doi.org/10.1111/dth.12225.
28. Criado PR, Pagliari C, Morita TCAB, Marques GF, Pincelli TPH, Valente NYS, Garcia MSC, de Carvalho JF, Abdalla BMZ, Sotto MN. Livedoid vasculopathy in 75 Brazilian patients in a single-center institution: clinical, histopathological and therapy evaluation. Dermatol Ther. 2021;34(2):e14810. https://doi.org/10.1111/dth.14810.
29. Criado PR, Rivitti EA, Sotto MN, Valente NY, Aoki V, Carvalho JF, et al. Livedoid vasculopathy: an intriguing cutaneous disease. An Bras Dermatol. 2011;86(5):961–77.

30. Majmundar VD, Baxi K. Livedoid vasculopathy. In: StatPearls. Treasure Island, FL: StatPearls Publishing; 2021.
31. Callen JP. Livedoid vasculopathy: what it is and how the patient should be evaluated and treated. Arch Dermatol. 2006;142:1481–2.
32. Gao Y, Jin H. Rivaroxaban for treatment of livedoid vasculopathy: a systematic review. Dermatol Ther. 2021;34(5):e15051. https://doi.org/10.1111/dth.15051.
33. Gao Y, Jin H. Efficacy of an anti-TNF-alpha agent in refractory livedoid vasculopathy: a retrospective analysis. J Dermatolog Treat. 2020;9:1–6. https://doi.org/10.1080/09546634.2020.1737634.
34. Song CH, Shin DS, Jang JW, Kim TL, Kim YG, Kim JS, Seo HM. A case of livedoid vasculopathy successfully treated with Sulodexide. Ann Dermatol. 2020;32(6):508–11. https://doi.org/10.5021/ad.2020.32.6.508.
35. Provenza JR, Pedri LE, Provenza GM. Livedoid vasculopathy. Rev Bras Reumatol. 2016;S0482–5004(16):00027–9. https://doi.org/10.1016/j.rbr.2015.09.011; English, Portuguese.
36. Alix JJ, Hadjivassiliou M, Ali R, Slater D, Messenger AG, Rao DG. Sensory ganglionopathy with livedoid vasculopathy controlled by immunotherapy. Muscle Nerve. 2015;51(2):296–301.
37. Mendiratta V, Malik M, Yadav P, Nangia A. Cilostazol: a novel agent in recalcitrant livedoid vasculopathy. Indian J Dermatol Venereol Leprol. 2016;82(2):222–4.
38. Eswaran H, Googe P, Vedak P, Marston WA, Moll S. Livedoid vasculopathy: a review with focus on terminology and pathogenesis. Vasc Med. 2022;27(6):593–603.
39. Franco Marques G, Criado PR, Alves Batista Morita TC, Cajas García MS. The management of livedoid vasculopathy focused on direct oral anticoagulants (DOACs): four case reports successfully treated with rivaroxaban. Int J Dermatol. 2018;57(6):732–41.

Ulcers in Hypercoagulable States

6

Ritika Khanna and Rahul Khanna

6.1 Introduction

A hypercoagulable state is a predisposition to clot/thrombus formation and is also called as thrombophilia. The most common and sometimes life-threatening manifestation of hypercoagulable state is deep venous thrombosis of leg veins. Skin ulceration is usually an atypical and nonspecific clinical feature. Thrombophilia can be congenital or hereditary variety and acquired variety [1].

Congenital/hereditary thrombophilia: This variety can be due to a deficiency of natural anticoagulants (Type I defect) or overactivity of coagulation factors (Type II defect). The Type II defects are more severe compared to Type I defects in their tendency to cause thrombosis [2].

Type I defects:

1. Antithrombin III deficiency.
2. Protein C and Protein S deficiency.
3. Factor XIII mutation.
4. Dysfibrinogenemia.
5. Congenital deficiency of plasminogen.

Type II defects

1. Factor V Leiden.
2. Prothrombin mutation.

R. Khanna · R. Khanna (✉)
Department of Dermatology and Surgery, Institute of Medical Sciences, Banaras Hindu University, Varanasi, India

A. K. Khanna, S. K. Tiwary (eds.), *Uncommon Ulcers of the Extremities*, https://doi.org/10.1007/978-981-99-1782-2_6

Acquired thrombophilia: Several acquired conditions are known to increase the risk of arterial as well as venous thrombosis. Important causes are:

1. Antiphospholipid antibody syndrome [3].
2. Heparin-induced thrombocytopenia [4].
3. Paroxysmal nocturnal hemoglobinuria.
4. Sickle cell disease.
5. Myeloproliferative disorders specially polycythemia vera and essential thrombocytosis [5].
6. Metastatic cancer and paraneoplastic syndromes [6].
7. Nephrotic syndrome.
8. Hypercoagulability of pregnancy [7].
9. Oral contraceptive pills and hormone replacement therapy.
10. Obesity.

Unsettled thrombophilia: There are a few conditions predisposing to a hypercoagulable state whose etiology is uncertain. They are elevated levels of factor VIII, factor X, fibrinogen, and thrombosis activatable fibrinolysis inhibitors. Activated protein C resistance not caused by factor V mutation and elevated homocysteine levels are other such uncertain situations [8].

Diagnostic tests for hypercoagulable states: Because a large number of biochemical investigations are available, the most relevant tests are advised on the basis of clinical evaluation. Mandatory tests will include complete blood count (including platelet count), prothrombin time/international normalized ratio, activated partial thromboplastin time, and thrombin time. Additional investigations as clinically indicated are lupus antibody, anticardiolipin and anti-β_2 glycoprotein 1 antibody, activated protein C resistance, fibrinogen levels, factor V Leiden and prothrombin mutation, and basal homocysteine levels. Real-time assessment of coagulation parameters is now possible with thromboelastography or rotational thromboelastometry. It can assess platelet function, enzymatic derangements, and fibrinolysis thus providing information on complete hemostatic function. The real-time information obtained on thromboelastography enables goal-directed therapy.

Hypercoagulable states are common in critical illness and often a cause for life-threatening complications. They need to be recognized early before complications set in and pose complex management issues. They result in excessive intravascular clotting of blood with serious organ derangements or ischemic ulcerations.

Hypercoagulable states predispose the patient to development of venous and/or arterial thrombus. Skin manifestations can be an important factor in diagnosing a patient's hypercoagulable state by the appearance of lesions such as purpura, purpura fulminans, livedo reticularis, livedo vasculopathy (atrophie blanche), anetoderma, and superficial venous thrombosis. Although the cutaneous manifestations are nonspecific, their appearance is an indicator for further workup for underlying thrombophilic disorder [9].

Cutaneous ulcers secondary to thrombophilia producing diseases have atypical presentation and present with pain and inflammation to begin with before ulceration occurs. They account for about 20–30% of leg ulcers [10]. These ulcers can occur at unusual sites such as trunk or thighs and do not respond to antibiotic therapy. Often they are mistaken for pyoderma gangrenosum.

6.2 General Pathogenesis of Cutaneous Ulcers in Hypercoagulable States

Although it has not been conclusively proven, thrombophilia-associated ulcers are thought to be a result of localized tissue hypoxia secondary to occlusion of capillary network by micro-thrombi. This leads to a painful lesion which ultimately ulcerates due to cutaneous necrosis. Nearly similar micro-thrombi-linked pathogenesis occurs in various causes of thrombophilia including abnormalities of red blood cell structure, vasospasm, emboli, cold-related and immune complex deposition diseases.

6.3 General Clinical Features of Thrombophilia Associated Ulcers

Ulcers located at unusual locations such as trunk or back or thighs should arouse suspicion of thrombophilia-associated ulcers. These are sites where diabetic, atherosclerotic-associated ischemic ulcers, neuropathic ulcers, or venous ulcers will not occur. Preceding the ulcer there is usually an erythematous swelling with pain out of proportion to the clinical findings. This is followed by development of a typical livedoid patch which over a few days converts into a black eschar. The eschar when it sheds off leaves behind a small and shallow ulcers with a pale floor. Poor or no response to antibiotic therapy gives further weight to a thrombophilia-associated etiology. Livedoid reticularis before the ulceration is very typical of such ulcers and is due to collection of venous blood giving rise to typical purplish color [11]. Typically such ulcers can best be described as chronic non-inflammatory ulcers located at atypical sites which are poorly responsive to antibiotic therapy.

6.4 Severity Index of Cutaneous Ulcers

The severity of leg ulcers is based on size, duration, and depth. Ulcers persisting beyond 6 months are said to be chronic. Depending on the depth cutaneous ulcers can be classified as follows:

Stage 1: Characterized by skin discoloration and non-blanchable erythema. The skin is intact but warm, edematous, and indurated.

Stage 2: Superficial ulcer presenting as abrasion, blister, or shallow ulcer. The skin loss is partial thickness involving epidermis and dermis.

Stage 3: Deep ulcers with or without undermining of adjacent tissue. The skin loss is full thickness and may extend down to but not through the underlying fascia.

Stage 4: The skin ulcers are deep with undermining and sometimes with sinus tracks. Skin loss is full thickness with necrosis or destruction of muscle, bone supporting structures such as tendon or joint capsule.

6.5 Antiphospholipid Antibody (APLA) Syndrome Associated Ulcers

APLA syndrome is an autoimmune disease characterized by antibody production against cell membrane phospholipid, thereby disrupting the vessel wall integrity [12]. APLA syndrome can be a primary condition or it can be secondary to other diseases such as systemic lupus erythematosus (SLE). When a thrombotic event occurs in the presence of APLAs it is called as APLA syndrome.

The pathogenesis of cutaneous ulcers in APLA is fibrin deposition leading to occlusion of superficial dermal vessels. The procoagulant state seen in APLA syndrome is attributed to APLAs interacting with phospholipid binding proteins, thus impeding the coagulation cascade. The alternative mechanisms proposed are platelet activation, inhibition of activated protein C, induction of tissue factors and antithrombin pathways [13].

Cutaneous lesions in APLA syndrome occur often but are nonspecific. The ulcers are multiple, painful, shallow, and recurrent. Their size varies from 5 to 200 mm. The pain can be severe enough to interfere with normal daily activities. The diagnosis is made only if there is a high index of clinical suspicion and associated other clinical features which are the hallmark of APLA syndrome and SLE are present.

6.5.1 Treatment of Cutaneous Ulcers in APLA Syndrome

Patients with APLA-associated ulcers should receive long-term oral anticoagulants. The intensity of anticoagulation is guided according to the nature of thrombotic event (venous or arterial). In mild cases aspirin with or without low molecular weight heparin is adequate therapy. Severe APLA syndrome requires high-dose intravenous steroids and parenteral anticoagulation. Associated catastrophic events will need supplemental intravenous gamma globulin and repeated plasma exchanges with fresh frozen plasma early in the course of the event [14].

6.6 Cryoglobulinemia and Cryofibrinogenemia Associated Ulcers

Both these conditions are diseases which are precipitated by exposure to cold weather. In cryoglobulinemia immunoglobulin aggregates at low temperature and precipitates within blood vessels leading to compromised circulation to tissues. There is also immune complex formation and complement fixation which causes vasculitis with micro-thrombi formation. The ulcer formation and gangrene typically occur in the distal most part of upper or lower limbs [15].

Cryofibrinogenemia is characterized by cryoprecipitates composed of fibrin, fibronectin, and fibrin degradation products. This process can be primary or secondary to infection, vasculitis, myeloproliferative disorders, solid organ malignancies, or diabetes mellitus. The cryofibrinogen leads to intravascular clot formation and capillary occlusion.

6.6.1 Treatment of Cryoglobulinemia and Cryofibrinogenemia Associated Ulcers

Antiviral medication such as sofosbuvir and ledipasvir are used for management of hepatitis C virus-associated cryoglobulinemia vasculitis. Immunosuppressive medication such as glucocorticoids, cyclophosphamide, and rituximab may be used. Avoidance of exposure to cold weather specially of the extremities is required. The ulcers will heal when the underlying hypercoagulable state brought on by the increased viscosity and vasculitis is controlled.

6.7 Sickle Cell Disease Associated Ulcers

Patients with sickle cell disease have rigid red blood cells because of irregular polymerization of hemoglobin. This leads to poor microvascular blood flow and local tissue ischemia. Chronic leg ulcers are seen in 25 to 75% of patients with sickle cell disease [16].

These ulcers are more common in males, in patients with more severe hemolysis and low hemoglobin levels. The ulcers occur in areas of the leg with less subcutaneous fat, thin skin, and decreased blood flow. The commonest sites are over medial and lateral malleoli. If not adequately treated they may become circumferential. The ulcers are indolent, intractable, and heal over months to years. The pain is severe and requires oral or sometimes parenteral opioid analgesics. Ulcers which are associated with priapism and pulmonary hypertension are indicative of advanced sickle cell vasculopathy.

6.7.1 Treatment of Sickle Cell Disease Associated Ulcers

Small ulcers may heal over months with good wound care. Chronic ulcers beyond 6 months will require additional therapy such as blood transfusion, skin grafting, Unna boots, zinc sulfate, and hyperbaric oxygen.

6.8 Livedoid Vasculopathy

This is a condition characterized by increased thrombotic activity, decreased fibrinolytic activity, and endothelial injury resulting in micro-thrombi in the capillary network [17]. It is also known as segmental hyalinizing vasculitis and Milian's atrophie blanche. Livedoid vasculopathy is a cutaneous manifestation of several prothrombotic states that impact the components of Virchow's triad.

6.8.1 Conditions Predisposing to Livedoid Vasculopathy

Hyperviscosity producing diseases	Endothelial injury producing diseases	Hypercoagulability producing diseases
Chronic myeloid leukemia	Systemic lupus erythematosus	Leiden factor V mutation
Heavy chain diseases	Rheumatoid arthritis	Protein C, S, Z and antithrombin deficiency
Cryoglobulinemia	Scleroderma	Elevated levels of plasminogen activator inhibitors (PAI-1)
	Hyperhomocysteinemia	

The clinical features of livedoid vasculopathy start with focal non-inflammatory thrombus of veins of superficial dermis mainly of the legs. The condition is bilateral, recurrent, and may involve the upper limbs. The accumulation of blood in the capillaries due to micro-thrombi leads to the appearance of livedoid reticularis. As cutaneous hypoxia increases the cutaneous manifestation evolves into painful papule, vesicles, bullae, and purpuric plaque. These lesions increase and merge to cause painful ulcers. Over 3–4 months the ulcers transform into white atrophic scar tissue with punctate telangiectasia which is called Milian's atrophie blanche.

The differential diagnosis includes pyoderma gangrenosum, factitious dermatitis, and cutaneous polyarteritis nodosa. The diagnosis is established by histopathology of skin biopsy specimen. The characteristic features are intravascular thrombi in the absence of perivascular inflammation and leukocytoclasia. At the periphery of the capillaries hyalinized fibrin rings can be seen which are characteristic of the condition.

6.9 Warfarin and Heparin Induced Skin Ulcers

In the initial stages of warfarin or heparin therapy particularly if a high loading dose has been given, coagulation factors imbalances can lead to a paradoxical hypercoagulable state and thrombosis. This phenomenon is attributed to a stronger inhibition of protein C and factor VII compared to other vitamin K-dependent factors such as II, IX, and X in the starting one or 2 days of therapy. The decrease of protein C leads to micro-thrombi in the cutaneous circulation and has occasionally led to massive thrombosis and gangrene of limbs. The patient can have a therapeutic range PT/INR but still be in a thrombophilic state because the PT/INR depends mainly on factor VII.

Obese middle-aged women are at highest risk for this condition. Painful and erythematous cutaneous eruptions typically appear around the third to tenth day of start of warfarin. The lesions may resolve or progress to form purpuric bullae which eventually necroses, forms eschar, and ulcerates [18]. The common sites are regions with substantial subcutaneous fat such as breasts, thighs, buttocks, and penis. If not clinically suspected it is mistaken for pyoderma gangrenosum or necrotizing fasciitis.

Treatment is early cessation of warfarin. Some patients may require fresh frozen plasma or pure activated protein C infusion. Large ulcers may ultimately require debridement and skin grafting.

6.10 Hydroxyurea Associated Ulcers

Hydroxyurea is a chemotherapeutic agent used for myeloproliferative disorders including myeloid leukemia. Besides the usual chemotherapy-associated side effects it is known to produce leg ulcers in about 9% of users [19]. The ulcers are typically located in the malleolar region, are painful, and surrounded by atrophie blanche (white stellate scarring). The proposed mechanism is disruption of S phase of cell cycle resulting in damage to basal keratinocytes and diminished collagen production. Treatment is by cessation of hydroxyurea therapy and moist wound dressing.

6.11 Cholesterol Emboli Associated Ulcers

Cholesterol crystals can dislodge from atheromatous plaques in large caliber arteries and even aorta and embolize into distal smaller arteries and capillaries. This can happen in the form of a few large emboli or as a shower of micro-emboli [20]. The organs at risk of ischemic injury are kidneys, intestine, and skeletal muscles. Cutaneous manifestations take the form of livedo reticularis and blue toe syndrome. Legs are the commonest site for cutaneous ulceration but are known to occur in the skin of the trunk.

6.11.1 Clinical Features

Although livedo reticularis specially of the lower limbs is the commonest manifestation it is not specific for cholesterol emboli. The ulcers are associated with other signs of ischemia such as blue toes or cyanosis. The peripheral pulses are palpable because the crystals lodge in arterioles and capillaries.

The diagnosis is suspected mainly on the basis of involvement of associated other organs specially heart and brain by atherosclerosis. Hypereosinophilia is found in 80% of patients.

6.11.2 Treatment

Like with all thrombophilic ulcers the primary pathology has to be addressed by thrombolytic therapy and anticoagulants. Supportive wound care with regular dressing and debridement is required for skin ulcers.

6.12 Calciphylaxis

Calciphylaxis, also known as calcific uremic arteriolopathy, is a rare disease seen in patients of chronic renal disease and in patients on dialysis. It is a result of calcification in the small blood vessels of deeper layers of skin. Calciphylaxis is a result of extraskeletal calcification [21]. Similar extraskeletal calcification is seen in patients with milk-alkali syndrome, sarcoidosis, primary hyperparathyroidism, and hypervitaminosis D.

6.12.1 Clinical Features

The initial manifestation of localized skin ischemia is livedo reticularis which is typical of most thrombophilic ulcers. As tissue necrosis progresses black leathery eschar in an untidy ulcer will occur. The ulcers are most common in the lower extremities, abdomen, buttocks, and penis. They are very painful and surrounded by indurated skin. Diagnosis is confirmed by biopsy which will reveal calcification of tunica media in small vessels.

6.12.2 Treatment

Timely control of phosphate and calcium balance can prevent calciphylaxis. Thrombolysis with tissue plasminogen activator may be considered early in course of disease. Parathyroidectomy may be helpful if there is evidence of primary hyperparathyroidism. Cinacalcet is an alternative agent to parathyroidectomy. Prognosis is very poor with average survival of 1 year.

6.13 Martorell's Hypertensive Ischemic Leg Ulcers

Martorell's ulcers are a sequelae of poorly controlled hypertension. They are most frequent in women between the ages of 50 to 70 years. The pathogenesis of these ulcers stems from uncontrolled systemic hypertension causing arteriosclerotic changes such as hyperplasia of middle layer of arterioles, a process described as hyalinosis [22]. The resulting luminal narrowing leads to reduced overlying skin perfusion.

6.13.1 Clinical Features

Women in the age group 50 to 70 years are most commonly affected. The ulcers are typically located on distal inner side of lower limbs and may be symmetrical. The ulcer base is necrotic with violaceous edges. They are very painful and ordinary analgesics are ineffective.

6.13.2 Treatment

The mainstay of treatment is antihypertensive medication. Drugs that reduce vasoconstriction such as calcium channel blockers and angiotensin converting enzyme inhibitors are useful. Besides local wound care with debridement and dressing changes will be required.

6.14 Summary

Cutaneous ulcers at atypical sites such as trunk, abdomen, breasts, thighs, and penis should arouse suspicion of an underlying hypercoagulable state or thrombophilia. Further they may appear non-inflammatory and are non-responsive to antibiotic therapy. Such ulcers are always preceded by livedo reticularis and/or atrophie blanche. A vigorous evaluation for the causative disease condition if not already diagnosed should be performed. Because of the similar clinical presentation the commonest differential diagnosis is pyoderma gangrenosum. Treatment is control of the underlying cause along with supportive wound care for the ulcer.

References

1. Baglin T, Gray E, Greaves M, et al. Clinical guidelines for testing for heritable thrombophilia. Br J Haematol. 2010;149(2):209–20.
2. Mehta R, Shapiro AD. Plasminogen deficiency. Haemophilia. 2008;14(6):1261–8.
3. Ruiz-Irastarza G, Crawther M, Branch W, Khamashta MA. Antiphospholipid syndrome. Lancet. 2010;376(9751):1498–509.
4. Keeling D, Davidson S, Watren H. The management of heparin induced thrombocytopenia. Br J Haematol. 2006;133(3):259–69.
5. Papadakis E, Hoffman R, Brenner B. Thrombohemorrhagic complications of myeloproliferative disorders. Blood Rev. 2010;24(6):227–32.
6. Prandoni P, Falanga A, Piccioli A. Cancer and venous thromboembolism. Lancet Oncol. 2005;6(6):401–10.

7. Daughety MM, Bannow S, Bethany T. Hemostasis and thrombosis in pregnancy. Hemost Thromb. 2019:197–206.
8. Crowther MA, Kelton JG. Congenital thrombophilia states associated with venous thrombosis; a qualitative overview and proposed classification system. Ann Intern Med. 2003;138(2):128–34.
9. Thornsberry LA, LoSicco KI, English JC III. The skin and hypercoagulable states. J Am Acad Dermatol. 2013;69(3):450–62.
10. Gottrup F, Karlsmark T. Leg ulcers: uncommon presentation. Clin Dermatol. 2005;23(6):601–11.
11. Young S, Narang J, Kumar S, Kwizera E, Malik P, Billings SD, Ko JS, Fernandez AP. Large sacral/ buttocks ulceration in the setting of coagulopathy: a case series establishing the skin as a target organ of significant damage and potential morbidity in patients with severe COVID-19. Int Wound J. 2020;17:2033–7.
12. Santos G, Joäo A, Sousa L. Leg ulcers in antiphospholipid syndrome secondary to systemic lupus erythematosus treated with intravenous immunoglobulin. J Dermatol Case Rep. 2014;8(2):38–41.
13. Takahashi K, Ikeda T, Yokoyama K, Kawakami T. Cutaneous ulcer resembling pyoderma gangrenosum in a patient with antiphospholipid syndrome. J Cutan Immunol Allergy. 2021;4:17–8.
14. Asherson RA, Francès C, Iaccarino L, Khamashta MA, Malacarne F, Piette JC, Tincani A, Daria A. The antiphospholipid antibody syndrome: diagnosis, skin manifestation and current therapy. Clin Exp Rheumatol. 2006;24(1supple 40):546–51.
15. Giuggioli D, Manfredi A, Lumetti F, Sebastiani M, Ferri C. Cryoglobulinemic vasculitis and skin ulcers. Our therapeutic strategy and review of the literature. Semin Arthritis Rheum. 2015;44(5):518–26.
16. Minniti CP, Eckman J, Sebastiani P, Steinberg MH, Bellas SK. Leg ulcers in sickle cell disease. Am J Hematol. 2010;85(10):821–33.
17. Freitas TQ, Halpern I, Criado PR. Livedoid vasculopathy: a compelling diagnosis. Autops Case Rep. 2018;8(3):e2018034.
18. Chan YC, Valenti D, Mansfield AO, Stansby G. Warfarin induced skin necrosis. Br J Surg. 2000;87(3):266–72.
19. Dissemond J, Körber A. Hydroxyurea induced ulcers on the leg. CMAJ. 2009;180(11):1132.
20. Kronzon I, Saric MDM. Cholesterol embolization syndrome. Circulation. 2010;122:631–41.
21. Nigwekar SU, Thadhani R, Brandenburg VM. Calciphylaxis. N Engl J Med. 2018;378(18):1704–14.
22. Pinto APFL, Silva JRNA, Osorio CT, Rivera LM, Carneiro S, Ramos-e-Silva M, Bica BERG. Martorell's ulcer: diagnostic and therapeutic challenge. Case Rep Dermatol. 2015;7(2):199–206.

Septic Emboli

7

Amrita Rath and Abhinay Jayanthi

7.1 Introduction

Septic embolism (SE) constitutes an important yet often under-reported class of infectious complications. The incidence of septic embolism is on the rise now a days secondary to widespread use of injectable drugs and indwelling catheters. Septic embolism is typically caused by occlusion of a blood vessel by an infected thrombus which travels in bloodstream from a distant infectious source. Septic embolism as was classically described results from infective endocarditis.

Osler nodes (the tender, purplish-coloured papules), which are pathognomonic of infective endocarditis, are indeed evidence of embolism [1].

SE can be associated with a wide range of both early and late sequelae. Among immediate complications is the occlusion of the downstream vascular tree, including devastating sequelae such as cerebral, bowel, or myocardial infarction [2]. Among late complications are mycotic aneurysms [3] and abscesses [4].

7.2 Epidemiology

The incidence of septic emboli among patients with infective endocarditis varies widely among studies. In a study including 437 patients with surgical endocarditis, septic emboli were present in 10.52% of patients with infective endocarditis [5]. Also, systemic embolization complicates about 20% to 50% of cases of infective endocarditis of left-sided heart valves [6]. In a systematic review and metanalysis, the pooled prevalence of septic embolism in patients with infective endocarditis

A. Rath (✉) · A. Jayanthi
Department of Anesthesiology, Institute of Medical Sciences, Banaras Hindu University, Varanasi, India

A. K. Khanna, S. K. Tiwary (eds.), *Uncommon Ulcers of the Extremities*,
https://doi.org/10.1007/978-981-99-1782-2_7

accounted for 25% [7]. Septic embolization occurs in at least 30% of patients with infective endocarditis referred for cardiac valve replacement [8].

The distribution of embolism was as follows: cerebral (26.3%), splenic (6.8%), pulmonary (6.1%), renal (2.9%), peripheral (2.2%), coronary (n = 4), mesenteric (n = 3) [9].

7.3 Aetiology

Various causes of septic embolism has been put forward. The following are some of the common causes:

(a) **Infected prosthetic valves**: Infected prosthetic valves develop vegetations on them, which can dislodge and travel through the bloodstream and occlude different blood vessels based on the size and the location.
(b) **Septic pelvic thrombophlebitis** occurring secondary to septic abortion and post puerperal uterine infection is an important attributer in females.
(c) **Indwelling catheters and intravenous drug use**: Currently, chronic intravenous drug use and chronic indwelling vascular catheters are considered more common risk factors for the development of septic emboli. In patients with endovascular devices/cannulations who present with recurrent or persistent bacteraemia, septic embolism should be suspected.
(d) **Presence of CIED:** Cardiac implantable electronic devices (CIED) infections occur in about 0.5% of de novo CIED implants and approximately 2% of CIED replacements [10]. Septic thrombophlebitis involving the internal jugular vein due to *Staphylococcus aureus* has been found after insertion of implantable cardioverter defibrillator [11].

Leading pathogens are *Staphylococcus aureus* (33.6%), *Streptococcus viridans* (18.7%), *Enterococci* (16.1%), and *Coagulase-negative Staphylococci* (11.6%).

7.4 Pathophysiology

Septic emboli result in two insults:

(a) Early embolic/ischaemic insult due to vascular occlusion that may lead to ischaemia, or even infarction.
(b) The infectious insult that leads to inflammation and possible abscess formation [12].

The pathophysiology and clinical course of septic emboli depend on various factors.

7.4.1 Anatomical Location

The origin of septic emboli depends on the anatomical location and the vasculature of the infected area. For example, orbital cellulitis caused by *Streptococcus constellates* was complicated with cavernous sinus thrombosis [13].

7.4.2 Presence of Right to Left Shunt

Patent foramen ovale (PFO), a congenital cardiac anomaly, may provide a conduit resulting in paradoxical embolism. This is one of the frequent causes of cryptogenic strokes [10].

7.4.3 Blood Stream as the Inlet

Septic pulmonary emboli from the right atrial thrombus related to tunnelled haemodialysis catheters [11].

Infection at the peripherally inserted central catheter (PICC) line in a neutropenic patient with MRSA bloodstream infection has resulted in septic superior vena cava thrombus [14].

7.4.4 Side of the Heart

Right-sided endocarditis vegetations usually embolize to the lungs and cause septic pulmonary emboli.

Left-sided endocarditis vegetations usually embolize to the brain (occlusion of cerebral vessels) leading to strokes.

7.4.5 Virulence of the Organism

The more virulent pathogens, *S. aureus* and *E. coli*, cause immediate and dramatic infections of the arterial wall, with aneurysm and haemorrhage. In contrast, streptococci usually cause progressive lesions, beginning in areas of infarction or ischaemia [4].

7.4.6 Immunity Status of the Host

Immunosuppressed patients may be at higher risk of SE in that their presentation as well as microbiologic findings may be atypical and/or clinically misleading [15, 16].

Microscopically, there is fibrinoid necrosis as well as neutrophilic infiltrate, both in the vessel walls and surrounding the vessels. There is presence of dense pauci-cellular fibrinoid material mixed/interspersed with clusters of bacterial cocci [17].

7.5 Clinical Presentation and Complications

Septic emboli have an extensive range of presentation from being asymptomatic to severe complications and sequelae with high mortality. Manifestations depend on the region of occlusion and can be as follows:

Right-sided endocarditis vegetations embolize to the lungs causing septic pulmonary emboli present with fever, dyspnoea, pleuritic chest pain, cough, and occasionally haemoptysis.

Left-sided endocarditis may result in systemic emboli in different organs with different clinical presentations:

(a) **Septic cerebral emboli**: Signs of neurological deficits depends on the stroke location, the extent of infarcted/inflamed area, and the number of the affected areas [18].

    The clinical presentation can be:

    - Focal Neurological: Hemiparesis, facial droop, diplopia, aphasia, vertigo.
    - Non-focal presentations: Headaches, seizures, altered mental status.
    - In severe cases, it can present as meningitis, brain abscess, encephalopathy, mycotic aneurysms, and cerebral haemorrhage.
    - These are usually diagnosed with the help of MRI with and without gadolinium, SPECT/CT, and [18F]FDG PET/CT.

(b) **Septic coronary artery embolization**: Coronary arterial SE should be considered in cases of known or suspected left-sided IE and evidence of concurrent acute myocardial ischaemia (e.g. abnormal ECG or elevated cardiac enzymes).

    Echocardiography (preferably TEE) can reliably demonstrate the presence of valvular vegetations, in addition to documenting other changes characteristics of myocardial ischaemia [19]. Trans-oesophageal echocardiography has a better yield for the detection of vegetations than transthoracic echocardiography.

    Coronary occlusion secondary to SE can also be confirmed via coronary angiography, with the potential for percutaneous coronary intervention at the same time [20].

(c) **Septic pulmonary embolism**: Right-sided IE usually manifests as persistent fevers, bacteraemia, and multiple septic pulmonary emboli. SPE may cause pleuritic chest pain, cough, and/or haemoptysis and may be complicated by pulmonary infarction, abscess, pneumothorax, pulmonary infiltrates, and purulent pulmonary effusion and mycotic aneurysm [21, 22]. Mycotic pulmonary artery aneurysms can rupture into the airways and be acutely fatal.

    Chest X-ray imaging usually shows nonspecific findings for septic pulmonary emboli.

CECT chest usually demonstrates bilateral nodules or multifocal infiltrates, often involving peripheral lung zones and associated cavitary lesions [23]. CT shows (a) multiple peripheral nodules, (b) feeding vessel sign, (c) pleura-abutting, wedge-shaped peripheral lesions, (d) cavity formation, and (e) pleural effusion [24].

The "feeding vessel" sign, or the finding of a vessel which projects into a peripheral lung lesion, is fairly specific for SPE [25, 26].

A ventilation/perfusion scan of the lung can help in diagnosis especially in patients in whom contrast cannot be administered.

(d) **Septic splenic emboli**: The two primary manifestations are splenic infarction (most common) and splenic abscess. Although often asymptomatic, splenic infarct may be associated with acute abdominal (usually left upper quadrant) pain and can be complicated by abscess formation (the primary source of subsequent morbidity and mortality) [27, 28].

A CT abdomen and an abdominal ultrasound may detect hypoechoic lesions in the spleen.

Streptococci and staphylococci are among the most common offending microorganisms, accounting for >80% of cases [28, 29]. The spleen is the most common abdominal site for systemic septic emboli that often complicate infective endocarditis [30].

(e) **Septic mesenteric emboli**: It manifests as severe and unrelenting abdominal pain, nausea, vomiting, and urgent urge to evacuate the bowel. Classically, the severity of abdominal pain is out of proportion to the physical findings. Dehydration and excessive fluid loss from third-spacing of fluid lead to mental confusion, tachycardia, tachypnoea, and circulatory collapse.

Septic mesenteric embolism can also result in ischaemia and infarctions in the corresponding anatomic distributions and end-organ structures [31].

In terms of vascular distribution, the inferior mesenteric artery (IMA) involvement is much less common than SE to the superior mesenteric artery (SMA, approximately 3% versus <1%, respectively) [32].

CT abdomen and abdominal ultrasound may provide insight into the diagnosis.

(f) **Renal septic emboli:** Three types of severe renal manifestations may be seen: renal infarcts, focal "embolic" glomerulonephritis, and acute diffuse glomerulonephritis [33]. Renal infarction or haemorrhages may lead to renal failure if a significant portion of the renal parenchyma is involved.

Most patients complain of an acute onset of fever and vomiting, abdominal, flank, or back pain. The pain is typically constant. Acute secondary hypertension from renin release can occur due to decreased arterial perfusion may be seen.

Laboratory findings may include leukocytosis, proteinuria, haematuria, elevated levels of lactate dehydrogenase, serum glutamic-oxaloacetic transaminase, serum glutamic-pyruvic transaminase, and alkaline phosphatase [34].

Ultrasound may detect hypoechoic lesions in the kidneys.

(g) **Pyogenic liver abscesses** could experience complications with metastatic infections, including septic embolism [35]. Larger hepatic abscesses may evolve over time from smaller, adjacent micro-abscesses [36]. In a variety of septic states, especially severe abdominal sepsis associated with clinico-pathologic entities such as diverticulitis or appendicitis, septic emboli may be released into the portal circulation. Larger abscesses may evolve and coalesce from smaller "seed" abscesses [37].

Such abscesses usually involve multiple bacterial species, with most common organisms being *Escherichia coli*, *Streptococcus* spp., and anaerobes [38, 39].

CT abdomen and abdominal ultrasound may provide insight into the diagnosis.

(h) **Pylephlebitis:** Portal vein thrombosis due to intrabdominal infection such as ascending cholangitis or diverticulitis usually presents with nonspecific symptoms like fever and abdominal pain and is diagnosed with CECT abdomen and abdominal ultrasound.

Arterial and venous duplex studies are needed to pursue arterial emboli and venous thrombophlebitis.

(i) **Septic emboli of the skin and mucosa**: Janeway lesions which occur secondary to bacterial endocarditis are due to SE. A biopsy of the lesion shows evidence of septic micro-emboli in it [40].

Lemierre syndrome is an acute oropharyngeal infection caused by *Fusobacterium necrophorum* with secondary septic thrombophlebitis of the internal jugular vein (IVJ). It involves the progression of the disease from a focal suppurative peritonsillar infection to local septic thrombophlebitis with haematogenous progression to distant septic emboli.

(j) **Septic emboli of the extremities:** Clinical manifestations can vary from extremity pain to limb-threatening ischaemia [8]. Transient ischaemia may be treated with antibiotics and anticoagulants to severe ischaemia necessitating limb amputation [41].

(k) **Septic retinal emboli** occur when emboli reach the retinal vessels [42].

7.6 Investigations

(a) Laboratory: Blood cultures are usually positive in patients with septic emboli. At least three blood cultures are needed to be obtained.
(b) Arterial and venous duplex studies are needed to pursue arterial emboli and venous thrombophlebitis.
(c) Echocardiography: TEE/TOE.
(d) Chest X-ray.
(e) CECT Chest and Abdomen.
(f) A ventilation/perfusion scan.
(g) Ultrasound.

(h) F-FDG-PET/CT has high diagnostic value for detecting peripheral emboli in patients with infective endocarditis and cardiac device infections.

The use of white blood cell SPECT/CT and [18F] FDG PET/CT allows for the early detection of septic emboli [43].

7.7 Treatment/Management

(a) Source control and prolonged antibiotic therapy are the mainstay in the management of septic emboli.
   - *Source Control*: It encompasses all measures undertaken to eliminate the source of infection.
   - Example: If an indwelling catheter is suspected to be the source of the infection, it should be removed.
   - Percutaneous abscess drainage is one of the treatment modalities in patients with liver abscess.
   - *Antibiotics*: The choice of antimicrobial therapy in the management of septic emboli depends on the causative organisms, the organ involved, and the pharmacokinetics and pharmacodynamics of the available drugs.
   - The antimicrobial therapy of infective endocarditis and subsequent septic emboli guidelines recommend 4–6 weeks of intravenous antimicrobial therapy [44].

(b) *Anticoagulation*: There is no definitive role of usage of anticoagulants in patients of septic emboli. However, anticoagulants can be continued in patients with left-sided infective endocarditis with a definitive pre-existing indication [45].

(c) Early surgery performed for the affected region within the first 2 days after diagnosis plays a pivotal role in treating these patients.

   Management of an embolic splenic abscess usually involves surgical splenectomy or image-guided drainage. The surgical indications include persistent sepsis (60% cases), large lesions (>2 cm), peripheral lesions (30%), and splenic rupture (10%) [46].

   Mycotic aneurysm of the superior mesenteric artery is successfully treated with surgical resection of the mycotic aneurysm, removal of the mycotic thrombi, and infected valve replacement [47].

(d) Endovascular management of acute ischaemic stroke secondary to septic emboli from bacterial endocarditis is case-specific and outside established guidelines.

7.8 Differential Diagnosis

(a) Marantic endocarditis, Libman-Sacks endocarditis, non-infectious, typically associated with cancer and collagen vascular diseases should be considered in patients with culture-negative endocarditis and elevated inflammatory markers.
(b) Metastatic disease and tumour embolism: require a high index of suspicion and history of underlying malignancy.
(c) Disseminated fungal or mycobacterial infections: It may require microbiologic diagnostic modalities such as tissue biopsy, cultures, antigen detection, and PCR testing.
(d) Non-infectious thromboembolic phenomena in patients with atrial fibrillation not on anticoagulation or other arrhythmias.

7.9 Prognosis

The prognosis varies significantly depending upon the affected organs and the combined toll of both ischaemic and infectious insults.

Independent predictors of mortality include ***Charlson comorbidity index*** which consists of the following parameters:

1. Creatinine greater than 2 mg/dL.
2. Congestive heart failure.
3. Vegetation length over 10 mm.
4. Cerebral complications.
5. Abscess.
6. Failure to undertake surgery when indicated [48].

7.10 Postoperative and Rehabilitation Care

Aggressive acute rehabilitation is very important in certain cases to reduce disability. For example, Cerebral septic emboli often result in stroke syndromes that require rehabilitation.

Septic pulmonary emboli may result in acute hypoxemic respiratory failure requiring mechanical ventilation and prolonged ICU stay may require pulmonary rehabilitation (deep breathing exercises, incentive spirometry, chest physiotherapy).

Acute limb ischaemia from septic emboli if severe may result in limb amputation due to critical limb ischaemia, and physical rehabilitation is required after that.

7.11 Conclusions

Septic emboli frequently pose a diagnostic dilemma due to variable organs affected with variable presentations. In addition to high index of suspicion and early clinical recognition, prompt identification of the source, multidisciplinary approach, and the institution of immediate goal-directed antibiotic therapy are all critical to successful outcomes. More widespread awareness of risk factors, clinical presentations, and management of SE is needed, with added focus on preventing embolic events and the management of associated complications.

References

1. Chan YH, Tse HF. Embolic origin of Osler nodes. Mayo Clin Proc. 2017;92(9):1459–60.
2. Caraballo V. Fatal myocardial infarction resulting from coronary artery septic embolism after abortion: unusual cause and complication of endocarditis. Ann Emerg Med. 1997;29:175–7.
3. Cassada DC, Stevens SL, Schuchmann GS, Freeman MB, Goldman MH. Mesenteric pseudoaneurysm resulting from septic embolism. Ann Vasc Surg. 1998;12:597–600.
4. Molinari GF. Septic cerebral embolism. Stroke. 1972;3:117–22.
5. Aalaei-Andabili SH, Martin T, Hess P, Hoh B, Anderson M, Klodell CT, Beaver TM. Management of Septic emboli in patients with infectious endocarditis. J Card Surg. 2017;32(5):274–80.
6. Bayer AS, Bolger AF, Taubert KA, Wilson W, Steckelberg J, Karchmer AW, Levison M, Chambers HF, Dajani AS, Gewitz MH, Newburger JW, Gerber MA, Shulman ST, Pallasch TJ, Gage TW, Ferrieri P. Diagnosis and management of infective endocarditis and its complications. Circulation. 1998;98(25):2936–48.
7. Abegaz TM, Bhagavathula AS, Gebreyohannes EA, Mekonnen AB, Abebe TB. Short- and long-term outcomes in infective endocarditis patients: a systematic review and meta-analysis. BMC Cardiovasc Disord. 2017;17(1):291.
8. Kitts D, Bongard FS, Klein SR. Septic embolism complicating infective endocarditis. J Vasc Surg. 1991;14(4):480–5; discussion 485–7.
9. Erdem H, Puca E, Ruch Y, Santos L, Ghanem-Zoubi N, Argemi X, Hansmann Y, Guner R, Tonziello G, Mazzucotelli JP, Como N, Kose S, Batirel A, Inan A, Tulek N, Pekok AU, Khan EA, Iyisoy A, Meric-Koc M, Kaya-Kalem A, Martins PP, Hasanoglu I, Silva-Pinto A, Oztoprak N, Duro R, Almajid F, Dogan M, Dauby N, Gunst JD, Tekin R, Konopnicki D, Petrosillo N, Bozkurt I, Wadi J, Popescu C, Balkan II, Ozer-Balin S, Zupanc TL, Cascio A, Dumitru IM, Erdem A, Ersoz G, Tasbakan M, Ajamieh OA, Sirmatel F, Florescu S, Gulsun S, Ozkaya HD, Sari S, Tosun S, Avci M, Cag Y, Celebi G, Sagmak-Tartar A, Karakus S, Sener A, Dedej A, Oncu S, Del Vecchio RF, Ozturk-Engin D, Agalar C. Portraying infective endocarditis: results of multinational ID-IRI study. Eur J Clin Microbiol Infect Dis. 2019;38(9):1753–63.
10. Thompson JJ, McDonnell KM, Reavey-Cantwell JF, Ellenbogen KA, Koneru JN. Paradoxical septic emboli secondary to pacemaker endocarditis: transvenous lead extraction with distal embolization protection. Circ Arrhythm Electrophysiol. 2014;7(6):1271–2.
11. Vyahalkar SV, Dedhia NM, Sheth GS, Pathan MAR. Tunneled hemodialysis catheter-associated right atrial thrombus presenting with septic pulmonary embolism. Indian J Nephrol. 2018;28(4):314–6.
12. Stawicki SP, Firstenberg MS, Lyaker MR, Russell SB, Evans DC, Bergese SD, Papadimos TJ. Septic embolism in the intensive care unit. Int J Crit Illn Inj Sci. 2013;3(1):58–63.
13. Allegrini D, Reposi S, Nocerino E, Pece A. Odontogenic orbital cellulitis associated with cavernous sinus thrombosis and pulmonary embolism: a case report. J Med Case Rep. 2017;11(1):164.

14. Schrenk KG, Frosinski J, Scholl S, Otto S, La Rosée P, Hochhaus A, Pletz MW. Successful treatment of neutropenic MRSA bacteremia with septic superior vena cava thrombus and cerebral embolism using high-dose daptomycin. Ann Hematol. 2016;95(2):355–7.
15. Avery RK, Barnes DS, Teran JC, Wiedemann HP, Hall G, Wacker T, et al. Listeria monocytogenes tricuspid valve endocarditis with septic pulmonary emboli in a liver transplant recipient. Transpl Infect Dis. 1999;1:284–7.
16. Miller FH, Ma JJ. Total splenic infarct due to aspergillus and AIDS. Clin Imaging. 2000;24:362–4.
17. Bhaskar S, Saab J, Cappelen-Smith C, Killingsworth M, Wu XJ, Cheung A, Manning N, Aouad P, McDougall A, Hodgkinson S, Cordato D. Clot histopathology in ischemic stroke with infective endocarditis. Can J Neurol Sci. 2019;46(3):331–6.
18. Cooper HA, Thompson EC, Laureno R, Fuisz A, Mark AS, Lin M, Goldstein SA. Subclinical brain embolization in left-sided infective endocarditis: results from the evaluation by MRI of the brains of patients with left-sided intracardiac solid masses (EMBOLISM) pilot study. Circulation. 2009;120(7):585–91.
19. Kessavane A, et al. Septic coronary embolism in aortic valvular endocarditis. J Heart Valve Dis. 2009;18(5):572–4.
20. Taniike M, et al. Acute myocardial infarction caused by a septic coronary embolism diagnosed and treated with a thrombectomy catheter. Heart. 2005;91(5):e34.
21. Miró JM, del Río A, Mestres CA. Infective endocarditis and cardiac surgery in intravenous drug abusers and HIV-1 infected patients. Cardiol Clin. 2003;21(2):167–84.
22. Rossi SE, Goodman PC, Franquet T. Nonthrombotic pulmonary emboli. Am J Roentgenol. 2000;174(6):1499–508.
23. Cook RJ, et al. Septic pulmonary embolism: presenting features and clinical course of 14 patients. Chest J. 2005;128(1):162–6.
24. Kuhlman JE, Fishman EK, Teigen C. Pulmonary septic emboli: diagnosis with CT. Radiology. 1990;174:211–3.
25. Wong K, et al. Clinical and radiographic spectrum of septic pulmonary embolism. Arch Dis Child. 2002;87(4):312–5.
26. Iwasaki Y, et al. Spiral CT findings in septic pulmonary emboli. Eur J Radiol. 2001;37(3):190–4.
27. Ting W, et al. Splenic septic emboli in endocarditis. Circulation. 1990;82(5 Suppl):IV105–9.
28. Beeson MS. Splenic infarct presenting as acute abdominal pain in an older patient. J Emerg Med. 1996;14(3):319–22.
29. Millaire A, et al. Incidence and prognosis of embolic events and metastatic infections in infective endocarditis. Eur Heart J. 1997;18(4):677–84.
30. Alnasser SA, Mindru C, Preventza O, Rosengart T, Cornwell L. Successful conservative management of a large splenic abscess secondary to infective endocarditis. Ann Thorac Surg. 2019;107(4):e235–7.
31. Misawa S, Sakano Y, Muraoka A, Yasuda Y, Misawa Y. Septic embolic occlusion of the superior mesenteric artery induced by mitral valve endocarditis. Ann Thorac Cardiovasc Surg. 2011;17:415–7.
32. Kirkwood ML, et al. Mycotic inferior mesenteric artery aneurysm secondary to native valve endocarditis caused by coagulase-negative staphylococcus. Ann Vasc Surg. 2014;28(5):1312.e13–5.
33. Mittal B. Renal lesions in infective endocarditis (an autopsy study of 55 cases). J Postgrad Med. 1987;33(4):193.
34. Lessman RK, et al. Renal artery embolism: clinical features and long-term follow-up of 17 cases. Ann Intern Med. 1978;89(4):477–82.
35. Keller JJ, Tsai MC, Lin CC, Lin YC, Lin HC. Risk of infections subsequent to pyogenic liver abscess: a nationwide population-based study. Clin Microbiol Infect. 2013;19(8):717–22.
36. Wang Y-J, et al. Liver abscess secondary to sigmoid diverticulitis: a case report. J Intern Med Taiwan. 2005;16:289–94.

37. Wang YJ, Wen SC, Chien ST, King J, Hsuea CW, Feng NH. Liver abscess secondary to sigmoid diverticulitis: a case report. J Intern Med Taiwan. 2005;16:289–94.
38. Sabbaj J. Anaerobes in liver abscess. Rev Infect Dis. 1984;6(Suppl 1):S152–6.
39. Chou FF, Sheen-Chen SM, Chen YS, Chen MC. Single and multiple pyogenic liver abscesses: clinical course, etiology, and results of treatment. World J Surg. 1997;21:384–8; discussion 388–98.
40. Vinson RP, Chung A, Elston DM, Keller RA. Septic microemboli in a Janeway lesion of bacterial endocarditis. J Am Acad Dermatol. 1996;35(6):984–5.
41. Ahmed M. Septic emboli resulting in an acutely ischaemic lower limb: a case report. Ann R Coll Surg Engl. 2012;94(2):e60–1.
42. Kilmartin DJ, Barry P. Recurrent septic retinal emboli following dental surgery. Br J Ophthalmol. 1996;80(12):1111–2.
43. Sollini M, Berchiolli R, Delgado Bolton RC, Rossi A, Kirienko M, Boni R, Lazzeri E, Slart R, Erba PA. The "3M" approach to cardiovascular infections: multimodality, multitracers, and multidisciplinary. Semin Nucl Med. 2018;48(3):199–224.
44. Baddour LM, Wilson WR, Bayer AS, Fowler VG Jr, Tleyjeh IM. Infective endocarditis in adults: diagnosis, antimicrobial therapy, and management of complications. Circulation. 2015;132(15):1435–86.
45. Davis KA, Huang G, Petty SA, Tan WA, Malaver D, Peacock JE. The effect of preexisting anticoagulation on cerebrovascular events in left-sided infective endocarditis. Am J Med. 2020;133(3):360–9.
46. Ting W, Silverman NA, Arzouman DA, Levitsky S. Splenic septic emboli in endocarditis. Circulation. 1990;82(Suppl 5):IV105–9.
47. Chai HT, Tan BL, Yen HT, Chen MC. Infective endocarditis caused by Streptococcus bovis complicated by a superior mesenteric artery mycotic aneurysm and systemic septic emboli in a patient with colon diverticulitis. Int J Infect Dis. 2010;14(Suppl 3):e317–8.
48. Habib G, Erba PA, Iung B, Donal E, Cosyns B, Laroche C, Popescu BA, Prendergast B, Tornos P, Sadeghpour A, Oliver L, Vaskelyte JJ, Sow R, Axler O, Maggioni AP, Lancellotti P. EURO-ENDO investigators. Clinical presentation, aetiology and outcome of infective endocarditis. Results of the ESC-EORP EURO-ENDO (European infective endocarditis) registry: a prospective cohort study. Eur Heart J. 2019;40(39):3222–32.

8 Ulcers Caused by Calciphylaxis

Alessandra Michelucci, Paolo Romanelli, Valentina Dini, and Marco Romanelli

8.1 Introduction

Calciphylaxis, also known as calcific uremic arteriolopathy (CUA), is a rare and life-threatening disorder that usually occurs in patients with end-stage renal disease (ESRD) and less frequently in non-uremic patients [1–3].

The term calciphylaxis, first coined by Dr. Seyle in 1961, literally means "protection by calcification." Dr. Seyle described calciphylaxis in rats as an adaptive (phylatic) response that leads to calcium deposition in the affected tissues [4]. In 1963, Eisenberg and Bartholow reported a case of extensive metastatic calcification in a patient with chronic renal failure, which represented the human counterpart of calciphylaxis [5]. Over the course of the following years several cases of calciphylaxis have been described [6–10].

The histologic aspect of the disease explains the meaning of the term: the calcification process involving the blood vessels of the dermis and subcutaneous tissue leads to their occlusion with consequent infarction of the irrigated tissues and the appearance of painful ulcers. Calciphylaxis injuries are mainly localized at adipose tissue-rich regions, such as the lower limbs and trunk [11].

To date, the etiopathogenesis, risk factors, and natural history of the disease are not fully clarified [12, 13].

In addition, the diagnosis is difficult and the therapeutic management of calciphylaxis does not refer to recognized guidelines, but rather relies on expert opinion from literature, thus representing a great challenge for the clinician [14].

A. Michelucci · V. Dini · M. Romanelli (✉)
Department of Dermatology, University of Pisa, Pisa, Italy

P. Romanelli
Department of Dermatology and Cutaneous Surgery, University of Miami Miller School of Medicine, Miami, FL, USA

A. K. Khanna, S. K. Tiwary (eds.), *Uncommon Ulcers of the Extremities*,
https://doi.org/10.1007/978-981-99-1782-2_8

8.2 Epidemiology

It is estimated that the incidence of calciphylaxis in dialysis patients is 1–4% per year. It generally occurs 35–105 months after dialysis' beginning, with a greater involvement toward the female, obese, and diabetic population. Recently, an increase in the incidence of the disease has been detected. Nevertheless, it is not known for sure whether it is due to a real increase in cases or to a greater awareness of the disease, resulting in a higher number of diagnoses. However, the enhanced use of calcium phosphate as well as the increase of patients in dialysis certainly represent factors that could explain the rising number of cases [11, 15–17].

A recent study conducted in the dialysis units of Fresenius Medical Care North America (FMCNA) counted 1030 newly diagnosed cases of calciphylaxis in the FMCNA cohort (>250,000 chronic hemodialysis patients) during an extended 5-year study period from January 2010 to December 2014, revealing an incidence rate of 3.49 per 1000 patient-years among ESRD patients on chronic hemodialysis [18].

Instead, a Japanese study identified a prevalence rate of less than 3/1000 cases in chronic hemodialysis patients per year, reporting a lower rate than studies conducted in Western countries [19].

Calciphylaxis without ESRD essentially affects obese, hypertensive, and type II diabetes population, and it has recently been defined as the proximal form of Martorell hypertensive ischemic leg ulcer (HYTILU) [20–24].

8.3 Pathogenesis

The pathogenesis of calciphylaxis remains poorly understood. The deposition of calcium within the medial layer of the arterioles as well as the fibrotic process underneath the intima and the proliferation of endothelial cells are considered the main causes of the consequent blood vessels' obstruction [25].

Calciphylaxis is characterized by ectopic bone formation that involves vessel walls and can be related to different mechanisms.

The smooth muscle cells of the middle tunica respond to the altered microenvironment (hyperphosphatemia, hypercalcemia, and hyperglycemia) by transforming into osteoblast-like cells responsible for the deposition of hydroxyapatite crystals [26, 27].

The greater involvement of fat-rich tissues can also be explained by in vitro evidence that adipocytes are able, when exposed to high doses of phosphate, to induce calcification of smooth muscle cells, through some mediators such as leptin [28].

In addition, ectopic bone formation is enhanced by the deficiency of molecular factors that inhibit the calcification process of vessel walls, including a potent inhibitor of calcification called Gla protein (MGP) [29, 30], which is usually released from endothelial cells and smooth muscle cells and activated by vitamin K [26].

In the patient with ESDR, vitamin K levels are lower than normal:

- They are forced into a diet low in foods rich in vitamin K, such as green leafy vegetables and dairy products, in order to reduce sodium and potassium intake [31].
- About 40% of patients are on warfarin therapy, a vitamin K antagonist [32].

The higher frequency of calciphylaxis in the patient with ESDR is also due to the altered chemical microenvironment with abnormal levels of calcium, phosphate, and PTH. Patients with ESRD also develop hyperparathyroidism secondary to renal failure, resulting in hypophosphatemia, hypercalcemia, and increased calcium deposition in extraosseous sites such as vascular walls [33–35].

An additional role is that one played by bone morphogenic proteins (BMP), involved in the process of bone formation, osteoclast differentiation, and extraosseous calcification [36–39].

Among these we mention bone morphogenetic protein 4 (BMP_4), capable of promoting the calcification process through the action of ROS that activates nuclear factor kappa b (NF-kb) [40, 41]. This transcription factor is very important for several cellular functions, including normal bone development, osteoclast differentiation, and bone mineral resorption. Elevated NF-kb activity is related to autoimmune inflammatory states, atherosclerosis, and bone mineral loss [42].

BMP 2 + 4 are procalcifying proteins, inhibited by the action of MGP, which is deficient in patients with ESRD [43].

In addition, patients with ESRD on hemodialysis have low levels of fetuin A, a human circulating factor capable of inhibiting calcification [44, 45].

In conclusion, we can state that hypercalcemia-related skin lesions are related to both thrombotic occlusion of vessels and thickening of vessel walls, which follows the process of fibrosis underneath the intima and calcification of the middle tunica [46].

This process can occur after surgery or trauma; events that evoke the Virchow's triad (hypercoagulability, stasis, and endothelial damage); and a period of sensitization induced by factors that promote calcification [47].

8.4 Risk Factors

Calciphylaxis has a wide spectrum of risk factors and triggers (Table 8.1). Among these, the one that certainly plays the most recognized role is ESRD. However, other risk factors reported in literature include female sex, white race, diabetes mellitus, obesity, autoimmune diseases, thrombophilia disorders, life-threatening diseases, hypoalbuminemia, hypercalcemia, hyperphosphatemia, hyperparathyroidism and adynamic bone disease, dependence of dialysis for more than 2 years, hypercoagulable states, such as protein C and S deficiency or antiphospholipid antibody syndrome, therapy with vitamin K antagonists (warfarin), calcium supplements, calcium-based phosphate binders, vitamin D analogs, iron therapy, corticosteroids, a syndrome called polyneuropathy syndrome, organomegaly, endocrinopathy, M protein, and skin changes (POEMS) [2, 3, 11, 48–55].

Table 8.1 Calciphylaxis risk factors

Calciphylaxis risk factors
Gender: Female
Ethnicity: White
Hypoalbuminemia
Metabolic diseases: Diabetes, ESRD (especially dependence on dialysis for >2 years, recent transition onto dialysis, or insufficient dialysis [i.e., missed sessions])
Nutritional disorders: Gastric bypass surgery, malnutrition, obesity
Skin trauma: Subcutaneous insulin or heparin injection, skin biopsy, other direct trauma to the skin
Autoimmune disease: Systemic lupus erythematosus
Coagulation disorders: Lupus anticoagulant, protein C deficiency, antithrombin III deficiency
Environmental factors: Exposure to heavy metals (e.g., aluminum) and UV light
Disturbed calcium/phosphate homeostasis: Hypercalcemia, hyperphosphatemia, secondary hyperparathyroidism, vitamin D
Malignancy: Metastatic cancer (e.g., colon, lungs), POEMS syndrome
Genetic polymorphisms: CD73 (rs4431401, rs9444348), FGF23 and vitamin D receptor (rs 7,310,492, ra11063118, rs 13,312,747, and rs 17,882,106)
Drugs: Calcium-containing drugs (e.g., phosphate binders), corticosteroids, iron supplements, recombinant human parathyroid hormone, warfarin, vitamins D and E

ESRD end-stage renal disease, *POEMS* polyneuropathy organomegaly endocrinopathy monoclonal gammopathy skin changes

It is supposed that Martorell HYTILU and calciphylaxis without ESRD are characterized by the same risk factors that include obesity, primary arterial hypertension, diabetes mellitus type II, and use of vitamin K antagonists [21, 23, 56].

8.5 Clinical Features

Calciphylaxis has different clinical and morphological features, most typically occurring with the appearance of painful ulcerative skin lesions that do not heal [38]. In the early stages of the disease, however, clinical features can be quite heterogeneous, such as livedo reticularis lesions, subcutaneous nodules, or indurated erythematous plaques resembling cellulitis [57].

Livedo reticularis usually occurs in the early stage and it is the clinical appearance of the altered skin vascularization. Plaques and nodules are the most frequent clinical presentation of the disorder and may precede the appearance of skin ulcers. Ulceration occurs in 1/3 of plaques and generally presents bilaterally, either like a unique large lesion (Fig. 8.1) or like a crop of different small ulcers [11].

Weenig classifies in his review [58] the wide range of possible clinical manifestations into 5 subtypes:

- necrotic ulcers,
- livedo racemosa-like purpura,
- hemorrhagic patches,

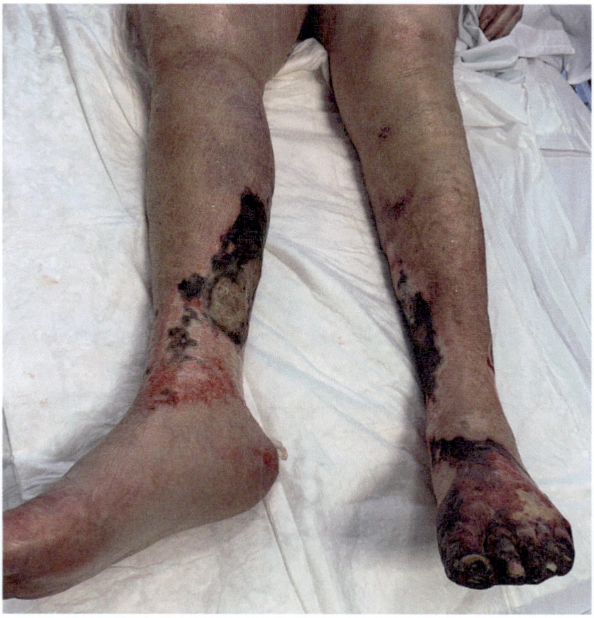

Fig. 8.1 Patient with chronic renal insufficiency and severe ulcers due to calciphylaxis

- hemorrhagic bullae,
- indurated plaques.

Calciphylaxis lesions generally affect areas rich in adipose tissue such as trunk, breasts, abdomen, hips, buttocks, and proximal lower extremities) [38], but more rarely in literature are also described involvements of genital and digital regions [59–61]. In addition to the classical form of skin infarction, a "not classical distal form" with the involvement of laterodorsal leg, Achilles tendon, finger, toe, and penis is recognized [62, 63].

Calciphylaxis lesions usually occur in areas of repeated skin trauma, such as abdomen or thigh in diabetic patients treated with daily insulin injection [18]. The patients experience an intense pain of both ischemic and neuropathic origin, refractory to opioid treatment, that usually precedes the occurrence of skin lesions [11, 23, 64]. More rarely, serious hemorrhages of the gastrointestinal tract or proximal myopathy have been shown in cases of extracutaneous vascular calcifications [7, 65].

8.6 Diagnosis

The diagnosis, which is essentially clinical, should always be preceded by a history of the patient's comorbidities and an objective examination of the entire skin surface [3]. However, its diagnosis is challenging and the occurrence of intensely painful ulcerative lesions or fixed subcutaneous nodules in an ESRD patient should suggest a diagnosis of calciphylaxis [3, 66].

Incisional biopsy of the skin lesion remains the gold standard for the confirmation of the diagnosis, especially in atypical manifestations of the disease and enables us to rule out any differential diagnoses [3, 67] (Table 8.2). Biopsy examination is mainly useful in non-uremic calciphylaxis [11], while its role for uremic calciphylaxis is still controversial [68]. The main reasons for this disagreement rely on the possibility of negative biopsy examinations and on the risk of procedure-related complications. A biopsy performed in an extensive necrotic area leads frequently to a negative biopsy, thus having a low diagnostic yield and the need to repeat the exam. Therefore, high clinical suspicion must be maintained in patients with risk factors even in case of negative biopsy [69]. Moreover, this procedure is not immune to risks such as infection, delayed healing, propagation of new lesions [11, 25] and increased risk of bleeding, ulceration, necrosis and, most rarely, sepsis, or death [70].

The best biopsy procedure is a punch biopsy with a double trephine technique [11, 71]. First, an 8-mm circular core of superficial tissue is taken with an 8-mm punch tool, within which at a later time an instrument of 4–6 mm is positioned, in order to reach deep subcutaneous fat. This strategy allows to identify the calcium within the walls of the dermis and subcutaneous blood vessels (Fig. 8.2a, b).

An excisional biopsy should not be performed because of the elevated risk of necrosis and bleeding [68, 72].

There are no specific laboratory tests to confirm diagnosis, but they are performed in order to assess the presence and severity of any risk factors. The most commonly required tests include renal function indices, degree of bone mineralization, coagulation indices, infection and inflammation parameters, tumor markers, and autoantibodies [3]. However, some patients do not have hyperphosphatemia, hypercalcemia, and hypo/hyperparathyroidism: consequently, low calcium and phosphate levels do not allow us to rule out calciphylaxis [73].

Table 8.2 Differential diagnoses

Differential diagnoses
Atherosclerosis (peripheral vascular disease)
Calcinosis cutis
Cellulitis
Hematoma
Infection ulcer
Livedoid vasculopathy
Pyoderma gangrenosum
Small-to-medium vessel vasculitis
Venous stasis ulcer
Antiphospholipid syndrome (or other hypercoagulable state)
Cholesterol embolism

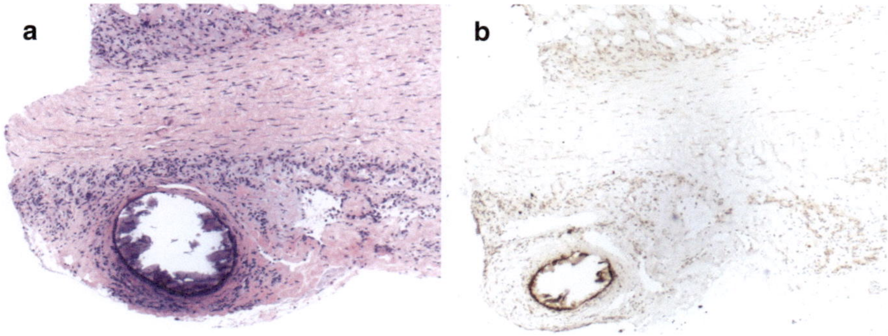

Fig. 8.2 (**a**, **b**) Wound biopsy of an ulcerative lesion due to calciphylaxis: (**a**) Hematoxylin and eosin staining, showing calcium deposits in the vascular wall; (**b**) Immunohistochemical staining with osteopontin, a bone matrix protein produced by osteoblasts, with an increased expression in tissues at risk or known to calcify

Calcified regions in the dermis and subcutaneous tissue as well as vascular calcification can be investigated by imaging procedures such as radiographs, bone scintigraphy, and evaluation of biomarkers like circulating levels of fetuin A [73–77].

In addition, the literature reports that triphasic bone scintigraphy with technetium Tc99m methylene diphosphate can reveal with a high degree of specificity and sensitivity the early stages of disease [78, 79].

8.7 Histopathology

On histologic examination of biopsy specimens, signs of ulceration of the epidermis, focal necrosis of the dermis, and calcium deposits within the vessel walls can be found [80, 81]. Calcium deposits are recognized with hematoxylin and eosin staining, due to intense basophilia, and appear black with Von Kossa silver staining [82]. The biopsy must be so deep as to involve the subcutaneous tissue where these histopathologic changes are most evident [44]. Other common findings include intimal hyperplasia, inflammatory responses, endovascular fibrosis, thrombosis, fat necrosis, acute and chronic calcifying panniculitis, and extravascular calcium deposition [58, 80, 83, 84].

8.8 Treatment

Treatment of calciphylaxis involves a multidisciplinary approach integrating dermatology, nephrology, pathology, wound care, pain and nutrition management, in a comprehensive care plan [85] (Fig. 8.3).

There are no evidence-based clinical practice guidelines and disease management is based on expert experience from literature, case reports, case series, and retrospective cohort studies [86].

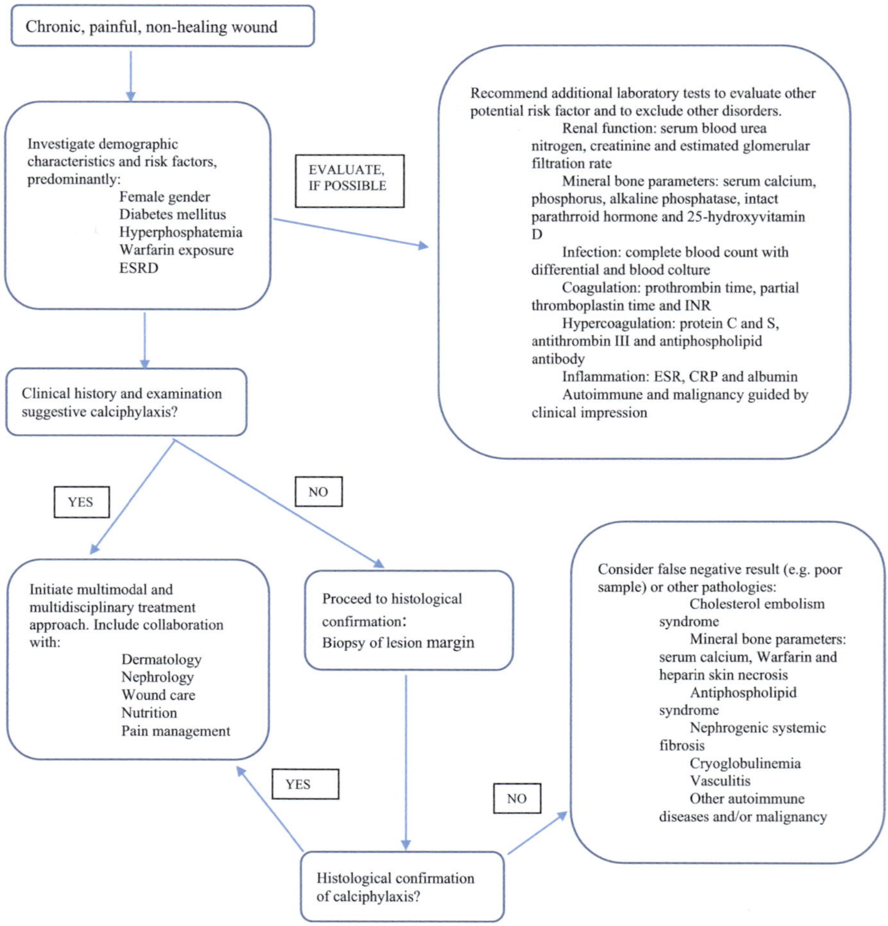

Fig. 8.3 Calciphylaxis management plan

Treatment involves blocking the process of vascular calcification or decalcifying the occluded vessels to reestablish flow. The aim of the treatment includes wound care management, metabolic control, prevention from local and systemic infection, and pain relief [68, 73].

8.8.1 Metabolic Control

Metabolic control to prevent vascular calcification acts on different fronts.

Phosphate should be maintained at serum levels of 3 mg/dL. Hyperphosphatemia is managed by trying to promote phosphate excretion, increasing the frequency of hemodialysis in dialysis patients by 4–5 times a week, and reducing dietary phosphate intake by helping with phosphate-binding factors. The target level of calcium in blood is 8 mg/dL. Hypercalcemia is managed by increasing the frequency of dialysis and reducing calcium intake, avoiding the use of calcium-based phosphate binders [87]. Finally, serum parathormone levels should remain neither too high nor too low: it is possible to suppress its excessive secretion by cinacalcet or in extreme cases by parathyroidectomy. Warfarin should be replaced by an alternative anticoagulant, and vitamin D supplements should be avoided [2, 18]. Patients who develop calciphylaxis should switch from peritoneal dialysis to hemodialysis, both because the latter one allows better control of calcium and phosphate levels and because it permits simultaneous administration of sodium thiosulfate.

Finally, bisphosphonates demonstrate efficacy in case series of "classical" forms of calciphylaxis in patients with ESRD [88].

8.8.2 Decalcification Strategies

Sodium thiosulfate (STS) is an inorganic salt that can chelate calcium, facilitating its expulsion by dialysis, and able to neutralize, through its antioxidant function, reactive oxygen species, in order to reduce the degree of inflammation and vascular thrombosis [89]. STS revealed the ability in vitro to limit the calcification of vascular smooth cells provoked by the adipocytes [86].

STS is generally administered in the last hour of hemodialysis as 25 g in 100 mL of normal saline for a period that generally lasts 6 months or until complete healing of the lesions [18]. Its use has been found to be effective both in treating the lesions and in reducing the mortality rate (from 55% before the advent of STS to 35% in patients treated with STS) [90].

Evidence that vitamin K is capable of activating a potent inhibitor of calcification has prompted several ongoing trials regarding the potential use of vitamin K in patients with calciphylaxis, at a dose of 10 mg orally three times a week for 12 weeks (ClinicalTrials.gov no. 02278692).

8.8.3 Wound Management

Recommendations for local management of ulcerative calciphylaxis injuries, as described by the wound care and dermatology physician and nurse teams, are reported in Table 8.3. The main goals of local management include removal of devitalized and necrotic tissue from the wound floor, control of exudate, and prevention from infection, thus promoting wound healing [91–93].

If dry eschar is present, in the absence of infection and with little tissue damage, physicians should prefer autolytic debridement with hydrocolloid or hydrogel dressings, rather than surgical one.

Surgical debridement may enlarge the necrotic area if the wound bed is minimally vascularized. However, the selection of the type of debridement should be done on a case-by-case basis, as in a retrospective study including 63 patients from the Mayo clinic, the 1-year survival rate of patients with calciphylaxis treated with

Table 8.3 Treatment options for ulcers caused by calciphylaxis

Wound care
Hyperbaric oxygen (second-line therapy): 2.5 atm of high-flow oxygen therapy (10–15 L/min) 90 min per day for 25 sessions[a]
Debridement
Surgical debridement
Maggot debridement
Chemical debridement
Other
Prevention of infection
Antibiotics in the presence of infection
Negative pressure wound therapy
Skin grafting

[a]Some authors recommend 20–40 sessions

surgical debridement was 61.6%, compared with 27.4% for patients who underwent enzymatic debridement [58].

The gold standard for the management of this kind of ulcer involves the choice of proper debridement, the use of negative pressure and skin grafts [94]. Surgery has not demonstrated its role in the treatment of central form of calciphylaxis [23].

Cases of treatment with hyperbaric oxygen therapy are frequently reported in literature [95, 96].

Moreover, several studies revealed the role of oxygen therapy in the improvement of wound bed perfusion, the reduction of inflammatory cytokines, and the promotion of angiogenesis and collagen deposition [97, 98].

A second-line treatment, which reported only a few cases in literature, is treatment with Lucilla fly larvae [99, 100].

Although the use of antibiotics in calciphylaxis ulcers is not a routine practice, in cases where the local appearance and systemic symptoms suggest it, it is appropriate to start with a low dose of antibiotic [23].

8.8.4 Pain Management

Pain relief represents the most important but at the same time the most challenging aspect in controlling the symptoms of calciphylaxis, also in relation to the strong impact on quality of life and non-responsiveness to common analgesics [101].

Pain in patients with calciphylaxis has a not completely understood etiopathogenesis, but most likely connected to either ischemic damage, due to arterial vessel infarction, or neuropathic damage, due to nerve inflammation [64].

The apparent disproportion between the pain experienced and the extent of tissue damage, as well as the tendency to increase during dressing changes suggest the use of preventive analgesia or simultaneous infusion of drug combinations, such as opioid benzodiazepines and ketamine [102, 103].

Opioid analgesics are necessary for the management of severe pain: methadone and fentanyl appear to be safe; hydromorphone and oxycodone can be used despite impaired renal function but require strict monitoring; morphine and codeine cannot be used in the dialysis patient because of excessive accumulation of neurotoxic metabolites [104].

It is therefore necessary to involve a specialized palliative care team both for pain management, through complex analgesic regimens, and as a bridge to terminal care, considering the poor prognosis of this condition.

8.9 Prognosis

The prognosis of patients affected by calciphylaxis with ESRD is poor, with a less than 50% survival rate at 1 year and less than 20% at 2 years [2, 58, 72]. The 1-year mortality rate in patients without ESRD is 25% and reaches 80% in case of ulceration [11, 105].

On the other hand, morbidity is mainly related to ulcerative lesions, severe pain, and high risk of recurrent hospitalizations, thus having a great impact on patients' quality of life [5, 58, 106, 107].

Sepsis secondary to infection of ulcerative lesions is the leading cause of death in these patients. The mortality rate is elevated and the success in wound healing remains low [14]. Obesity and female sex are related to worse prognosis [108].

8.10 Conclusions

Calcification is a clinical condition defined as a debilitating and very life-threatening ischemic vasculopathy. The etiology is multifactorial, but the main risk factor is ESRD. No standardized approach for the treatment of this condition is reported in the literature. But early diagnosis as well as multidisciplinary intervention involving dermatology, nephrology, wound care, nutrition, and pain management can improve the survival rate of patients with calciphylaxis.

References

1. Brandenburg VM, Cozzolino M, Mazzaferro S. Calcific uremic arteriolopathy: a call for action. Semin Nephrol. 2014;34:641–7.
2. Nigwekar SU, Kroshinsky D, Nazarian RM, et al. Calciphylaxis: risk factors, diagnosis, and treatment. Am J Kidney Dis. 2015;66:133–46.
3. Nigwekar SU. Multidisciplinary approach to calcific uremic arteriolopathy. Curr Opin Nephrol Hypertens. 2015;24:531–7.
4. Selye H, Gentile G, Prioreschi P. Cutaneous molt induced by calciphylaxis in the rat. Science. 1961;134(3493):1876–7.
5. Eisenberg E, Bartholow PV Jr. Reversible calcinosis cutis: calciphylaxis in man. N Engl J Med. 1963;268(22):1216–20.

6. Rees JK, Coles GA. Calciphylaxis in man. BMJ. 1969;2(5658):670–2.
7. Edelstein CL, Wickham MK, Kirby PA. Systemic calciphylaxis presenting as a painful, proximal myopathy. Postgrad Med J. 1992;68(797):209–11.
8. Bargman JM, Prichard SS. A usual peritoneal dialysis patient with an unusual skin disease. Perit Dial Int. 1995;15(6):252–8.
9. Budisavljevic MN, Cheek D, Ploth DW. Calciphylaxis in chronic renal failure. J Am Soc Nephrol. 1996;7(7):978–82.
10. Richens G, Piepkorn MW, Krueger GG. Calcifying panniculitis associated with renal failure. A case of Selye's calciphylaxis in man. J Am Acad Dermatol. 1982;6(4 Pt 1):537–9.
11. Nigwekar SU, Thadhani R, Brandenburg VM. Calciphylaxis. N Engl J Med. 2018;378(18):1704–14.
12. Fine A, Zacharias J. Calciphylaxis is usually non-ulcerating:riskfactors, outcome and therapy. Kidney Int. 2002;61(6):2210–7.
13. Anderson DC, Stewart WK, Piercy DM. Calcifying panniculitis with fat and skin necrosis in a case of uraemia with autonomous hyper parathyroidism. Lancet. 1968;2:323–5.
14. Kodumudi V, Jeha GM, Mydlo N, Kaye AD. Management of cutaneous calciphylaxis. Adv Ther. 2020;37(12):4797–807.
15. Westphal SG, Plumb T. Calciphylaxis. In: StatPearls. Treasure Island, FL: StatPearls Publishing; 2018; https://www.ncbi.nlm.nih.gov/books/NBK519020. Accessed 12 Nov 2018.
16. Nigwekar SU. Calciphylaxis. Curr Opin Nephrol Hypertens. 2017;26:276–81.
17. Angelis M, Wong LL, Myers SA, Wong LM. Calciphylaxis in patients on hemodialysis: a prevalence study. Surgery. 1997;122(6):1083–9; discussion 1089–90.
18. Nigwekar SU, Zhao S, Wenger J, et al. A nationally representative study of calcific uremic arteriolopathy risk factors. J Am Soc Nephrol. 2016;27:3421–9.
19. Hayashi M, Takamatsu I, Kanno Y, et al. A case-control study of calciphylaxis in Japanese end-stage renal disease patients. Nephrol Dial Transplant. 2012;27:1580–4.
20. Kalajian AH, Malhotra PS, Callen JP, Parker LP. Calciphylaxis with normal renal and parathyroid function: not as rare as previously believed. Arch Dermatol. 2009;145(4):451–8.
21. Nigwekar SU, Wolf M, Sterns RH, Hix JK. Calciphylaxis from nonuremic causes: a systematic review. Clin J Am Soc Nephrol. 2008;3(4):1139–43.
22. Ramsey-Stewart G. Eutrophication: spontaneous progressive dermatoliponecrosis. A fatal complication of gross morbid obesity. Obes Surg. 1992;2(3):263–4.
23. Isoherranen K, O'Brien JJ, Barker J, Dissemond J, Hafner J, Jemec GBE, Kamarachev J, Läuchli S, Montero EC, Nobbe S, Sunderkötter C, Velasco ML. Atypical wounds. Best clinical practice and challenges. J Wound Care. 2019;28(Sup6):S1–S92.
24. Bertranou EG, Gonoraky SE, Otero AE. Martorell hypertensive arteriolar ulcer: outpatient outcome on 366 cases. Phlebologie. 2001;54:267–72; [Articles in French].
25. Baby D, Upadhyay M, Joseph MD, Asopa SJ, Choudhury BK, Rajguru JP, Gupta S. Calciphylaxis and its diagnosis: a review. J Family Med Prim Care. 2019;8(9):2763–7.
26. Schurgers LJ, Uitto J, Reutelingsperger CP. Vitamin K-dependent carboxylation of matrix Gla-protein: a crucial switch to control ectopic mineralization. Trends Mol Med. 2013;19:217–26.
27. Bessueille L, Fakhry M, Hamade E, Badran B, Magne D. Glucose stimulates chondrocyte differentiation of vascular smooth muscle cells and calcification: a possible role for IL-1β. FEBS Lett. 2015;589(19 Pt B):2797–804.
28. Chen NX, O'Neill K, Akl NK, Moe SM. Adipocyte induced arterial calcification is prevented with sodium thiosulfate. Biochem Biophys Res Commun. 2014;449:151–6.
29. Kramann R, Brandenburg VM, Schurgers LJ, et al. Novel insights into osteogenesis and matrix remodelling associated with calcific uraemic arteriolopathy. Nephrol Dial Transplant. 2013;28(4):856–68.
30. Luo G, Ducy P, McKee MD, et al. Spontaneous calcification of arteries and cartilage in mice lacking matrix GLA protein. Nature. 1997;386:78–81.
31. Cranenburg EC, Schurgers LJ, Uiterwijk HH, et al. Vitamin K intake and status are low in hemodialysis patients. Kidney Int. 2012;82(5):605–10.

32. Brandenburg VM, Kramann R, Rothe H, et al. Calcific uraemic arteriolopathy (calciphylaxis): data from a large nationwide registry. Nephrol Dial Transplant. 2017;32:126–32.
33. London GM, Guerin AP, Marchais SJ, Metivier F, Pannier B, Adda H. Arterial media calcification in end-stage renal disease: impact on all-cause and cardiovascular mortality. Nephrol Dial Transpl. 2003;18(9):1731–40.
34. London GM, Marty C, Marchais SJ, Guerin AP, Metivier F, de Vernejoul MC. Arterial calcifications and bone histomorphometry in end-stage renal disease. J Am Soc Nephrol. 2004;15(7):1943–51.
35. Ishida M, Yao N, Yachiku S, Anzai T, Kobayashi T, Ishida H. Management of calcium, phosphorus and bone metabolism in dialysis patients using sevelamer hydrochloride and vitamin D therapy. Ther Apheresis Dial. 2005;9(Suppl 1):S16–21.
36. Moe SM, Chen NX. Mechanisms of vascular calcification in chronic kidney disease. J Am Soc Nephrol. 2008;19(2):213–6.
37. Hayden MR, Tyagi SC, Kolb L, Sowers JR, Khanna R. Vascular ossification-calcification in metabolic syndrome, type 2 diabetes mellitus, chronic kidney disease, and calciphylaxis-calcific uremic arteriolopathy: the emerging role of sodium thiosulfate. Cardiovasc Diabetol. 2005;4:4.
38. Rogers NM, Teubner DJ, Coates PT. Calcific uremic arteriolopathy: advances in pathogenesis and treatment. Semin Dial. 2007;20(2):150–7.
39. Wozney JM, Rosen V, Celeste AJ, Mitsock LM, Whitters MJ, Kriz RW, et al. Novel regulators of bone formation: molecular clones and activities. Science. 1988;242(4885):1528–34.
40. Griethe W, Schmitt R, Jurgensen JS, Bachmann S, Eckardt KU, Schindler R. Bone morphogenic protein-4 expression in vascular lesions of calciphylaxis. J Nephrol. 2003;16(5):728–32.
41. Feng JQ, Xing L, Zhang JH, Zhao M, Horn D, Chan J, et al. NF- kappaB specifically activates BMP-2 gene expression in growth plate chondrocytes in vivo and in a chondrocyte cell line in vitro. J Biol Chem. 2003;278(31):29130–5.
42. Weenig RH. Pathogenesis of calciphylaxis: Hans Selye to nuclear factor kappa-B. J Am Acad Dermatol. 2008;58(3):458–71.
43. Mikhaylova L, Malmquist J, Nurminskaya M. Regulation of in vitro vascular calcification by BMP4, VEGF and Wnt3a. Calcif Tissue Int. 2007;81(5):372–81.
44. Yerram P, Chaudhary K. Calcific uremic arteriolopathy in end stage renal disease: pathophysiology and management. Ochsner J. 2014;14(3):380–5.
45. Schafer C, Heiss A, Schwarz A, Westenfeld R, Ketteler M, Floege J, et al. The serum protein alpha 2-Heremans-Schmid glycoprotein/fetuin-a is a systemically acting inhibitor of ectopic calcification. J Clin Investig. 2003;112(3):357–66.
46. Jeong HS, Dominguez AR. Calciphylaxis: controversies in pathogenesis, diagnosis and treatment. Am J Med Sci. 2016;351(2):217–27.
47. Wilmer WA, Magro CM. Calciphylaxis: emerging concepts in prevention, diagnosis, and treatment. Semin Dial. 2002;15(3):172–86.
48. Yu WY, Bhutani T, Kornik R, et al. Warfarin-associated nonuremic calciphylaxis. JAMA Dermatol. 2017;153:309–14.
49. Nigwekar SU, Bhan I, Turchin A, et al. Statin use and calcific uremic arteriolopathy: a matched case-control study. Am J Nephrol. 2013;37:325–32.
50. Storan ER, O'Gorman SM, Murphy A, Laing M. Case report of calciphylaxis secondary to calcium and vitamin D3 supplementation. J Cutan Med Surg. 2017;21:162–3.
51. Araki N, Misawa S, Shibuya K, et al. POEMS syndrome and calciphylaxis: an unrecognized cause of abnormal small vessel calcification. Orphanet J Rare Dis. 2016;11:35.
52. Monegal A, Peris P, Alsina M, et al. Development of multiorganic calciphylaxis during teriparatide, vitamin D, and calcium treatment. Osteoporos Int. 2016;27:2631–4.
53. Davis JM. The relationship between obesity and calciphylaxis: a review of the literature. Ostomy Wound Manage. 2016;62:12–8.
54. Nigwekar SU. An unusual case of nonhealing leg ulcer in a diabetic patient. Southern Med J. 2007;100:851–2.

55. Nigwekar SU, Bloch DB, Nazarian RM, et al. Vitamin K-dependent carboxylation of matrix gla protein influences the risk of calciphylaxis. J Am Soc Nephrol. 2017;28:1717.
56. Hafner J. Calciphylaxis and Martorell hypertensive ischemic leg ulcer: same pattern - one pathophysiology. Dermatology. 2016;232(5):523–33.
57. Ghosh T, Winchester DS, Davis MDP, El-Azhary R, Comfere NI. Early clinical presentations and progression of calciphylaxis. Int J Dermatol. 2017;56(8):856–61.
58. Weenig RH, Sewell LD, Davis MD, McCarthy JT, Pittelkow MR. Calciphylaxis: natural history, risk factor analysis, and outcome. J Am Acad Dermatol. 2007;56(4):569–79.
59. Handa SP, Strzelczak D. Uremic small artery disease: calciphylaxis with penis involvement. Clin Nephrol. 1998;50(4):258–61.
60. Barbera V, Di Lullo L, Gorini A, Otranto G, Floccari F, Malaguti M, et al. Penile calciphylaxis in end stage renal disease. Case Rep Urol. 2013;2013:968916, 1.
61. Kazanji N, Falatko J, Neupane S, Reddy G. Calciphylaxis presenting as digital ischemia. Intern Emerg Med. 2015;10(4):529–30.
62. Hafner J, Nobbe S, Partsch H, et al. Martorell hypertensive ischemic leg ulcer: a model of ischemic subcutaneous arteriolosclerosis. Arch Dermatol. 2010;146(9):961–8.
63. Schnier BR, Sheps SG, Juergens JL. Hypertensive ischemic ulcer. Am J Cardiol. 1966;17(4):560–5.
64. Polizzotto MN, Bryan T, Ashby MA, Martin P. Symptomatic management of calciphylaxis: a case series and review of the literature. J Pain Symptom Manag. 2006;32:186–90.
65. Gupta N, Haq KF, Mahajan S, et al. Gastrointestinal bleeding secondary to calciphylaxis. Am J Case Rep. 2015;16:818–22.
66. Brewster UC. Dermatological disease in patients with CKD. Am J Kidney Dis. 2008;51(2):331–44.
67. Dauden E, Onate MJ. Calciphylaxis. Dermatol Clin. 2008;26(4):557–68. ix
68. Brandenburg VM, Evenepoel P, Floege J, et al. Lack of evidence does not justify neglect: how can we address unmet medical needs in calciphylaxis? Nephrol Dial Transplant. 2016;31(8):1211–9.
69. Stavros K, Motiwala R, Zhou L, Sejdiu F, Shin S. Calciphylaxis in a dialysis patient diagnosed by muscle biopsy. J Clin Neuromuscul Dis. 2014;15(3):108–11.
70. Sreedhar A, Sheikh HA, Scagliotti CJ, Nair R. Advanced-stage calciphylaxis: think before you punch. Cleve Clin J Med. 2016;83(8):562–4.
71. Ha CT, Nousari HC. Surgical pearl: double-trephine punch biopsy technique for sampling subcutaneous tissue. J Am Acad Dermatol. 2003;48:609–10.
72. Fine A, Zacharias J. Calciphylaxis is usually non-ulcerating: risk factors, outcome and therapy. Kidney Int. 2002;61(6):2210–7.
73. Chang JJ. Calciphylaxis: diagnosis, pathogenesis, and treatment. Adv Skin Wound Care. 2019;32(5):205–15.
74. Burdorf BT. Calciphylaxis: the potential diagnostic role of radiologists. Radiol Case Rep. 2020;16(3):415–8.
75. Shmidt E, Murthy NS, Knudsen JM, Weenig RH, Jacobs MA, Starnes AM, et al. Net-like pattern of calcification on plain soft- tissue radiographs in patients with calciphylaxis. J Am Acad Dermatol. 2012;67(6):1296–301.
76. Han MM, Pang J, Shinkai K, Franc B, Hawkins R, Aparici CM. Calciphylaxis and bone scintigraphy: case report with histological confirmation and review of the literature. Ann Nucl Med. 2007;21(4):235–8.
77. Norris B, Vaysman V, Line BR. Bone scintigraphy of calciphylaxis: a syndrome of vascular calcification and skin necrosis. Clin Nucl Med. 2005;30(11):725–7.
78. Martineau P, Pelletier-Galarneau M, Bazarjani S. The role of bone scintigraphy with single-photon emission computed tomography-computed tomography in the diagnosis and evaluation of calciphylaxis. World J Nuclear Med. 2017;16(2):172–4.
79. Paul S, Rabito CA, Vedak P, Nigwekar SU, Kroshinsky D. The role of bone scintigraphy in the diagnosis of calciphylaxis. JAMA Dermatol. 2017;153(1):101–3.

80. Sowers KM, Hayden MR. Calcific uremic arteriolopathy: pathophysiology, reactive oxygen species and therapeutic approaches. Oxidative Med Cell Longev. 2010;3(2):109–21.
81. Dahl PR, Winkelmann RK, Connolly SM. The vascular calcification-cutaneous necrosis syndrome. J Am Acad Dermatol. 1995;33(1):53–8.
82. Magro CM, Simman R, Jackson S. Calciphylaxis: a review. J Am Coll Certif Wound Spec. 2010;2(4):66–72.
83. Essary LR, Wick MR. Cutaneous calciphylaxis. An underrecognized clinicopathologic entity. Am J Clin Pathol. 2000;113(2):280–7.
84. Zembowicz A, Navarro P, Walters S, Lyle SR, Moschella SL, Miller D. Subcutaneous thrombotic vasculopathy syndrome: an ominous condition reminiscent of calciphylaxis: calciphylaxis sine calcifications? Am J Dermatopathol. 2011;33(8):796–802.
85. Vedvyas C, Winterfield LS, Vleugels RA. Calciphylaxis: a systematic review of existing and emerging therapies. J Am Acad Dermatol. 2012;67(6):e253–60.
86. Erfurt-Berge C, Renner R. Management of patients with calciphylaxis: current perspectives. Chronic Wound Care Manag Res. 2019;6:109–15.
87. Sprague SM. Painful skin ulcers in a hemodialysis patient. Clin J Am Soc Nephrol. 2014;9:166–73.
88. Torregrosa JV, Sánchez-Escuredo A, Barros X, et al. Clinical management of calcific uremic arteriolopathy before and after therapeutic inclusion of bisphosphonates. Clin Nephrol. 2015;83(4):231–4.
89. Pasch A, Schaffner T, Huynh-Do U, Frey BM, Frey FJ, Farese S. Sodium thiosulfate prevents vascular calcifications in uremic rats. Kidney Int. 2008;74(11):1444–53.
90. Nigwekar SU, Brunelli SM, Meade D, Wang W, Hymes J, Lacson E Jr. Sodium thiosulfate therapy for calcific uremic arteriolopathy. Clin J Am Soc Nephrol. 2013;8:1162–70.
91. Baldwin C, Farah M, Leung M, et al. Multi-intervention management of calciphylaxis: a report of 7 cases. Am J Kidney Dis. 2011;58(6):988–91.
92. Martin R. Mysterious calciphylaxis: wounds with eschar—to debride or not to debride? Ostomy Wound Manage. 2004;50(4):64–6, 68–70; discussion 71.
93. Bechara FG, Altmeyer P, Kreuter A. Should we perform surgical debridement in calciphylaxis? Dermatol Surg. 2009;35(3):554–5.
94. Wollina U, Helm C, Hansel G, et al. Deep ulcer shaving combined with split-skin transplantation in distal calciphylaxis. Int J Lower Extremity Wounds. 2008;7(2):102–7.
95. Basile C, Montanaro A, Masi M, Pati G, De Maio P, Gismondi A. Hyperbaric oxygen therapy for calcific uremic arteriolopathy: a case series. J Nephrol. 2002;15(6):676–80.
96. Podymow T, Wherrett C, Burns KD. Hyperbaric oxygen in the treatment of calciphylaxis: a case series. Nephrol Dial Transplant. 2001;16(11):2176–80.
97. Cole W, Yoder CM, Coe S. The use of topical oxygen therapy to treat a Calciphylaxis wound during a global pandemic: a case report. Wounds. 2020;32(11):294–8.
98. Sayadi LR, Banyard DA, Ziegler ME, Obagi Z, Prussak J, Klopfer MJ, Evans GR, Widgerow AD. Topical oxygen therapy & micro/nanobubbles: a new modality for tissue oxygen delivery. Int Wound J. 2018;15(3):363–74.
99. Tittelbach J, Graefe T, Wollina U. Painful ulcers in calciphylaxis—combined treatment with maggot therapy and oral pentoxyfillin. J Dermatolog Treat. 2001;12(4):211–4.
100. Picazo M, Bover J, de la Fuente J, Sans R, Cuxart M, Matas M. Sterile maggots as adjuvant procedure for local treatment in a patient with proximal calciphylaxis. Nefrologia. 2005;25(5):559–62.
101. Davison SN. The prevalence and management of chronic pain in end-stage renal disease. J Palliat Med. 2007;10(6):1277–87.
102. Cleary JF. Incident pain. Palliat Med. 2005;19(1):1e2.14.
103. Good P, Tullio F, Jackson K, Goodchild C, Ashby M. Prospective audit of short term concurrent ketamine, opioid and anti-inflammatory ('triple-agent') therapy for episodes of acute on chronic pain. Intern Med J. 2005;35:39e44.
104. Dean M. Opioids in renal failure and dialysis patients. J Pain Symptom Manag. 2004;28(5):497–504.

105. Santos PW, He J, Tuffaha A, Wetmore JB. Clinical characteristics and risk factors associated with mortality in calcific uremic arteriolopathy. Int Urol Nephrol. 2017;49(12):2247–56.
106. JT MC, El-Azhary RA, Patzelt MT, et al. Survival, risk factors, and effect of treatment in 101 patients with calciphylaxis. Mayo Clin Proc. 2016;91:1384–94.
107. Riemer CA, El-Azhary RA, Wu KL, et al. Underreported use of palliative care and patient-reported outcome measures to address reduced quality of life in patients with calciphylaxis: a systematic review. Br J Dermatol. 2017;177:1510–8.
108. Lal G, Nowell AG, Liao J, Sugg SL, Weigel RJ, Howe JR. Determinants of survival in patients with calciphylaxis: a multi-variate analysis. Surgery. 2009;146(6):1028–34.

Unusual Ulcers of the Extremities: Cryofibrinogenemia and Cryoglobulinemia

9

M. Vautier and D. Saadoun

9.1 Plan

9.1.1 Introduction

Cryoproteins are blood protein that can be precipitated by cooling and redissolved by warming. We distinguish cryoglobulins that precipitate in serum's patient and cryofibrinogenemia that precipitate in plasma with cold (Table 9.1).

The prevalence of cryoglobulinemia vasculitis has been reported as approximately 10 per million inhabitants [1]. However, the prevalence and incidence of cryoglobulinemia vasculitis is difficult to estimate because of the numerous cause and clinical presentation.

Cryofibrinogenemia represents 10% of cryoproteins. Essential cryofibrinogenemia is rare but its prevalence remains unknown. A study in 36,000 hospitalized patients reported a prevalence of 3.4% of cryofibrinogenemia [2]. In a recent study, among 2312 cryofibrinogenemia requests between 1996 and 2006, 515 were positive, of which 455 (88.3%) were associated with cryoglobulin. Sixty patients (11.7%) had isolated cryofibrinogenemia and 36 (7%) had essential cryofibrinogenemia [3].

The main clinical presentation of cryoproteins includes skin involvement with often difficult to treat ulcers.

M. Vautier · D. Saadoun (✉)
Department of Internal Medicine and Clinical Immunology, Sorbonne Universités, AP-HP, Groupe Hospitalier Pitié-Salpêtrière, Paris, France
e-mail: david.saadoun@aphp.fr

A. K. Khanna, S. K. Tiwary (eds.), *Uncommon Ulcers of the Extremities*, https://doi.org/10.1007/978-981-99-1782-2_9

Table 9.1 Differences according to cryoprecipitate type

	Type I cryoglobulin	Mixed (type II/III) cryoglobulin	Cryofibrinogenemia
Mechanism	Occlusion of the capillary lumen Vasculitis is uncommon	Small-vessel vasculitis++ Occlusion of the capillary lumen is less common	Thrombotic occlusions in small and medium vessel
Clinical manifestations	Skin necrosis, distal ischemia+++	Purpura, arthralgia, glomerulonephritis, peripheral neuropathy	Purpura, ulceration, gangrene, and ischemic necrosis Arterial and venous thrombotic events
Cold-induced symptoms	+++	+/−	+++
Laboratory tests	RF activity is rare Hypocomplementemia is inconsistent	RF activity C4 consumption	0
Cryoprecipitate	Monoclonal IgM > IgG > IgA	Polyclonal immunoglobulins with or without monoclonal IgM+++ (kappa » lambda)	Fibrinogen, fibrin, fibronectin, factor VIII

RF rheumatoid factor, *Ig* immunoglobulin, *C4* complement component 4

9.1.2 Cryoprotein and Classifications

Cryofibrinogenemia is a cryoprotein originally characterized in 1955 by Korst and Kratochvil [4] and defined by the presence of cold precipitable proteins in the plasma. The cryoprecipitate is made of fibrinogen, fibrin, fibronectin, factor VIII, and smaller amounts of various plasma proteins [5]. Cryofibrinogenemia is able to precipitate in cooled plasma (4 °C) and to redissolve after increasing the sample temperature (37 °C). The cooled temperature-induced precipitation of proteins in plasma, but not in serum, allows the distinction between cryofibrinogenemia and cryoglobulinemia. Cryofibrinogenemia can be classified as 2 types: a primary (essential) or a secondary form [6]. Thus, cryofibrinogenemia is potentially associated with a variety of diseases, such as autoimmune disorders, malignancy, cardiovascular thrombosis, and active sepsis.

Cryoglobulinemia is defined as the persistent presence of abnormal immunoglobulins (Ig) in the serum that precipitate when cold and re-solubilize when warm. We distinguish 3 types of cryoglobulinemia [7], according to components:

- Type I cryoglobulinemia is composed of a single monoclonal immunoglobulin, most often IgM or IgG.
- Type II cryoglobulinemia is composed of polyclonal immunoglobulins that are associated with one or more monoclonal components, thus forming an immune

complex. Most often, the monoclonal Ig is IgM associated with polyclonal IgG (mixed monoclonal cryoglobulinemia).

- Type III cryoglobulinemia is composed only of polyclonal immunoglobins and may be composed of a combination of polyclonal IgM and IgG (mixed polyclonal cryoglobulinemia).

This immunochemical classification is used to assist in the diagnosis (etiology of cryoglobulin) and treatment. Type I cryoglobulinemia (10–15% of symptomatic vasculitides) is often associated with a hematological disease (MGUS, myeloma, or B lymphoma). Mixed cryoglobulinemia (80–85%) is associated with infectious diseases (especially chronic hepatitis C infection), B lymphoid hemopathies, but also autoimmune diseases (Sjögren's syndrome, lupus). For some mixed cryoglobulinemias, no cause is found and the cryoglobulinemia is said to be "essential" (15%).

9.1.3 Physiopathology

9.1.3.1 Cryofibrinogenemia

We have demonstrated significant abnormalities of fibrinolysis in essential cryofibrinogenemia [3]. We observed a significant increase in fibrinolysis inhibitors (PAI-1, 2-macroglobulin) at diagnosis as well as lysis time of euglobulins [3]. The 1-antitrypsin present in the plasma of patients with cryofibrinogenemia is also an inhibitor of fibrinolysis (via its inhibitory action on plasmin) [2, 8]. These abnormalities could allow accumulation of cryofibrinogenemia and deposition with thrombin leading to thrombotic occlusions in small and medium vessel. Under antifibrinolytic treatment, these abnormalities of fibrinolysis regressed in parallel with the disappearance of cryofibrinogenemia and clinical recovery [3]. These thrombotic phenomena can lead to distal ischemic lesions and even to the development of gangrene [2, 9].

9.1.3.2 Cryoglobulin

The mechanism of cryoprecipitation is not well known. It depends on many parameters such as Ig concentration, pH, ionic strength, temperature, but also on the electrical charge directly related to the amino acid sequences and carbohydrate components of the immunoglobulin. Ischemic lesions may be related to vascular obstruction by cryoglobulin precipitation, mainly in type 1 cryoglobulins. Mixed cryoglobulinemias are responsible for true immune complex vasculitides. The parameters that explain the presence of symptomatic vasculitis in only some patients are not fully understood. Some recent studies highlight the importance of the physicochemical properties (stereotactic properties, glycosylation of heavy chains, etc.) of immunoglobulins in the genesis of lesions. Indeed, the different types of Ig have, according to their physicochemical properties, a more or less important propensity to form immune complexes (different solubility, variable rigidity, and possibility of cleavage of certain immunoglobulins limiting the formation of voluminous immune complexes), to precipitate and to induce an inflammatory response (recruitment of the complement and the Fc receptor of the macrophages).

9.1.4 Clinical Manifestation

9.1.4.1 Cryofibrinogenemia (Fig. 9.1)

There appeared to be a female predominance with a sex ratio of 1.6. The average age at diagnosis is 50–60 years. The skin is the most common target organ, inaugural of cryofibrinogenemia in over 80% of cases. Cutaneous manifestations are variable, including cold sensitivity, purpura, livedo reticularis, and Raynaud's phenomenon. In more severe clinical forms, ulceration, gangrene, and ischemic necrosis are described. These lesions typically appear at the distal extremities with lower temperature: buttocks, hands, feet, ears, and nose.

Arterial or venous thrombotic events occurred in 20–40% of cases and appear to be correlated with cryofibrinogenemia levels. Arterial thrombosis most often affect small and medium-sized arteries. Rare cases of cerebral, myocardial, mesenteric, or retinal thrombosis have been reported [6].

9.1.4.2 Cryoglobulinemia (Figs. 9.2 and 9.3)

Vascular purpura is often the inaugural manifestation. The lower limbs are affected first but the lesions may then extend to the abdomen. The purpura follows an intermittent relapsing course. The lesions are infiltrated by non-pruriginous petechiae or papules. Necrosis may develop, notably in patients with type I cryoglobulinemia. Distal necrosis at the upper or lower limbs is also most common in type I cryoglobulinemia. Cold-induced symptoms such as Raynaud's phenomenon occur in 25% of patients overall, with higher rates in patients who have type I cryoglobulinemia. Cold urticaria is a chronic systemic non-pruriginous urticarial rash with plaques that remain unchanged for more than 24 h. The trigger is exposure to cold. The rash can be induced by placing an ice cube on the forearm.

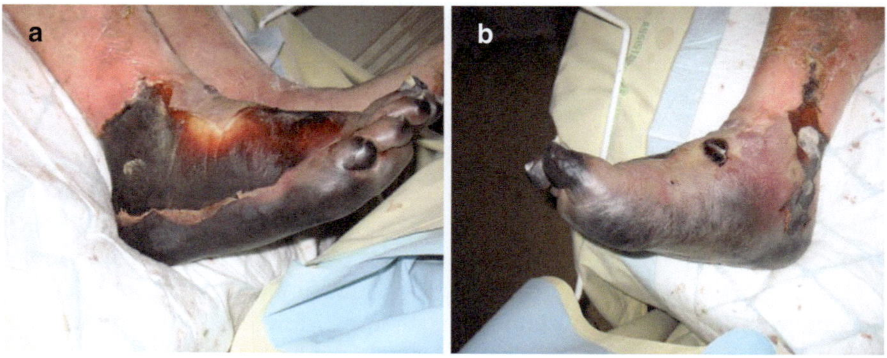

Fig. 9.1 (**a** and **b**) are examples of severe cryofibrinogenemia

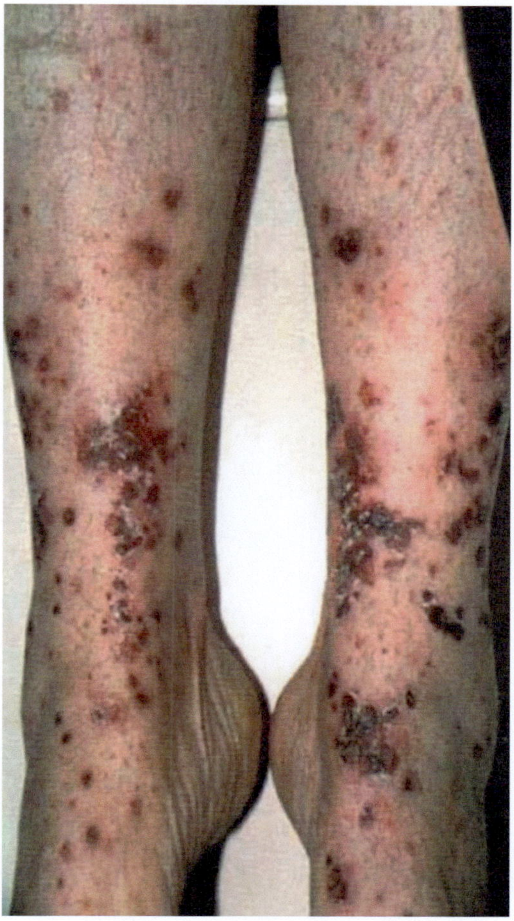

Fig. 9.2 Vascular purpura of the lower limbs during an outbreak of mixed cryoglobulinemic vasculitis

The joint manifestations (50%–75%) often consist of non-migratory pain that predominantly involves the hands and knees; the elbows and ankles are less often affected.

Renal involvement is usually a late manifestation. Proteinuria and microscopic hematuria are the main manifestations, although renal failure may develop. The renal biopsy evidences diffuse global membranoproliferative glomerulonephritis with mesangial proliferation, which may have a nodular appearance. Extra-capillary proliferation may be present. Immunofluorescence shows subendothelial and intraluminal deposits of immunoglobulins identical to those present in the cryoprecipitate; C3 is found only in the subendothelial deposits.

The peripheral nervous system is the main target of neurological involvement. Distal sensory or sensorimotor polyneuropathy predominating at the lower limbs occurs in two-thirds of patients and mononeuritis multiplex in one-third of patients. Common inaugural symptoms include neuropathic pain and paresthesia. Motor loss

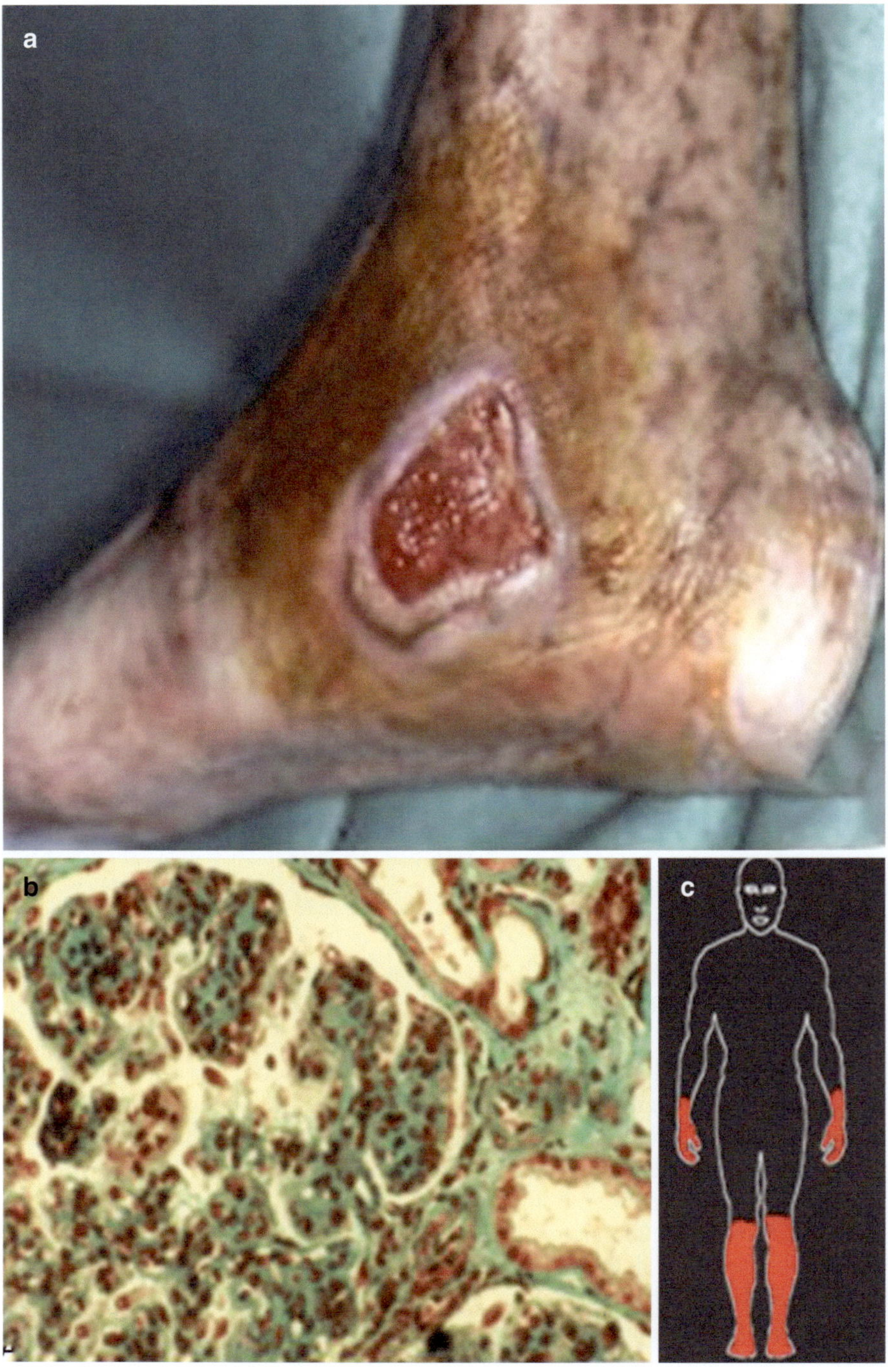

Fig. 9.3 Clinical manifestations of cryoglobulinemic vasculitis. (**a**) severe skin ulcer; (**b**) renal biopsy showing membranoproliferative glomerulonephritis; (**c**) distribution of the peripheral neurological involvement indicating length dependency

is less common, delayed by a few months to a few years, and sets in gradually; the anterolateral leg compartments are preferentially affected, often asymmetrically.

Gastrointestinal manifestations, due to distal vasculitis involving the mesenteric arterioles and capillaries, include abdominal pain, gastrointestinal tract bleeding, or perforation. Rarely, cryoglobulinemia may involve the central nervous system (acute or subacute neurological deficits, headaches, seizures, cranial nerve impairments…) and heart (acute pericarditis, heart failure). Lung disease is extremely rare. Bronchiolitis obliterans organizing pneumonia and alveolar hemorrhage syndromes are probably due to vasculitis.

9.1.5 Diagnosis

In practice, the search for cryofibrinogenemia should not be dissociated from that of cryoglobulinemia (Fig. 9.4). Thus, two samples are necessary: one on a dry tube (for the search for cryoglobulin) and the other on an anticoagulant (for the search for cryofibrinogenemia). The choice of anticoagulant is crucial. Indeed, fibrinogen is one of the least soluble and most easily precipitated plasma proteins, particularly in the presence of heparin. The blood sample should therefore be collected in tubes containing oxalate, citrate, or ethylene diamine tetraacetic acid (EDTA). Tubes containing heparin should not be used due to the risk of false-positive results due to the formation of cryoprecipitates known as the "heparin-precipitable fraction." Cryofibrinogenemia testing should be performed in specialized laboratories. It is detected by cooling the plasma to +4 °C for 24 to 72 h.

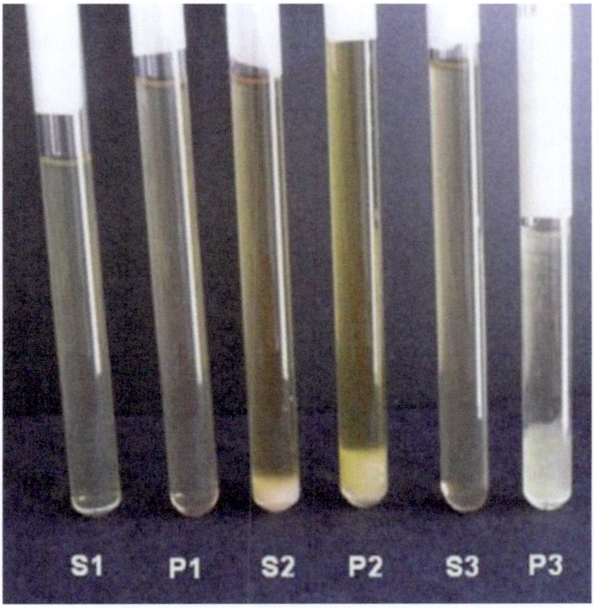

Fig. 9.4 Detection of cryofibrinogenemia. Patient 1: absence of cryoprecipitate in serum (S1) and plasma (P1). Patient 2: Cryoprecipitate present in serum (S2) and plasma (P2), corresponding to the concomitant presence of cryoglobulin and cryofibrinogen. Patient 3: absence of cryoprecipitate in serum (S3) but presence of cryoprecipitate in plasma (P3), corresponding to cryofibrinogen

It appears as a gel or flaky precipitate, which dissolves on heating to 37 °C, but reappears when cold. This reversible transformation by simple heating differs from that undergone by fibrinogen under the action of thrombin. The use of a protease inhibitor is not recommended [5]. If the sample is not centrifuged immediately it should be stored at 37 °C to prevent self-adsorption of cryofibrinogen onto red blood cells in cold. Compliance with strict rules for collection, transportation, coagulation, and centrifugation at 37 °C is essential. If the result is positive, the cryoprecipitate is then purified by a succession of washing and centrifugation at +4 °C. The immunochemical analysis of the cryoprecipitate can be performed either by immunofixation or by immunoblotting using anti-fibrinogen monospecific antisera. This identification is performed at 37 °C after solubilization of the cryoprecipitate at 37 °C. As with cryoglobulins, cryofibrinogen assay techniques are not very precise. The assay can be performed by the cryocrit technique, by differential determination of fibrinogen before and after cryoprecipitation, or by measuring the absorbance of the aromatic rings at 280 nm from purified cryoprecipitate. All of these methods lack precision, so that only rate variations of 30–50% are interpretable for monitoring a patient. Elevated serum levels of α1-antitrypsin, α2-macroglobulin, and inhibitors of fibrinolysis may also be observed [2, 3, 5]. Unlike cryoglobulinemia, there is no decrease in the C4 fraction of complement.

Several precautions are important to avoid false-negative results from cryoglobulin detection tests. To avoid premature cryoprecipitation, the blood sample must be kept at 37° during transport to the laboratory then during centrifugation. Cryoglobulins precipitate below 37 °C. After centrifugation, the serum sample is stored at 4 °C for 8 days to ensure the detection of delayed cryoprecipitation. The cryoprecipitate is dissolved by increasing the temperature. After purification, immunoelectrophoresis is performed to identify the type of cryoglobulin as I, II, or III, as described above. The cryoprecipitate is quantified using immunofixation or western blotting. After lengthy debates, it was determined that a concentration above 50 mg/L is considered abnormal. Cryoglobulin detection can be technically difficult due to the considerable thermal instability of cryoglobulins, which precipitate readily if the temperature of the blood sample falls below 37 °C before processing at the laboratory (Fig. 9.5). Consequently, evaluation for other laboratory features that suggest cryoglobulinemia is important. Although inconsistently present, several complement abnormalities are fairly specific, such as decreases in early components (C1q, C2, and C4) and in CH50 and increased levels of the late components (C5 and C9) and of C1 inhibitor; the C3 level is usually normal. Rheumatoid factor activity is common in mixed cryoglobulinemia but is rarely found in type I cryoglobulinemia.

9.1.6 Differential Diagnosis

Patients with skin ulcers or gangrene have a limited number of differential diagnoses including cryoglobulinemia and cryofibrinogenemia. Other causes of thrombotic occlusion of small and medium arteries should be searched. Cryoglobulinemia

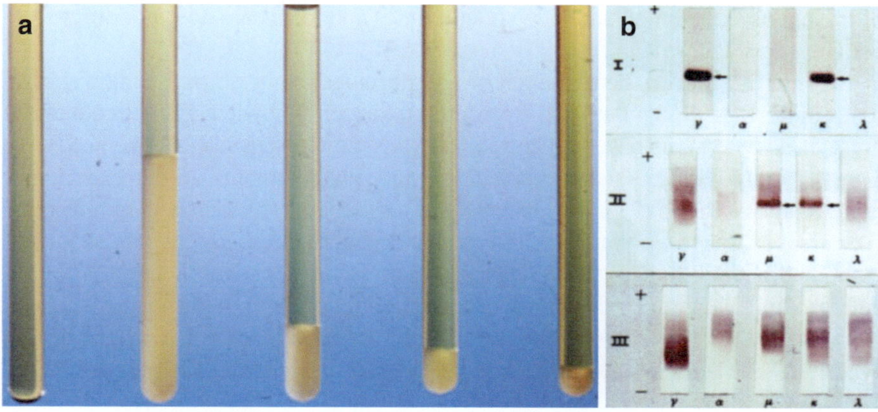

Fig. 9.5 Biological detection of cryoglobulin. (**a**) Detection of a cryoglobulin. One negative control tube on the left and four positive tubes on the right with an increasing concentration of yellowish cryoprecipitate at the bottom of the tube. (**b**) Immunochemical typing of cryoglobulins by immunoblot (types I, II, or III)

and cryofibrinogenemia must be distinguished from other causes of vasculopathy of small and medium vessels such as embolic arterial disease (endocarditis, emboli cholesterol), thrombotic microangiopathies, antiphospholipid syndrome, disseminated intravascular coagulation, vasculitis, and atheromatous septic or thrombotic peripheral arterial disease linked to a genetic hypercoagulable state.

Cryocrystalglobulinemia is an occlusive vasculopathy involving type 1 cryoglobulinemia classically associated with an underlying paraproteinemia. Diagnosis is histological with eosinophilic extracellular crystals, periodic acid–Schiff positive, and nonbirefringence under polarized light.

9.1.7 Prognosis and Treatment

9.1.7.1 Cryofibrinogenemia

Prognosis

With treatment, complete remission is observed in almost 80% of patients with essential cryofibrinogenemia [3]. However, relapse occurred in 40% of patient after a median time of 9 months (range 7–42 months) with the reappearance of purpura or arthralgia and detectable plasma cryofibrinogenemia. Complications of cryofibrinogenemia include gangrene potentially leading to leg amputation and septicemia. The main cause of death is infection [3, 10].

Treatment

Simple measures to avoid exposure to cold and to keep symptomatic patients in a warm environment should be implemented systematically. Symptomatic treatment of infectious skin complications with antibiotics and local care does not differ from the usual management.

Most of the data on the treatment of cryofibrinogenemia are from single clinical cases or small series of patients. According to current knowledge, the treatment of cryofibrinogenemia is based on antifibrinolytics, corticosteroids (prednisone 0.5 to 1 mg/kg daily with gradual decrease), and anti-platelet agents. In our experience, more than two-thirds (77%) of patients with essential cryofibrinogenemia respond (i.e., disappearance of symptoms and plasma cryofibrinogen) to oral corticosteroids combined with anti-aggregation (aspirin). In most cases, patients present with vascular purpura, superficial thrombosis, and inflammatory arthralgias. Anticoagulants are indicated in cases of associated venous thrombosis. However, a progression of symptoms has been reported with heparin [8] and anti-vitamin K drugs are inconsistently effective [3].

Fibrinolytics remain the cornerstone of treatment [3, 11]. In severe forms, low-dose intravenous fibrinolytics (alteplase 10 mg/24 h or streptokinase) are preferred to get through the initial phase. Then a relay with stanozolol (4 to 8 mg/day per os) can be used. Stanozolol is an androgenic steroid derived from testosterone which has profibrinolytic effects. However, its delay of action of several days limits its use in severe forms. Side effects such as hirsutism, fluid retention, acne, hepatic test disturbance, or hypertriglyceridemia may limit its prolonged use. We have shown by following a patient treated with fibrinolytics (alteplase 10 mg/24 h intravenous then stanozolol per os) for a severe form of essential cryofibrinogenemia that clinical recovery was associated with a disappearance of plasma cryofibrinogen and a normalization of fibrinolysis inhibitor levels (PAI-1, α2-macroglobulin) [3]. These data reinforce the rationale for the use of fibrinolytics in cryofibrinogenemia.

Immunosuppressants (especially azathioprine) may be beneficial, particularly in secondary forms (associated inflammatory disease) or in cases of severe extracutaneous involvement. By analogy with the treatment of cryoglobulinemia, some authors recommend use of plasmapheresis. However, there is not enough data in the literature to recommend this technique in cryofibrinogenemia [8, 12, 13].

9.1.7.2 Cryoglobulinemia

Prognosis

The course and outcome of cryoglobulinemia varies considerably across individuals. The prognosis depends chiefly on the severity of the organ involvement and more specifically of the renal, gastrointestinal, cardiac, and/or central nervous system manifestations. An underlying hematological malignancy is also a major prognostic factor.

In a retrospective study of 242 patients with non-infectious symptomatic mixed cryoglobulinemia, compared to the type III subgroup, the type II subgroup was characterized by higher prevalence of purpura, renal involvement, and peripheral neurological involvement; higher cryoglobulin concentrations; and lower C3 and C4 concentrations [14]. Among the manifestations of cryoglobulinemic vasculitis, the gastrointestinal and myocardial involvements lead to the highest risk of death.

Prognostic factors in early case series studies included age older than 65 years and renal involvement. In keeping with these data, a more recent study of non-infectious mixed cryoglobulinemic vasculitis found poorer outcomes in patients with pulmonary involvement, gastrointestinal involvement, a creatinine clearance below 60 mL/min, and age older than 65 years [14]. Survival rates after 1, 2, 5, and 10 years were 91%, 89%, 79%, and 65%, respectively.

The main causes of death in patients with HCV-related cryoglobulinemic vasculitis are infections related to immunosuppressive therapy, liver cirrhosis, cardiovascular involvement, and severe renal dysfunction. The main adverse prognostic factors reported to date are severe hepatic fibrosis (METAVIR Score $\geq$ 3) and involvement of the central nervous system, kidneys, or heart.

Type I Cryoglobulinemia

In patients with symptomatic cryoglobulinemia type I, the treatment strategy focuses on the underlying hematological malignancy. Thus, lymphoma requires combination chemotherapy and myeloma treatment with drugs such as bortezomib, thalidomide, lenalidomide, or alkylating agents [15]. Autologous bone marrow transplantation may be in order in myeloma-related cryoglobulinemia. IgG MGUS, which indicates plasma cell proliferation, is treated with those myeloma drugs that target the plasma cells, whereas rituximab is generally preferred for IgM MGUS, which indicates lymphoplasmacytic proliferation [16]. Plasma exchange therapy is warranted in selected patients with severe renal involvement or extensive leg necrosis [17]. Exposure to low temperatures exacerbates cryoglobulin formation and should therefore be avoided [17, 18].

Type II and III Cryoglobulinemia

HCV-related cryoglobulinemia vasculitis: Sustained suppression of HCV replication is associated with a significantly higher rate of complete clinical remission in patients with cryoglobulinemia vasculitis [19]. The introduction of direct-acting antivirals has radically transformed the management of HCV-related cryoglobulinemic vasculitis [20]. Direct-acting antivirals should be viewed as first-line treatments in patients with HCV-related cryoglobulinemic vasculitis. Selection of the antiviral combination is guided by the clinical manifestations of vasculitis, HCV genotype, and severity of fibrosis. Despite the marked efficacy of antivirals on the symptoms of HCV-related cryoglobulinemic vasculitis, immunosuppressive drugs remain a valid option in selected patients. Immunosuppressant therapy is indispensable in patients with severe vasculitis manifestations such as severe kidney dysfunction, skin necrosis, and/or involvement of the gastrointestinal tract or central nervous system. Rituximab targets the clonal B-cell population upstream from cryoglobulin production [21, 22]. Rituximab has demonstrated greater efficacy than conventional immunosuppressants or placebo therapy. In earlier studies, adding rituximab to Peg-IFN and ribavirin shortened the time to clinical remission and increased the renal response and cryoglobulin clearance rates. Plasma exchange is indicated in patients with refractory disease and/or severe organ involvement (rapidly progressive glomerulonephritis, gastrointestinal vasculitis, severe mononeuritis multiplex, or myocarditis) and/or severe cutaneous involvement (extensive ulcers, distal ischemia). Intravenous methylprednisolone and immunosuppressants, notably cyclophosphamide, also deserve consideration in these very severe forms.

Cryoglobulinemic vasculitis unrelated to HCV: Treatment at the case is the main focus in patients with symptomatic mixed cryoglobulinemia unrelated to the HCV. Infection should be managed with appropriate anti-infectious agents. Rituximab combined with glucocorticoid therapy is the first-line treatment in the event of autoimmune disease [14, 23]. Plasma exchange therapy may deserve consideration in patients at the severe end of the clinical spectrum.

References

1. Gorevic PD, Kassab HJ, Levo Y, Kohn R, Meltzer M, Prose P, et al. Mixed cryoglobulinemia: clinical aspects and long-term follow-up of 40 patients. Am J Med. 1980;69(2):287–308.
2. Smith SB, Arkin C. Cryofibrinogenemia: incidence, clinical correlations, and a review of the literature. Am J Clin Pathol. 1972;58(5):524–30.
3. Saadoun D, Elalamy I, Ghillani-Dalbin P, Sene D, Delluc A, Cacoub P. Cryofibrinogenemia: new insights into clinical and pathogenic features. Am J Med. 2009;122(12):1128–35.
4. Korst DR, Kratochvil CH. Cryofibrinogen in a case of lung neoplasm associated with thrombophlebitis migrans. Blood. 1955;10(9):945–53.
5. Stathakis NE, Karamanolis D, Koukoulis G, Tsianos E. Characterization of cryofibrinogen isolated from patients plasma. Haemostasis. 1981;10(4):195–202.
6. Amdo TD, Welker JA. An approach to the diagnosis and treatment of cryofibrinogenemia. Am J Med. 2004;116(5):332–7.
7. Brouet JC, Clauvel JP, Danon F, Klein M, Seligmann M. Biologic and clinical significance of cryoglobulins. A report of 86 cases. Am J Med. 1974;57(5):775–88.
8. Blain H, Cacoub P, Musset L, Costedoat-Chalumeau N, Silberstein C, Chosidow O, et al. Cryofibrinogenaemia: a study of 49 patients. Clin Exp Immunol. 2000;120(2):253–60.
9. Kalbfleisch JM, Bird RM. Cryofibrinogenemia. N Engl J Med. 1960;263:881–6.
10. Belizna CC, Tron F, Joly P, Godin M, Hamidou M, Lévesque H. Outcome of essential cryofibrinogenaemia in a series of 61 patients. Rheumatology (Oxford). 2008;47(2):205–7.
11. Rachmilewitz EA, Sacks MI, Zlotnick A. Essential cryofibrinogenemia. Clinical, pathological and immunological studies. Isr J Med Sci. 1970;6(1):32–43.
12. Euler HH, Zeuner RA, Béress R, Gutschmidt HJ, Christophers E, Schroeder JO. Monoclonal cryo-antifibrinogenemia. Arthritis Rheum. 1996;39(6):1066–9.
13. Copeman PW. Cryofibrinogenaemia and skin ulcers: treatment with plasmapheresis. Br J Dermatol. 1979;101(Suppl 17):57–8.
14. Terrier B, Krastinova E, Marie I, Launay D, Lacraz A, Belenotti P, et al. Management of noninfectious mixed cryoglobulinemia vasculitis: data from 242 cases included in the CryoVas survey. Blood. 2012;119(25):5996–6004.
15. Terrier B, Karras A, Kahn J-E, Le Guenno G, Marie I, Benarous L, et al. The Spectrum of type I Cryoglobulinemia vasculitis: new insights based on 64 cases. Medicine. 2013;92(2):61–8.
16. Fermand J-P, Bridoux F, Kyle RA, Kastritis E, Weiss BM, Cook MA, et al. How I treat monoclonal gammopathy of renal significance (MGRS). Blood. 2013;122(22):3583–90.
17. Harel S, Mohr M, Jahn I, Aucouturier F, Galicier L, Asli B, et al. Clinico-biological characteristics and treatment of type I monoclonal cryoglobulinaemia: a study of 64 cases. Br J Haematol. 2015;168(5):671–8.
18. Sidana S, Rajkumar SV, Dispenzieri A, Lacy MQ, Gertz MA, Buadi FK, et al. Clinical presentation and outcomes of patients with type 1 monoclonal cryoglobulinemia. Am J Hematol. 2017;92(7):668–73.

19. Cacoub P, Desbois AC, Comarmond C, Saadoun D. Impact of sustained virological response on the extrahepatic manifestations of chronic hepatitis C: a meta-analysis. Gut. 2018;67(11):2025–34.
20. Cacoub P, Vautier M, Desbois AC, Lafuma A, Saadoun D. Effectiveness and cost of hepatitis C virus cryoglobulinaemia vasculitis treatment: from interferon-based to direct-acting antivirals era. Liver Int. 2017;37(12):1805–13.
21. Cacoub P, Delluc A, Saadoun D, Landau DA, Sene D. Anti-CD20 monoclonal antibody (rituximab) treatment for cryoglobulinemic vasculitis: where do we stand? Ann Rheum Dis. 2008;67(3):283–7.
22. Saadoun D, Resche Rigon M, Sene D, Terrier B, Karras A, Perard L, et al. Rituximab plus peg-interferon-alpha/ribavirin compared with peg-interferon-alpha/ribavirin in hepatitis C-related mixed cryoglobulinemia. Blood. 2010;116(3):326–34; quiz 504–5.
23. Terrier B, Marie I, Launay D, Lacraz A, Belenotti P, de Saint-Martin L, et al. Predictors of early relapse in patients with non-infectious mixed cryoglobulinemia vasculitis: results from the French nationwide CryoVas survey. Autoimmun Rev. 2014;13(6):630–4.

Buruli Ulcer

10

Adriana Lozano-Platonoff and Teresa Alonso-León

10.1 Introduction

Buruli ulcer (BU), caused by *Mycobacterium ulcerans*, is a necrotizing cutaneous infection, causing a chronic debilitating disease that affects mainly the skin and sometimes bone.

BU is the third most common mycobacterial infection and is considered an emerging infection caused by *Mycobacterium ulcerans* [1].

BU affects predominantly the lower extremities and is presented as painless, necrotizing skin lesions.

The pathogenesis of the ulcers is mediated by mycolactone, a unique toxin secreted by *M. ulcerans*.

Early diagnosis and treatment are crucial to minimize morbidity and disability.

BU is one of the 19 neglected tropical diseases addressed by the World Health Organization (WHO) in its "Global plan to combat neglected tropical diseases 2008–2015" [2].

10.2 History

The first cases described in the literature are from the 1930s, in Australia [3].

A. Lozano-Platonoff (✉)
Division of Dermatology, Wound and Ostomy Care Center, Hospital General "Dr. Manuel Gea González", Mexico City, Mexico

T. Alonso-León
Division of Dermatology, Hospital General "Dr. Manuel Gea González", Mexico City, Mexico

A. K. Khanna, S. K. Tiwary (eds.), *Uncommon Ulcers of the Extremities*, https://doi.org/10.1007/978-981-99-1782-2_10

In 1897, Albert Cook, a medical missionary who worked in Uganda, was the first who described a progressively destructive skin disease [4]. In 1947, *Mycobacterium ulcerans* was identified as the cause of Buruli Ulcer by P. Mac Callum (BU) [3, 5].

The first study was *held* in Northwestern Uganda by Lunn et al., who proposed that contact with water was important but could not isolate the organism from water or any aquatic animal [4].

In 1962, the disease was named Buruli Ulcer by Dodge and Lunn, after Buruli County, Uganda, where a large number of cases were *reported* in the 1960s [1, 2, 6].

Mycobacteria are aerobic rod-shaped bacteria that do not form spores and that are lipid rich with long-chain mycolic acids in their cell walls, which are largely responsible for their acid fastness [3].

10.3 Epidemiology

Tuberculosis and leprosy are the most common mycobacterial infections in humans, followed by BU [1].

In 1998, the World Health Organization (WHO) recognized BU as a reemerging infectious disease in West and Central Africa, with important public health impact [5].

Tuberculosis and leprosy nearly always involve human-to-human transmission or other animal-to-host transmission, but on the other hand, BU is almost always associated with an environmental source [4].

BU is a mycobacterial disease identified predominantly in rural tropical areas, especially those with wetlands (ponds, swamps, marshes, slow-moving rivers, flooding zones). The most possible mode of transmission is local skin trauma that allows inoculation of *M. ulcerans* [1, 3].

According to WHO, BU has been reported in 33 countries in Africa, America, Asia, and Western Pacific. Africa appears to be the worst affected region, followed by Australia, French Guyana, Peru, and, in recent years, Japan [2], Tourism is also responsible for the increase in recent years, because a brief contact may be sufficient to become infected [2]. A great number of cases have been documented in international travelers from nonendemic areas such as Europe or North America [6].

The rapid reemergence of BU in the early 1980s may be attributable to environmental alterations such as deforestation and global warming that change global temperature and precipitation patterns, beyond others [1].

According to the last data published by the World Health Organization (May 2021), the annual number of suspected BU cases reported globally decreased from around 5000 until 2010 to 1961 cases per year in 2016, but then started to rise again, reporting 2271 cases in 2019.

BU affects people of all ages, but it depends also on the geographical regions; in general children (5–15 years old) are the group with the highest incidence of BU (75%) [1]. Among those affected in Africa 48% are <15 years, and in Australia only 10% are <15 years [2].

In Africa, BU is more *prevalent* in men (52%), but in Japan it is more frequent in women (66%) [2].

Those who suffered from this condition usually live in remote rural areas, where there is limited access to health services. This is the reason that BU is considered a neglected tropical disease [4].

Up to 60% of patients with BU suffer a degree of sequelae with disability, scarring, contractures, or bone destruction [1].

10.4 Microbiology of *M. ulcerans*

M. ulcerans is a gram-positive bacillus and a slowly growing mycobacterium. The incubation period is 5 to 8 weeks, but can be as long as 6 months [3].

M. ulcerans grows at a temperature between 29 and 33 °C and needs a low (2.5%) oxygen concentration. It may be cultured in Löwenstein-Jensen media; colonies are yellowish, rough, and distinct from one another [3].

The organism produces a unique toxin—mycolactone—which causes tissue damage and inhibits the immune response [2].

The exact mode of transmission remains unclear [5].

10.5 Physiopathology

The pathogenesis of cutaneous mycobacterial infections is the result of the interaction between the pathogen and humans, with the subsequent hematogenous dissemination or local spread from another site/infection, or direct inoculation to the skin. In *M. ulcerans,* transmission may possibly be vector-borne or through environmental exposures [3].

The exact mode of transmission remains unclear, but it *is likely* to occur when a host interacts with contaminated water, particularly stagnant water, and suffers insect bites, puncturing injuries, or skin trauma [3]. In Australia, some investigators propose that BU is a zoonosis transmitted by mosquitoes such as *Aedes camptorhynchus* and aquatic organisms in West Africa like *Naucoridae*; however it is unknown if their bodies act as reservoirs [1].

M. ulcerans produces a necrotizing, immunosuppressive macrolide toxin (polyketide)—mycolactone. There are SigA-like gene promoters, involved in the virulence, that encode for the synthesis of mycolactone [1].

Mycolactone causes significant tissue destruction and necrosis, particularly in subcutaneous fat [6]. The toxin also produces immunosuppression, by suppressing innate and adaptive cell-mediated immunity. It Inhibits macrophages, monocytes, B cells, and T cells, thereby inhibiting interleukin production. The toxin also induces hypoesthesia, by altering angiotensin II receptors pathways, causing an hyperpolarization of neurons [1, 3].

10.6 Clinical Feature

Buruli ulcers can appear everywhere, but they are more common in lower extremities (>55%), following upper extremities (35%), or other body parts, predominantly [3].

Its wide morphology is described. The ulcers can be first described as "pre-ulcerative lesions" or the "active form," characterized as painless nodules, as large, indurated plaques, or as diffuse painless swellings, like edema [7]. The disease progresses without pain and fever, leading to necrosis, and after 4 weeks, the first lesion evolves into an ulcer with a cotton wool-like appearance, undermined borders, and spreading laterally [3, 7]. The underlying bone is affected, leading to variable deformities [2]. The inactive form is characterized by scars with or without sequelae [7].

M. ulcerans induces painless skin necrosis, secondary to mycolactone and its role in analgesia [5] (Fig. 10.1).

Buruli ulcers can be divided into three categories depending on the degree of cutaneous involvement, and therefore severity [3].

Stage 1: Single small lesion, <5 cm in diameter (32%).
Stage 2: Nonulcerative or ulcerative plaques and edematous forms, 5–15 cm (35%).
Stage 3: Severe disease, with dissemination: osteitis, osteomyelitis, or joint involvement (33%).
- 3a: Single lesion, >15 cm in diameter, without osteomyelitis.
- 3b: Lesion(s) at critical sites: eye, breast, genitalia.
- 3c: Small multiple lesions.

If the patient does not receive treatment, the toxin persists, causing extensive, deep ulcerations, developing scarring contractures, deformity, osteonecrosis, and finally limb loss [3].

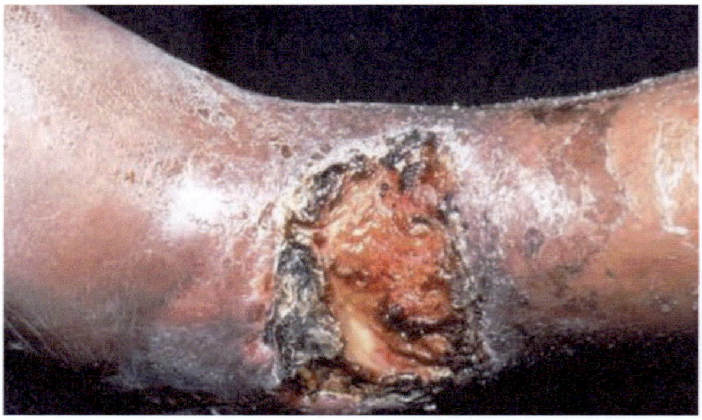

Fig. 10.1 Buruli ulcer. Localized in left ankle, painless ulcer with necrotic borders. Important swelling and edema around the ulcer. (Photo kindly provided by Dr. Roberto Arenas Guzman)

10.7 Diagnosis

With experienced health professionals, the diagnosis is mostly clinical, based on age and geographic area, but training is essential [3].

The clinical diagnosis of BUs can be confirmed by four standard laboratory methods: direct microscopy of the lesion, histopathology, culture, and molecular detection methods (PCR IS2404) [3].

The real-time polymerase chain reaction (PCR) techniques to identify the agent detect two sequences insertions characteristic of *M. ulcerans*: IS2404 and IS2606. PCR is only available in research laboratories and is considered the gold standard to confirm the diagnosis [5].

In high endemicity areas, a rapid diagnostic test to detect mycolactone is being developed.

10.8 Differential Diagnosis

The diagnosis of mycobacterial infections of the skin has a broad spectrum of clinical presentations, so having into account differential diagnosis when a BU is suspected is important.

The most important differential diagnoses are: tropical ulcers, cutaneous tuberculosis, vascular ulceration (venous or arterial), diabetic foot ulcerations, pyoderma gangrenosum, cutaneous leishmaniasis, fungal infections, lipomas, ganglions, lymph node tuberculosis, onchocerciasis nodules, cellulitis (the lesions are painful, and the patient is ill).

HIV infection increases the risk of BU and complicates and changes the typical clinical progression, with a more aggressive progression and poor treatment outcomes [2].

10.9 Treatment

Early diagnosis and treatment are important to minimize morbidity and progression of the clinical stages.

Historically the treatment of BU was surgical excision of the affected area, correction of wound defects, and rehabilitation physiotherapy.

Nowadays the treatment of BU is based on a combination of antimycobacterial drugs and supportive treatments like wound care, surgery including skin grafting, and heat therapy.

The antimicrobial regimens lasting 8 weeks or longer, which include rifampin (10 mg/kg once daily) and clarithromycin (7.5 mg/kg twice daily), are now recommended as the first line of treatment. The *second-line options consist of the combination* of rifampin (10 mg/kg) and intramuscular streptomycin (15 mg/kg) or rifampin and moxifloxacin [3]. Other described agents are dapsone, trimethoprim-sulfamethoxazole, and quinolones [7].

Until 2004 antibiotic therapy was used, and surgery was the mainstream treatment to remove all infected tissues [2]. Today, surgery is used to speed up healing and prevent disability, and the most performed surgery is wound debridement followed by closure. In the debridement procedure, the aim is to remove all necrotic tissue, respecting deep structures as tendons, nerves, joint capsules, and bone. If there are large skin defects, and primary *closure* is not feasible, then negative pressure wound therapy can be used to improve healing and reduce area requiring skin grafts [2]. The WHO recommends surgical intervention for category 2 and 3, with concomitant use of antibiotics [6].

Other described therapy is the heat therapy, which consists in applying continuous warming pads on the affected skin at 39 °C. The bacteria grow optimally at 28 °C, and its growth stops at higher temperatures. This technique has been avoided, because *of the good performance* of antibiotic therapy, but adjuvant therapy can be considered in extensive lesions, in cases where antibiotics are contraindicated, or surgery is not available for the patient [2].

Some guidelines describe the use of antibiotics depending on the clinical stage [8]:

Stage 1: Small lesions (<5 cm) → Antibiotics alone.

Stage 2: Moderate lesions (5–15 cm) → Antibiotics for 4 weeks, and then surgery, if necessary, *followed by another 4 weeks of antibiotics.*

Stage 3: Advanced disease → Antibiotics 1 week before surgery, *and then continue up to the eighth week.*

Telacebec is a new anti-tuberculous drug which has demonstrated extreme potent activity against *Mycobacterium ulcerans* in animal studies, reducing the duration from 8 weeks to 2 weeks [9, 10]. In January 2021, the US Food and Drug Administration granted orphan drug designation (OOD) to Telacebec, a Buruli ulcer treatment (*https://www.koreabiomed.com/news/articleView.html?idxno=10169).*

10.10 Conclusion

Buruli ulcer is a disease of the skin and soft tissue caused by *Mycobacterium ulcerans*.

It is more prevalent in rural wetland zones, where a humid and hot climate predominates. The gender varies according to the geographic zone. *It generally* affects predominantly young people, <15 years. The mode of transmission remains unclear, but the main risk factor for infection is contact with bacteria in a traumatic skin lesion. The most affected areas are lower extremities, but almost every part can be affected. The morphology of lesions can start differently, but after 4 weeks, the lesion ulcerates without pain. The diagnosis can be clinical in high prevalence areas. The IS2404 PCR is the gold standard. Treatment consists of an 8-week course of antibiotics, with other supportive therapies like wound care, surgery, or heat therapy.

References

1. Walsh DS, Portaels F, Meyers WM. Buruli ulcer: advances in understanding mycobacterium ulcerans infection. Dermatol Clin. 2011;29(1):1–8. https://doi.org/10.1016/j.det.2010.09.006.
2. Kumar S, Basu S, Bhartiya SK, Shukla VK. The Buruli ulcer. Int J Low Extrem Wounds. 2015;14(3):217–23.
3. Franco-Paredes C, Marcos LA, Henao-Martínez AF, Rodríguez-Morales AJ, Villamil-Gómez WE, Gotuzzo E, et al. Cutaneous mycobacterial infections. Clin Microbiol Rev. 2019;32(1):1–25.
4. Parson W. Mycobacterium ulcerans. Lancet. 2011;354(9196):2171.
5. Manry J. Human genetics of Buruli ulcer. Hum Genet. 2020;139(6–7):847–53. https://doi.org/10.1007/s00439-020-02163-1.
6. Yotsu RR, Richardson M, Ishii N. Drugs for treating Buruli ulcer (Mycobacterium ulcerans disease). Cochrane Database Syst Rev. 2018;2018(8):1.
7. Al Ramahi JW, Annab H, Al Karmi M, Kirresh B, Wreikat M, Batarseh R, et al. Chronic cutaneous mycobacterial ulcers due to mycobacterium ulcerans (Buruli ulcer): the first indigenous case report from Jordan and a literature review. Int J Infect Dis. 2016;2017(58):77–81.
8. Chauty A, Ardant MF, Adeye A, Euverte H, Guédénon A, Johnson C, et al. Promising clinical efficacy of streptomycin-rifampin combination for treatment of Buruli ulcer (mycobacterium ulcerans disease). Antimicrob Agents Chemother. 2007;51(11):4029–35.
9. Almeida DV, Converse PJ, Omansen TF, Tyagi S, Tasneen R, Kim J, et al. Telacebec for ultrashort treatment of Buruli ulcer in a mouse model. Antimicrob Agents Chemother. 2020;64(6):1–10.
10. Thomas SS, Kalia NP, Ruf MT, Pluschke G, Pethe K. Toward a single-dose cure for Buruli ulcer. Antimicrob Agents Chemother. 2020;64(9):10.

11 Lepromatous Ulcer

Tulika Rai

11.1 Introduction

Leprosy also known as Hansen's disease is a chronic, infectious disease caused by *Mycobacterium leprae* bacillus, which affects mainly peripheral nerves and skin but may also affect sites such as the eyes, mucous membranes, bones, and testes and produces a spectrum of clinical phenotypes [1, 2]. Although the prevalence of disease is decreasing, Hansen's disease represents one of the major public health problems mainly in India and Brazil [3, 4].

The presentation of the disease is determined by many factors such as the host's immune response, and there is a spectrum of presentation from the tuberculoid end of leprosy to the lepromatous leprosy. Cutaneous lesions of leprosy usually present as hypoesthetic/anaesthetic hypochromic macules, papules, plaques, and diffuse infiltration of the skin with alopecia and xerosis [5]. The less frequent manifestations include spontaneous blisters on palms and soles, hyperpigmented patches, verrucous lesions, macrocheilia, facial infiltration, uveitis, orchitis, reactionary states, and pure neural leprosy [6–9].

The diagnosis is based on clinical findings followed by the bacteriological examination of slit-skin smears performed by an experienced technician. However, in resource poor settings clinical examination is performed for diagnosing leprosy. Therefore, clinical suspicion after careful examination of skin and peripheral nerves is of utmost importance for the diagnosis of leprosy. Unfortunately, delayed diagnosis and treatment are still an issue in our settings.

Ulcer can develop in leprosy patients during reactional states, Lucio's phenomenon (LP), or secondary to neuropathies. Neuropathic ulcers or trophic ulcers result due to an injury to an area which is compromised due to disease, vascular

T. Rai (✉)
Department of Dermatology, Institute of Medical Sciences, Banaras Hindu University, Varanasi, India

A. K. Khanna, S. K. Tiwary (eds.), *Uncommon Ulcers of the Extremities*, https://doi.org/10.1007/978-981-99-1782-2_11

insufficiency, or sensory loss. Leprosy has a wide range of neurocutaneous features. The cutaneous and sensory-motor manifestations usually appear after a long period of incubation in leprosy.

The nerve injury in Hansen's disease leads to sensory and motor changes which may cause deformities and the formation of skin ulcers. The pathogenesis is explained by the penetration of gram-positive alcohol-acid-resistant bacilli into the peripheral nerves, especially Schwann cells that damage the free nerve endings and induce changes in thermal, pain, and tactile sensitivity. The protective sensitivity is compromised by the disease along with the deformities of the foot resulting from the weakness of muscles, mechanical trauma, and use of inadequate footwear which further leads to hyperkeratosis, fissures, abrasions, blisters, erosions, and trophic ulcers on foot [10].

Various treatment modalities have been tried like total plaster cast immobilization, saline or collagen dressings, topical metronidazole application, topical growth factors like platelet-derived growth factor (becaplermin), epidermal growth factor, platelet-rich plasma therapy, and other reconstructive surgical procedures [11–14]. Few studies have shown promising results with platelet-rich fibrin therapy.

11.2 Trophic Ulcers

These ulcers usually develop on the sole of feet or fingertips, at sites exposed to repetitive high pressures during activities of daily living like walking or working. In patients with peripheral sensory deficits, the protective pain perception is absent, leading to repetitive trauma which may result in skin breakdown and ulceration. There may be modification of the gait due to a motor weakness and muscle mass decrease in many patients of peripheral neuropathy. This may lead to a sharp increase of pressure under the forefoot with very high pressures localized under the metatarsal heads and the heel. This explains the anatomical location of trophic ulcers in Hansen's disease.

The World Health Organization (WHO) disability grading is used to define 3 groups:

Grade 0: No anesthesia, no visible deformity or damage, Grade 1: anesthesia present but no visible deformity or damage, Grade 2: visible deformity or damage present [15]. Most of the patients with trophic ulcers have other deformities at the time of presentation.

In a study, the lepromatous form of Leprosy had the greatest impact on physical disability and deformity, with a 16.5-fold greater chance of developing grade 2 versus other clinical forms. In the lower limb, the posterior tibial and fibular nerves were the most commonly affected and when affected, the patient had a predisposition to plantar lesion formation, which began with a superficial lesion and evolved to a deep ulcer, osteomyelitis, and septic arthritis and gangrene [10].

The basis of treatment regimens for the neuropathic or insensitive lower limb is derived from the work of Dr. Paul Brand. His work demonstrated that plantar

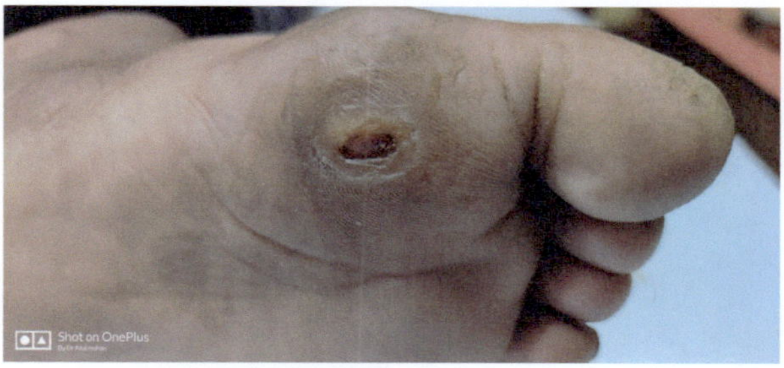

Fig. 11.1 Clinical photograph showing callosity on foot

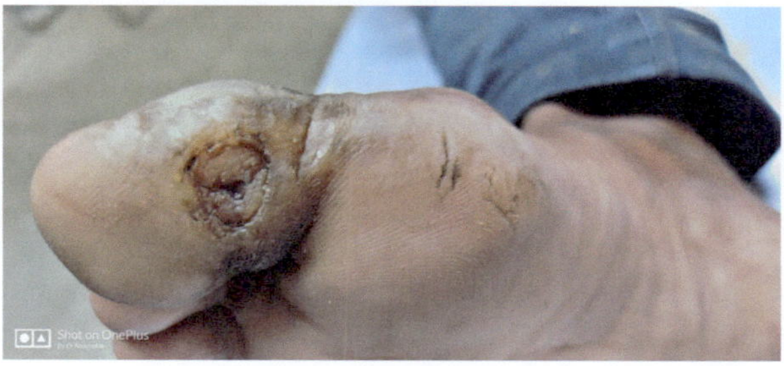

Fig. 11.2 Clinical photograph showing trophic ulcer on foot in a patient with Lepromatous Hansen's disease

ulceration results from a lack of protective sensation along with high plantar mechanical forces so offloading of affected limbs is important for wound healing.

The excessive pressure causes a hypertrophic reactive response of the local keratinocytes causing local hyperkeratosis and callosity at pressure bearing sites (Fig. 11.1). This callus may crack and break leading to ulceration (Figs. 11.2 and 11.3). Hence, the risk of an ulcer is even higher when a callus is present so it is important to shave callus at the margins of the ulcer and callus removal has shown reduction in dynamic plantar pressures in the forefoot by 30% during barefoot walking [16]. Topical keratolytic agents like urea and salicylic acid can be applied on callosity to soften the thick skin.

Wound management begins with surgical debridement and must include removal of all surrounding hard callus, hyperkeratotic skin, all dead necrotic tissue, and infected soft tissue and bone. The end result of debridement should be soft, non-keratotic wound edges with a well-vascularized tissue bed. During debridement a swab or a deep tissue culture should be taken. Any secondary infection should be treated.

Systemic antibiotics, oral or parenteral, are required only in the acute infective phase, in the presence of cellulitis or failure of a properly treated wound to heal. The treating physician should look for clinical signs of infection like purulent secretions, signs of inflammation (e.g., pain, redness, erythema, warmth, tenderness and induration), foul odor, and presence of necrotic tissue. Once debridement is done topical antimicrobial therapies are usually adequate to help eliminate bacteria in the foot ulcer. Radiographs may be done to rule out osteomyelitis. Other investigations like magnetic resonance imaging (MRI) may be done to know the extent of soft tissue involvement in selected cases.

Fig. 11.3 Clinical photograph showing trophic ulcer on the foot

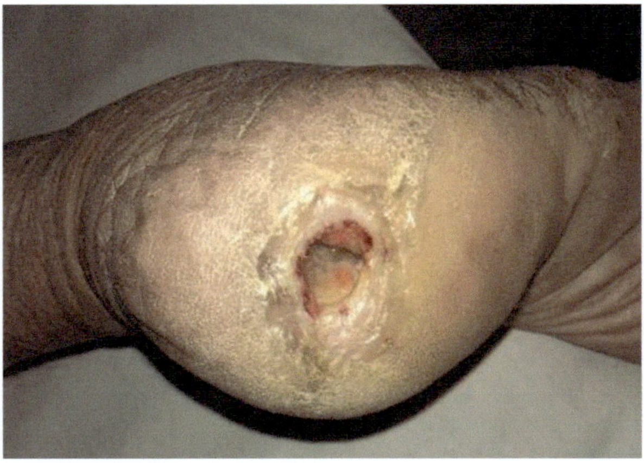

The most effective treatment of plantar ulceration in Leprosy is total contact cast and posterior walking splint. Visual inspection and touching the feet daily for any evidence of new trauma or injury are essential habits to develop in an effort to protect the feet from injury in all patients. Patient education is important to prevent development of plantar ulcers.

A Wound Management Program for all patients must include:

- Assessment.
- Treatment.
- Protection from further injury.
- Patient education.

In patients with leprosy, sometimes insensitive hands may have a series of small injuries or an insidious infection which can result in a gradual loss of soft tissue and bone reabsorption. The infection process is believed to be primarily responsible for the loss of finger length in insensitive hands. Patients must be taught to examine insensitive extremities routinely for redness or swelling and to identify objects and equipment they use which may cause injury. They should protect from hot water from a faucet or a hot object. Patients are taught to use areas where they do have "protective sensation" to test potentially damaging hot objects and to wear gloves when manipulating hot or sharp objects.

Splinting of wounds is often necessary for patients with insensitive hands in order to protect the affective area during healing. Patient education programs are important in prevention of further wounds and also for healing of wounds.

Dressings on ulcers may improve healing in chronic ulcers. A moist wound environment facilitates rapid migration of keratinocytes across the wound bed. As moist dressings have become available now, advanced moist wound therapy (AMWT) can be easily given with hydrogels (INTRASITE Gel, Smith and Nephew, Hydroheal, Dr. Reddys) and alginates. Few clinical trials have shown biomaterial-based treatment of leprosy wounds as an excellent affordable alternative for wound management [17].

Most patients experience recurrence of ulcers so patient education is very important. Most of the patients belong to low socio-economic status and deformities and chronic ulcers affect their livelihood. Rehabilitative programs by government and NGOs can improve their lives.

The treatment of such patients requires a multidisciplinary approach. The combined efforts of dermatologists, general surgeons, orthopedicians, plastic surgeons, field workers, and social workers are needed for complete rehabilitation of the patients.

11.3 Non-Trophic Ulcers

Patients of leprosy frequently experience lepra reactions. Type I lepra reactions are seen in borderline leprosy patients. Type II lepra reactions are seen in lepromatous leprosy (LLHD) and borderline lepromatous leprosy (BLHD) patients. Type II lepra reaction, also known as erythema nodosum leprosum (ENL), is a type III hypersensitivity reaction which commonly manifests as sudden appearance of crops of erythematous, edematous, evanescent, and tender nodules and plaques associated with fever and joint pain. ENL is associated with involvement of multiple organs leading to various complications [18]. ENL is an immune complex-mediated type III hypersensitivity reaction involving antigen, antibody, and complements. Neutrophilic activation and T cell dysfunction occur [19].

Many morphological patterns of ENL have been described such as nodular, bullous, pustular, and necrotic. The nodular form is the most common presentation along with fever, malaise, and joint pain. There is immune complex-mediated damage which can lead to the involvement of various organs leading to uveitis, lymphadenitis, synovitis, mastitis, epididymo-orchitis, arthritis, glomerulonephritis, and hepatitis [20]. Necrotic ENL represents a severe form of ENL and is less common and is associated with systemic complications (Figs. 11.4 and 11.5).

The close differential diagnosis of a patient with leprosy with multiple, necrotic ulcers is lucio phenomenon (LP) which occurs in patients with diffuse form of leprosy and presents with purpuric lesions followed by ulcers with irregular margins. There is absence of constitutional and systemic symptoms.

LP is also known as erythema necroticans. This was first described by Lucio and Alvarado and later confirmed by Latapi and Zamoraas. This is a vasculitis which occurs in the diffuse form of leprosy. It is a rare presentation in untreated lepromatous (LLHD) and borderline lepromatous leprosy (BLHD). This is endemic in Mexico and cases have been reported from the USA, Spain, Brazil, and Asia [21].

Lucio phenomenon usually appears in untreated or inadequately treated non-nodular lepromatous leprosy (LLHD) patients after a median of 1 to 3 years after the first manifestations of the disease and presents with painful, erythematous areas over the extremities which evolve into necrotic ulcers [22].

On histopathology in LP there is ischemic epidermal necrosis, necrotizing vasculitis, endothelial proliferation, and presence of a large number of AFB in endothelial cells. Lucio phenomenon responds to MDT [23].

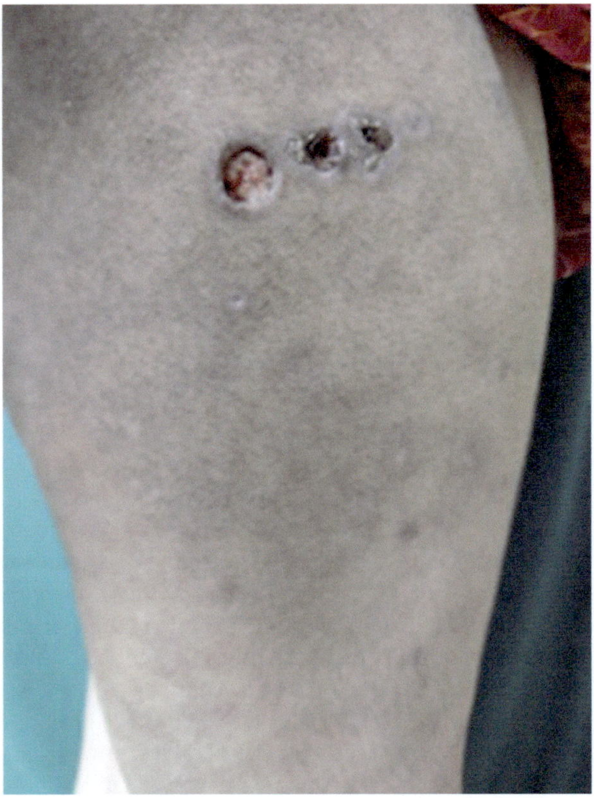

Fig. 11.4 A 35-year-old female on MB-MDT for 6 months presenting with necrotic erythema nodosum leprosum with multiple ulcers distributed on buttocks and thighs

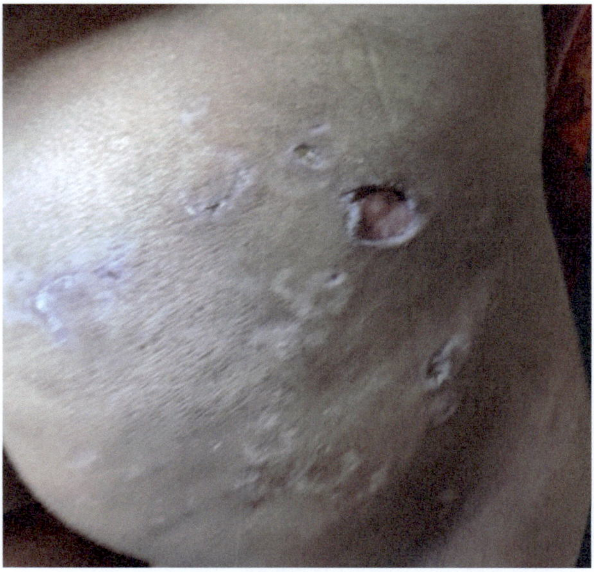

Fig. 11.5 A 35-year-old female on MB-MDT for 6 months presenting with necrotic erythema nodosum leprosum with punched out ulcer on buttocks with a violaceous border. Multiple ulcers were present

Non-trophic ulcers are rare and very few cases of necrotic ENL with ulcers and lucio phenomenon have been reported from India.

11.4 Conclusion

Patients with lepromatous leprosy frequently present with trophic ulcers and many of these patients experience lepra reactions. Trophic ulcers are difficult to treat and patient education plays an important role in the prevention of ulcers. These patients are from low socio-economic status and need rehabilitation. More efforts are needed to diagnose leprosy and treat these patients early to prevent deformities.

References

1. Graham A, Furlong S, Margoles LM, Owusu K, Franco-Paredes C. Clinical management of leprosy reactions. Infect Dis Clin Pract. 2010;18:235–8.
2. Polycarpou A, Walker SL, Lockwood DNJ. New findings in the pathogenesis of leprosy and implications for the management of leprosy. Curr Opin Infect Dis. 2013;26:413–9.
3. Andrade V, Militao de Albuquerque MD, Chagastelles SP. The importance of operational factors for the interpretation of indicators in the Hansen's disease endemic in Brazil. Acta Leprol. 1997;10:131–9.
4. Noordeen SK. Elimination of leprosy as a public health problem: progress and prospects. Bull World Health Organ. 1995;73:1–6.
5. Britton WJ, Lockwood DNJ. Leprosy. Lancet. 2004;363(9416):1209–19.
6. Handa S, Saraswat A, Radotra BD, Kumar B. Chronic macrocheilia: a clinicopathological study of 28 patients. Clin Exp Dermatol. 2003;28(3):245–50.

7. Ghorpade A. Multiple superficial sporotrichoid nerve abscesses with a hyperpigmented lesion in a tuberculoid leprosy patient: a rare and unusual presentation. J Eur Acad Dermatol Venereol. 2006;20(3):357–8.
8. Agarwal US, Mehta S, Kumar R, Besarwal RK, Agarwal P. Bullous lesions in leprosy: a rare phenomenon. Indian J Dermatol Venereol Leprol. 2013;79(1):107–9.
9. Medeiros MZ, Hans Filho G, Takita LC, Vicari CFS, Barbosa AB, Couto DV. Verrucous lepromatous leprosy: a rare form of presentation—report on two cases. An Bras Dermatol. 2014;89(3):481–4.
10. Moschioni C, Antunes CM, Grossi MA, Lambertucci JR. Risk factors for physical disability at diagnosis of 19,283 new cases of leprosy. Rev Soc Bras Med Trop. 2010;43:19–22.
11. Mishra S, Singh PC, Mishra M. Metronidazole in management of trophic ulcers in [2] leprosy. Indian J Dermatol Venereol Leprol. 1995;61:19–20.
12. Wieman TJ, Smiell JM, Su Y. Efficacy and safety of a topical gel formulation [3] of recombinant platelet-derived growth factor-BB (becaplermin) in patients with chronic neuropathic diabetic ulcers: a phase III randomized placebo-controlled double-blind study. Diabetes Care. 1998;21:822–7.
13. Birang R, Torabi A, Shahabooei M, Rismanchian M. Effect of platelet-rich in [4] platelet derived growth factors on peri-implant bone healing: an experimental study in canines. Dent Res J (Isfahan). 2012;9(1):93–9.
14. Suryanarayan S, Budamakuntla L, Khadri SI, Sarvajnamurthy S. Efficacy of [8] autologous platelet-rich plasma in the treatment of chronic nonhealing leg ulcers. Plast Aesthet Res. 2014;1:65–9.
15. Brandsma JW, Van Brakel WH. WHO disability grading: operational definitions. Lepr Rev. 2003;74:366–73.
16. Young MJ, Cavanagh PR, Thomas G, Johnson MM, Murray H, Boulton AJ. The effect of callus removal on dynamic plantar foot pressures in diabetic patients. Diabet Med. 1992;9:55–7.
17. Sivasubramanian S, Mohana S, Maheswari P, Victoria V, Thangam R, Mahalingam J, et al. Leprosy-associated chronic wound management using biomaterials. J Global Infect Dis. 2018;10:99–107.
18. Pradhan S, Prasad Nayak B, Padhi T, Sethy M. Bullous erythema Nodosum Leprosum masquerading as systemic onset juvenile idiopathic arthritis: a case report. Lepr Rev. 2015;86:387–90.
19. Kar HK, Raina A, Sharma PK, Bhardwaj M. Annular vesiculobullous eruptions in type 2 reaction in borderline lepromatous leprosy: a case report. Indian J Lepr. 2009;81:205–8.
20. Walker SL, Balagon M, Darlong J, Doni SN, Hagge DA, Halwai V, et al. ENLIST 1: an international multi-centre cross-sectional study of the clinical features of erythema Nodosum Leprosum. PLoS Negl Trop Dis. 2015;9:e0004065.
21. Furtado TA. The Lucio-Alvarado form of leprosy. A case observed in Brazil. Int J Lepr. 1959;27:110–5.
22. Sehgal VN. Lucio's phenomenon/erythema necroticans. Int J Dermatol. 2005;44:602–5.
23. Leticia F, Elemir MS, Maria LC, Paulo ENFV. Vasculonecrotic reactions in leprosy. Brazilian J Infect Dis. 2007;11:378–82.

Lupus Vulgaris

12

Varadraj V. Pai

Cutaneous tuberculosis (TB) is a relatively uncommon form of extrapulmonary tuberculosis with diverse clinical manifestations which can frequently result in diagnostic challenges. The wide clinical spectrum of cutaneous tuberculosis is dependent on the route of infection (endogevnous or exogenous), the immune status of the patient and whether or not there has been previous sensitization with tuberculosis.

Cutaneous tuberculosis is classified into

- Multibacillary form which includes conditions like tuberculosis chancre (due to inoculation), orofacial tuberculosis, scrofuloderma, acute military cutaneous tuberculosis, tuberculosis gumma.
- Paucibacillary form which include warty tuberculosis, lupus vulgaris and tuberculids.

In India, scrofuloderma and lichen scrofulosorum were the most frequently found types in childhood, whereas lupus vulgaris was the commonest form in adults [1–3].

12.1 History

Tuberculosis has plagued humankind throughout known history and human prehistory. The genus *Mycobacterium* originated more than 150,000,000 years ago from which the different species diverged over the course of millions of years [4]. References to tuberculosis have been made in Sanskrit works, namely the Rigveda

V. V. Pai (✉)
Department of Dermatology, Goa Medical College, Bambolim, Goa, India

A. K. Khanna, S. K. Tiwary (eds.), *Uncommon Ulcers of the Extremities*,
https://doi.org/10.1007/978-981-99-1782-2_12

(1500 BC), Ayurveda (700 BC) and in the Laws of Manu (1000 BC). It has also been mentioned in Indian mythologies as *Rajayakshma*. The Charaka Samhita (second century BCE) mentions the disease and also the various treatment modalities of that era. Hippocrates (460–376 BC) gives an intelligent description of this disease as 'phthisis', which meant to dry up [5].

12.2 Epidemiology

The incidence of cutaneous tuberculosis parallels that of pulmonary TB and is more commonly seen in developing countries and impoverished populations [6]. Cutaneous tuberculosis is relatively uncommon, comprising 1–1.5% of all extrapulmonary tuberculosis manifestations, which manifests only in 8.4–13.7% of all tuberculosis cases [7].

The overall prevalence of cutaneous TB in various Indian studies is 0.25%–0.6% [2, 8].

Lupus vulgaris is the most common form of cutaneous tuberculosis in adults in the Indian subcontinent and South Africa [9]. All age groups are equally affected with females two to three times more than males [10].

12.3 Pathogenesis

Mycobacterium tuberculosis is the predominant causative agent in cutaneous TB. Very rarely *M. Bovis* or Bacillus Calmette-Guerin [BCG], an attenuated strain of BCG, can cause skin lesions. The mode of transmission is primarily through aerosol route; rarely transmission can occur through inoculation or ingestion [6]. Lupus vulgaris is caused by haematogenous, lymphatic or contiguous spread from elsewhere in the body. Lupus vulgaris originates from an underlying focus of tuberculosis, typically in a bone, joint or lymph node, and arises by either contiguous extension of the disease from underlying affected tissue or by haematogenous or lymphatic spread [1]. In patients where the underlying focus is not apparent it has been postulated that it may be due to the reactivation of a latent cutaneous focus secondary to previous silent bacteraemia It can also arise after exogenous inoculation or as a complication of BCG vaccination [8].

Granulomas are the characteristic histopathological reaction seen in TB. These granulomas were previously considered as host protective, are now in studies using zebra fish infected with *M. marinum* have found to actually contribute to bacterial growth and facilitate its spread. Virulent mycobacteria release the early secreted target 6 protein, which stimulates epithelial cells to produce metalloproteinase 9 (MMP-9). MMP-9 secretion promotes the recruitment of new macrophages to the granuloma where they become infected and expand the granuloma. The host responds by producing CD4 and CD8 T cells that attempt to control bacterial growth. The mature granuloma therefore represents an equilibrium between mycobacterial growth and the host immune response [1, 6].

12.4 Clinical Features

The various types of cutaneous TB, mode of spread and their relation to the host immune response are given in Table 12.1 [11].

Lupus vulgaris (LV) is a chronic, progressive, post-primary, paucibacillary form of cutaneous tuberculosis, occurring in a person with a moderate or high degree of immunity. Lupus vulgaris is caused by haematogenous, lymphatic or contiguous spread from elsewhere in the body. Lesions of lupus vulgaris are usually solitary over a normal appearing skin, but sometimes can be few in number particularly in patients with pulmonary involvement [1, 10].

In Europe, over 80% of lesions are on the head and neck, particularly around the nose. Next in frequency are the arms and legs, but involvement of the trunk is uncommon. In India, cutaneous tuberculosis more commonly affects the buttocks and extremities rather than the face. Such a pattern is usually due to re-inoculation and may relate to playing without clothing or shoes [8, 12].

Classically the initial lesion of LV presents as a small, reddish brown, flat macule of soft, almost gelatinous, consistency. On diascopy, the diagnostic 'apple jelly'

Table 12.1 Types of Cutaneous TB

Clinical disease	Aetiology	Host immune status
Lupus vulgaris Scrofuloderma	Haematogenous spread	Can affect immunocompetent or immunocompromised people
Acute miliary TB Orofacial TB Metastatic tuberculous abscess (tuberculous Gumma)	Haematogenous spread	Usually seen in immunocompromised people
Primary inoculation TB	Inoculation of the skin with mycobacteria TB, e.g. by needle stick injury, or at site of trauma	No previous TB infection, immunocompetent
Tuberculosis verrucosa cutis	Inoculation of the skin with mycobacteria TB, e.g. by needle stick injury, or at site of trauma	Previous TB infection, immunocompetent
Normal primary complex-like reaction Post-vaccination lupus vulgaris Perforating regional adenitis	BCG inoculation	No previous TB infection
Lichen scrofulosorum Papulonecrotic tuberculid	True tuberculids—Thought to represent hypersensitivity reactions, rather than local TB infection of the skin	Not clear; likely some immunity due to previous exposure
Nodular vasculitis (erythema induratum of Bazin) Erythema nodosum	Facultative tuberculids—Mtb may be one of several aetiological agents causing this pathology	Not clear; likely some immunity due to previous exposure

nodules may be demonstrated. Progression is characterized by elevation, a deeper brownish colour and formation of a plaque. Later it shows the characteristic scarring and involution in one area with progression in another often results in a gyrate outline border [1].

The clinical forms vary widely and fall into five different general patterns, depending on the local tissue response to the infection [1]:

1. In plaque form, the lesions have irregular or serpiginous edge and large plaques show irregular areas of scarring with islands of active lupus tissue. The edge often becomes thickened and hyperkeratotic (Figs. 12.1, 12.2 and 12.3).
2. In ulcerative and mutilating forms, scarring and ulceration predominate with crusts forming over areas of necrosis. The deep tissues and cartilage are invaded and contractures and deformities can occur (Fig. 12.4).
3. Vegetating form is characterized by marked infiltration, ulceration and necrosis with minimal scarring. Mucous membranes are invaded and cartilage is slowly destroyed. When the nasal or auricular cartilage is involved, extensive destruction and disfigurement occur.
4. Tumour-like forms present either as soft tumour-like nodules or as epithelial hyperplasia with the production of hyperkeratotic masses.
5. In papular and nodular forms, multiple lesions occur simultaneously in disseminated lupus—true 'miliary lupus' and usually occurs after immunosuppression.

The nasal, buccal or conjunctival mucosa may also become involved, either primarily by a papule, nodule or ulcer, or by spread from a contiguous skin lesion.

The differential diagnoses in the early stages to be considered are leprosy, sarcoidosis, lymphocytoma, Spitz naevus and lupus erythematosus, and in older patients syphilis must be excluded. The histopathologic and culture reports help to differentiate lupus vulgaris from the deep mycoses, which closely resemble the vegetating and crusted type. Leprosy and sarcoidosis are the chief causes of diagnostic

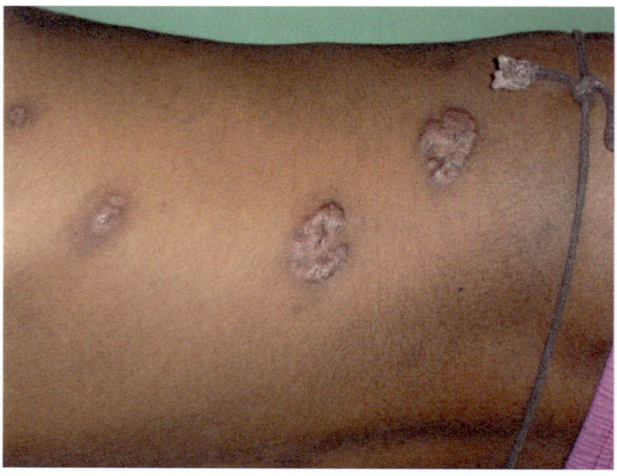

Fig. 12.1 Plaque type

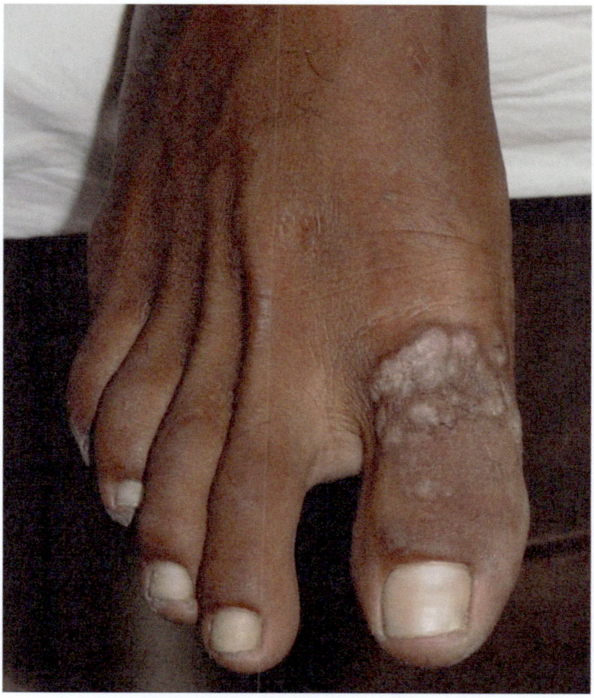

Fig. 12.2 Plaque type

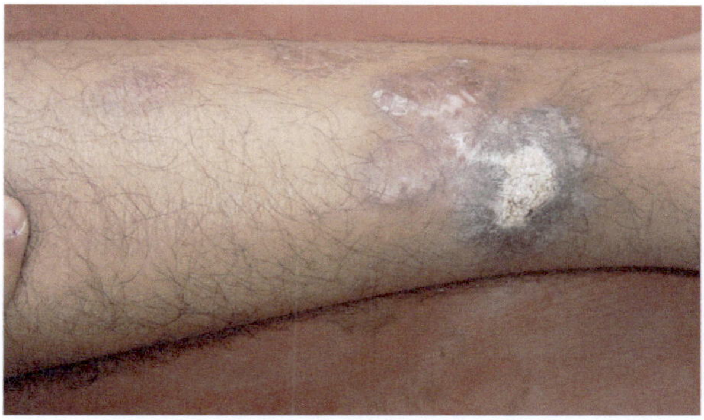

Fig. 12.3 Classical feature of scarring on one edge and progression on the other

difficulty. The nodules in leprosy are firmer with other positive signs of leprosy, and the nodules of sarcoidosis resemble grains of sand rather than 'apple jelly' on palpation [1].

Diagnostic tests for lupus vulgaris [11]:

- Chest X-ray—All patients presenting with symptoms consistent with TB should have a chest X-ray to look for previous or active pulmonary TB.
- HIV testing—Extrapulmonary TB is associated with HIV infection. All patients should be offered integrated counselling and testing.

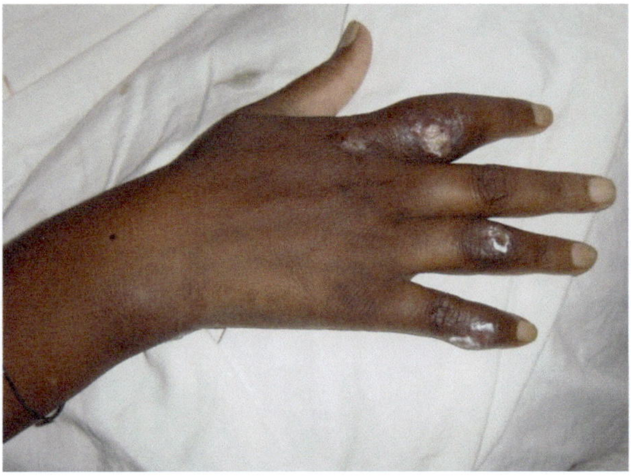

Fig. 12.4 Ulcerative form

– Tuberculin skin test.

The TST is a delayed-type hypersensitivity to mycobacterial antigens, following an intradermal injection of purified protein derivative (PPD). Tuberculin testing should be done by the Mantoux method as this is the only technique that has been standardized and extensively validated. PPD (0.1 mL = 5 tuberculin units) is injected into the volar aspect of the forearm using a 27-gauge needle to raise a small weal. The diameter of the induration is measured after 48–72 h. Normally a cut-off of 5 mm induration is used to determine those at high risk of infection, for example close contacts of an active case, patients with radiographic abnormalities consistent with tuberculosis, those with HIV infection and those immunosuppressed with corticosteroids or other agents. A cut-off of 10 mm is used in migrants from endemic areas, healthcare workers, the homeless and residents of some urban areas, and those patients with diabetes, renal disease, silicosis and other conditions associated with an increased risk of latent tuberculosis. Finally a cut-off of 15 mm is used in those with no risk factors [1].

In Indian scenario, the Mantoux test is not usually part of the diagnosis of active TB infection. However, the Cutaneous TB Group agreed that in selected cases where diagnosis was equivocal, it might be used as an ancillary test. However, only a strongly positive result (with a diameter of 22 mm or more at reading) supports a diagnosis of cutaneous TB. A negative or weakly positive result does not rule out TB. Sensitivity and specificity estimates for this test vary widely across case series, and the result must be interpreted in the context of the other clinical findings [11].

– Interferon-γ release assays are T cell-based blood tests that measure the host response to *M. tuberculosis* by utilizing antigens that are much more specific for *M. tuberculosis* than tuberculin. These tests are more specific than the TST in the diagnosis of latent *M. tuberculosis* infection in adults and children; however the sensitivity is no better than that of the TST [1].

- Histopathology.

  In lupus vulgaris there are tuberculoid granulomas with a variable mantle of lymphocytes in the upper and mid dermis. The granulomas have a tendency to confluence. Caseation is sometimes present. Multinucleate giant cells are not always numerous. Langerhans cells are present in moderate numbers in the granulomas. The overlying epidermis may be atrophic or hyperplastic, but only rarely is there pseudoepitheliomatous hyperplasia. Staining and microscopy for AFB have very low sensitivity [1, 8].
- Culture has low sensitivity; but if positive, confirms the diagnosis of cutaneous TB and facilitates drug susceptibility testing. PCR-based tests are in use with variable diagnostic accuracy, but a lack of evidence from high-quality studies means they cannot be recommended for routine use currently [11].
- Gene-Xpert, a CBNAAT (cartridge-based nucleic acid amplification test), is a widely accepted diagnostic test for tuberculosis. This test is a rapid diagnostic test for tuberculosis detection as well as Rifampicin resistance in direct smear negative cases [11].

The diagnosis of skin tuberculosis in many cases can be challenging and may require more than pure clinical skills in areas where it is less frequently seen and in HIV-positive patients in whom the course of the disease is altered. Demonstration of a classical tubercular granuloma on histopathology is diagnostic but caseation necrosis is usually sparse or absent. The infiltrate can be nonspecific in up to one-third of the patients. Demonstration of AFB in Ziehl-Neelsen–stained tissue smears, histopathological sections, or their recovery in culture is disappointing in most instances. Since lupus vulgaris is a paucibacillary condition a diagnosis can be made based on the classical clinical, histopathological findings and demonstration of tuberculosis bacilli from smear, biopsy, PCR or CBNAAT [1, 5].

Other indications towards the diagnosis, which are by themselves unreliable, include the following:

1. The presence of active, proven tuberculosis elsewhere in the body.
2. The presence of acid-fast bacilli in the lesion itself—this will also be seen in infections with other mycobacteria.
3. A positive reaction to tuberculin—a strongly positive reaction of >15 mm in diameter may be considered of diagnostic value.
4. Positive IFN-γ release assay.
5. The effect of specific therapy—in areas of high tuberculous prevalence a therapeutic trial of anti-tuberculous therapy should be considered.

12.5 Course and Progression

The natural course of an untreated lesion is progressive leading to scarring, contractures and tissue destruction. The scars are usually thin, white and smooth, but are unstable and may break down or become keloidal. Active lupus vulgaris frequently reappears in scar tissue. Squamous cell and basal cell carcinomas or sarcomas can occur insidiously in up to 8% of patients and may be confused with renewed activity of the lupus itself [1].

12.6 Treatment [11]

All patients with the following results should be treated for cutaneous TB:

- Patients with histology diagnostic of cutaneous TB.
- Patients with positive culture of Mtb or microscopy for AFBs from skin biopsy.
- Patients with equivocal histology findings and negative microscopy and culture, but strongly positive Mantoux test.

The first-line therapy for adults and children with lupus vulgaris is 2HRZE/4RHE (2 months of Isoniazid, Rifampicin, pyrazinamide and ethambutol followed by 4 months of Isoniazid, Rifampicin and ethambutol). The patients have to be followed up at 4–6 weeks interval to note the response to therapy. Failure to respond to therapy may be due to misdiagnosis or drug resistance.

In conclusion, lupus vulgaris is most common among middle aged patients, commonly presenting as a plaque type, with frequent involvement of the extremities. Diagnosis is based on clinical features and histopathological examination. All patients should be treated with standard anti-tubercular regimen.

References

1. Yates VM, Walker SL. Mycobacterial infection. In: Griffiths C, Barker J, Bleiker T, Chalmers R, Creamer D, editors. Rook's textbook of dermatology. 9th ed. Oxford: Blackwell science Ltd; 2016. p. 27.1–27.45.
2. Patra AC, Gharami RC, Banerjee PK. A profile of cutaneous tuberculosis. Indian J Dermatol. 2006;51:105–7.
3. Khadka P, Koirala S, Thapaliya J. Cutaneous tuberculosis: Clinicopathologic arrays and diagnostic challenges. Dermatol Res Pract. 2018;2018:7201973, 2018, 1.
4. Daniel TM. The history of tuberculosis. Respir Med. 2006;100:1862–70.
5. Kumar B, Dogra S. Cutaneous tuberculosis. Skin infections: diagnosis and treatment. 2009: 59–75. https://doi.org/10.1017/CBO9780511576829.007.
6. Ramos-e-Silva M, Riberio de Castro MC. Mycobacterial infections. In: Bolognia JL, Jorizzo JL, Schaffer JV, editors. Dermatology. 3rd ed. Amsterdam: Elsevier; 2012. p. 1221–42.
7. Van Zyl L, du Plessis J, Viljoen J. Cutaneous tuberculosis overview and current treatment regimens. Tuberculosis. 2018;95:629–38.
8. Pai VV, Naveen KN, Athanikar SB, Dinesh US, Divyashree A, Gupta G. A clinico-histopathological study of lupus vulgaris: a 3 year experience at a tertiary care centre. Indian Dermatol Online J. 2014;5:461–5.
9. Kumar B, Muralidhar S. Cutaneous tuberculosis: a twenty-year prospective series. Int J Tuberc Lung Dis. 1999;3:494–500.
10. Tappeiner G. Tuberculosis and infections with atypical mycobacteria. In: Wolff K, Goldsmith LA, Katz SI, Gilchrist BA, Paller AS, Leffell DJ, editors. Fitzpatrick s dermatology in general medicine. 7th ed. New York, NY: McGraw Hill; 2008. p. 1771–2.

11. Index TB Guidelines. Guidelines on extra-pulmonary tuberculosis for India. World health Organization 2016. http://www.icmr.nic.in/guidelines/TB/Index-TB%20Guidelines%20-%20green%20colour%202594164.pdf. Accessed 21 Sep 2021.
12. Sehgal VN, Waugh SA. Cutaneous tuberculosis. Current concepts. Int J Dermatol. 1990;29:237–52.

13 Dermal Leishmaniasis

Jaya Chakravarty

13.1 Introduction

Leishmaniases are a group of vector-borne neglected tropical diseases caused by the protozoan parasite *Leishmania* and are transmitted by the bite of infected female phlebotomine sandflies. It presents in three forms—systemic form visceral leishmaniasis (VL) or kala-azar, mucocutaneous leishmaniasis (MCL), and cutaneous leishmaniasis (CL). Cutaneous leishmaniasis is the commonest form of the disease with approximately 600,000 to 1 million new cases occurring worldwide annually. As per WHO, in 2020 over 85% of new CL cases occurred in 10 countries: Afghanistan, Algeria, Brazil, Colombia, Iraq, Libya, Pakistan, Peru, the Syrian Arab Republic, and Tunisia [1]. Post-kala-azar dermal leishmaniasis (PKDL) is usually a sequel of visceral leishmaniasis that occurs mainly in East Africa and on the Indian subcontinent. The importance of PKDL lies in the fact that these patients are a source of *Leishmania* infection. As the Indian subcontinent plans to eliminate visceral leishmaniasis by 2023, early diagnosis and treatment of PKDL become very important [2]. The data from national vector-borne disease control program of India shows that the PKDL cases had a rising trend from 2012 to 2017 with subsequent decline [3].

13.2 Epidemiology

Based on the geographical distribution cutaneous leishmaniasis is divided into Old World cutaneous leishmaniasis (OWCL) and New World cutaneous leishmaniasis (NWCL). OWCL occurs in southern Europe, Middle East part of southwest Asia,

J. Chakravarty (✉)
Department of Medicine, Institute of Medical Sciences, Banaras Hindu University, Varanasi, India

A. K. Khanna, S. K. Tiwary (eds.), *Uncommon Ulcers of the Extremities*,
https://doi.org/10.1007/978-981-99-1782-2_13

Central Asia, and Africa and is caused by *L. aethiopica*, *L. donovani*, *L. infantum*, *L. major*, and *L. tropica*. In India, cutaneous leishmaniasis is known to be endemic to the Thar Desert of Bikaner in Rajasthan State mainly due to *L. tropica* and has been also reported from Himachal Pradesh where the causative agent is *L. donovani* [4–10]. NWCL is caused by many species of leishmania and is mainly found in Mexico and Latin America. New World species are more likely to cause MCL and rarer diffuse and disseminated cutaneous leishmaniasis (DCL). Over 90% of mucocutaneous leishmaniasis cases occur in Bolivia, Brazil, Ethiopia, and Peru [1]. A severe form called diffuse cutaneous leishmaniasis (DCL) is caused by *L. aethiopica* in the Old world and by *L. mexicana* and *L. amazonesis* in the New world. CL mostly has zoonotic transmission except for disease caused by *L. tropica* and post-kala-azar dermal leishmaniasis caused by *Leishmania donovani* is predominantly anthroponotic [11].

13.3 Clinical Features

The incubation period for symptomatic CL ranges from weeks to months; however mucosal involvement may occur years following initial infection. Asymptomatic infection may occur in about 10% of patients. As CL is caused by different species its clinical features vary between and within regions and immunological status of the host.

Old World species like *L. infantum*, *L. major*, and *L. tropica* cause self-limiting ulcers. It starts as a papule or nodule at the site of inoculation, taking at least 1 week to reach its final size. A central crust develops, which may lead to an ulcer up to 5 cm in diameter with a raised edge and variable surrounding induration, which heals gradually over months or years, leaving a depressed scar with altered pigmentation. Satellite nodules at the edge of the lesion are common. In nonimmune patients lesions are multiple. Secondary infection leads to slow healing leaving large, disfiguring or disabling scars.

Rarely CL due to *L. aethiopica* can cause oronasal leishmaniasis, which may distort the nostrils and lips, or diffuse cutaneous leishmaniasis. DCL is characterized by widely disseminated cutaneous macules, papules, nodules, or plaques, or by diffuse infiltration of the skin, especially on extensor surfaces of the limbs and on the face, causing thickening of the eyebrows and ear lobes mimicking lepromatous leprosy. It does not lead to ulceration. DCL is caused by polyparasitic disease and does not heal spontaneously, and relapses are frequent after treatment [11].

In the New world (Americas) *L.L. mexicana* infection generally produces small, chronic skin ulcers, usually one or few in number which heal spontaneously, while those caused by *L.V. braziliensis* are large, frequently with lymphocutaneous involvement. Lymphadenopathy, fever, and malaise may precede development of any lesion. Ulcers usually heal in 6 to 12 months but can be quite persistent and lead to mucosal leishmaniasis concurrently or subsequently. *L.L. mexicana*, and *L.L. amazonensis* can also cause DCL. Espundia or mucosal leishmaniasis occurs in the New World and is caused by the *Viannia* subgenus, especially *L.V. braziliensis*,

L.V. guyanensis, and *L.Voratister panamensis*, but also *L.L. amazonensis* [12–14]. It is an oligoparasitic disease associated with a marked cellular immune response.

Patients with immunosuppressing conditions like use of steroids, biologics, immunosuppressive agents, HIV/AIDS, organ transplant recipients, and pregnant patients are at increased risk for more severe CL.

Approximately 50% of patients with VL in East Africa particularly Sudan have PKDL while 5–20% develop PKDL in the Indian subcontinent. Although most patients with PKDL have a history of VL in India, approximately 5% may not have a history of visceral leishmaniasis. In East Africa, PKDL may occur soon after treatment for VL or even concurrently with the disease and is self-limiting while in India it usually occurs after a 2–3-year interval and is not self-resolving. The lesions appear as a macule, papule, or nodule, or a combination of these, typically on the face, but it may subsequently affect all parts of the body.

13.4 Differential Diagnosis

Cutaneous leishmaniasis—Fungal infection like histoplasmosis and coccidioidomycosis, sporotrichosis, cutaneous tuberculosis and atypical mycobacterial infection, leprosy and squamous cell carcinoma.

PKDL—For the macular form the differential diagnosis is leprosy, pityriasis versicolor, pityriasis alba, and vitiligo while the nodular form needs to be differentiated from leprosy, lupus vulgaris, and acne.

13.5 Diagnosis

Definitive diagnosis requires demonstration of the amastigote form of the parasite in a clinical specimen (usually skin) by histology, culture, or leishmania DNA by polymerase chain reaction (PCR). A full-thickness punch biopsy of the skin (4 to 5 mm) allows evaluation of histology and culture and to rule out other causes like acid-fast mycobacteria and fungi.

PKDL should be suspected in patients in endemic areas who present with skin lesions compatible with PKDL combined with previous or concomitant visceral leishmaniasis. Slit-skin smears or biopsy can be used to identify parasites to confirm the diagnosis of PKDL. Smears are more likely to show amastigotes if they are taken from nodular lesions rather than papular lesion, and macular lesions are least likely to show amastigotes. An rK39-based rapid test can be helpful when other diseases like leprosy are considered in the differential diagnosis, or if a history of visceral leishmaniasis is uncertain.

13.6 Treatment

13.6.1 Post-Kala-Azar Dermal Leishmaniasis

In India, miltefosine for 12 weeks and Amphotericin B 60–80 doses over 4 months are the recommended regimens. In East Africa, PKDL is not routinely treated, as the majority of cases (85%) heal spontaneously within 1 year. Only patients with severe or disfiguring disease, those with lesions that have remained for >6 months, those with concomitant anterior uveitis, and young children with oral lesions that interfere with feeding are treated, with either sodium stibogluconate (20 mg/kg/day per day) for up to 2 months or a 20-day course of L-AmB at 2.5 mg/kg/day.

13.6.2 Cutaneous Leishmaniasis

In the OWCL, local wound care with careful follow-up is indicated for patients with *L. major*; in those with fewer than four lesions requiring immediate treatment; lesions <5 cm in diameter; no potentially disfiguring or disabling lesion (face, joints, toes, and fingers); no immunosuppression and possibility for follow-up. If at least one criterion is absent, local therapy should be given. Lesions due to *L. tropica*, *L. aethiopica,* and *L. infantum* need local therapy.

The options for local therapy are Paromomycin ointments (15% PM/12% MBCL ointment b.i.d. for 20 days), intralesional antimonials (intralesional antimonials, 1–5 mL per session plus cryotherapy both every 3–7 days for 1–5 sessions), thermotherapy (1–2 sessions with localized heat 50 °C for 30 s), and cryotherapy [11, 13, 14]. Systemic therapy is given for severe and complex lesions like lesions on face, fingers, toes, or genitalia where local therapy cannot be given, failure of local therapy or in immunosuppressed host (Table 13.1).

For NWCL the decision to wait and watch or to give local or systemic treatment depends on factors like risk of developing MCL, presence of complicated or uncomplicated lesions. Complicated CL means infection with species associated with mucosal leishmaniasis, more than four lesions of significant size (e.g., >1 cm), individual lesions ≥5 cm, subcutaneous nodules, regional adenopathy >1 cm size, size or location of lesions for which local treatment is not feasible, lesions on face, fingers, toes, or genitalia, immunosuppressed host or clinical failure of local therapy after 2 to 3 months post-treatment [15]. Before starting treatment the clinician should know the high-risk areas and species causing MCL. Leishmania species with an increased risk of causing MCL include *L. (V.) braziliensis* mainly, but also *L. (V.) guyanensis* and *L. (V.) panamensis.* The Pan American Health Organization (PAHO) guidelines prefer treating NWCL either with local or systemic treatment [12] (Table 13.2).

Table 13.1 Recommended systemic treatment regimens for Old World CL

Systemic therapy
L. major • Fluconazole, 200 mg/day oral for 6 weeks[a] • Sbv, 20 mg Sb5+/kg/day intramuscularly or intravenously for 10–20 days[b] • Sbv, 20 mg Sb5+/kg/day intramuscularly or intravenously plus pentoxifylline, 400 mg t.i.d. for 10–20 days[a]
L. tropica and *L. infantum*[c] • Sbv, 20 mg Sb5+/kg/day intramuscularly or intravenously for 10–20 days[b] • Sbv, 15–20 mg Sb5+/kg/day intramuscularly or intravenously for 15 days plus oral allopurinol 20 mg/kg for 30 days, to treat leishmaniasis recidivans caused by *L. tropica*[d]
L. aethiopica • Sbv 20 mg Sb5+/kg/day intramuscularly or intravenously plus PM, 15 mg (11 mg base)/kg/day intramuscularly for 60 days or longer to treat diffuse CL

[a]Evidence obtained from at least one properly designed randomized controlled trial
[b]Expert opinion without consistent or conclusive studies
[c]Few data are available on therapy for CL caused by L. infantum and L. aethiopica
[d]Opinions of respected authorities, based on clinical experience, descriptive studies, or reports of expert committees
[B]Evidence obtained from well-designed trials without randomization

Table 13.2 Treatment options for cutaneous and mucosal leishmaniases in the Americas by clinical presentation and therapeutic indication. PAHO[a, b]

Clinical presentation	Therapeutic indication
Localized cutaneous leishmaniasis • Single lesion up to 900 mm² (3-cm diameter) in any location except head and periarticular regions, absence of immunosuppression, and possibility of monitoring	**Local** [a] • Thermotherapy • Intralesional pentavalent antimonials
	Systemic First-line • Pentavalent antimonials • Miltefosine (*L. guyanensis* and *L. panamensis*) • Pentamidine isethionate[b] • Ketoconazole (*L. mexicana* and *L. panamensis*)
	Second-line • Amphotericin B

(continued)

Table 13.2 (continued)

Clinical presentation	Therapeutic indication
Localized cutaneous leishmaniasis • Single lesion larger than 900 mm^2 in any location or • Single lesion of any size, on head or periarticular regions or • Multiple lesions • Single lesions previously treated locally that did not respond or relapsed	**Systemic** First-line • Pentavalent antimonials • Miltefosine • Pentamidine isethionate *(L. guyanensis and L. panamensis)* • Ketoconazole (*L. mexicana* and *L. panamensis*)
	Second-line • Pentamidine isethionate • Amphotericin B • Liposomal amphotericin B
Disseminated cutaneous Leishmaniasis	**Systemic** First-line • Pentavalent antimonials
	Second-line • Liposomal amphotericin B • Amphotericin B
Diffuse cutaneous leishmaniasis	**Systemic** • Pentavalent antimonials • Liposomal amphotericin B • Pentamidine isethionate • Amphotericin B deoxycholate
Mucosal leishmaniasis	**Systemic** • Pentavalent antimonials + pentoxifylline • Pentavalent antimonials Liposomal amphotericin B • Pentamidine isethionate • Amphotericin B deoxycholate

[a]Decisions on whether to add local treatments as a therapeutic option for cutaneous leishmaniasis should be based on the available evidence for each country
[b]Better results with *L. guyanensis*

13.7 Conclusion

PKDL patients are reservoirs of infection and can cause VL outbreaks making it very important to diagnose and treat it for the success of the VL elimination program. The most important barriers to the treatment of PKDL are the fact that patients are symptomless and the long and arduous treatment of 12 weeks duration is a major obstacle in completion of therapy. Thus active surveillance for PKDL, proper counseling regarding importance of completing treatment, and shorter regimen for PKDL are the need of the hour.

The treatment of CL depends on the infecting species, geographic region, risk of MCL, and response rate of drugs in that region. A wait and watch approach can be adopted if the lesion is healing spontaneously or if it is a well-localized lesion caused by *L. major* or *L. Mexicana*. Local therapy is recommended for non-self-curing uncomplicated CL and systemic therapy for complicated CL.

References

1. World Health Organization. Leishmaniasis. https://www.who.int/news-room/fact-sheets/detail/leishmaniasis.
2. https://www.who.int/news-room/fact-sheets/detail/leishmaniasis.
3. Saurabh S, Roy P, Pandey DK, Ray D, Tarak S, Pandey R, Kumar D, Jamil S, Paulraj A, Kumar A, Dutta S. Changing clinico-epidemiology of post-kala-azar dermal leishmaniasis (PKDL) in India: results of a survey in four endemic states. J Vector Borne Dis. 2020;57:161–9.
4. Aara N, Khandelwal K, Bumb RA, et al. Clinco-epidemiologic study of cutaneous leishmaniasis in Bikaner, Rajasthan, India. Am J Trop Med Hyg. 2013;89(1):111–5. https://doi.org/10.4269/ajtmh.12-0558.
5. Srivastava D, Vyas MC, Joshi CK. Clinico-epidemiological study of cutaneous leishmaniasis in Bikaner (Rajasthan). J Commun Dis. 1987;19:326–31.
6. Sharma MID, Suri JC, Krishna M, Swami PN. Epidemiological and entomological features of an out break of cutaneous leishmaniasis in Bikaner, Rajasthan during 1971. J Commun Dis. 1973;5:54–72.
7. Agrawal KS, Chadda VS. A study of epidemiology of human cutaneous leishmaniasis in Bikaner (Rajasthan). Indian J Dermatol Venereol Leprol. 1981;47:303–6.
8. Vyas MC, Kalla G, Shrivastav D, Bhardwaj AK. A clinico-epidemiological study of cutaneous leishmaniasis in Bikaner. Indian J Dermatol Venereol Leprol. 1994;60:197–9.
9. Kumar R, Bumb RA, Ansari NA, Mehta RD, Salotra P. Cutaneous leishmaniasis caused by *L. tropica* in Bikaner, India: parasite identification and characterization using molecular and immunologic tools. Am J Trop Med Hyg. 2007;76:896–901.
10. Sharma NL, Mahajan VK, Kanga A, Sood A, Katoch VM, Mauricio I, Singh CD, Parwan UC, Sharma VK, Sharma RC. Localized cutaneous leishmaniasis due to *Leishmania donovani* and *Leishmania tropica*: preliminary findings of the study of 161 new cases from a new endemic focus in Himachal Pradesh, India. Am J Trop Med Hyg. 2005;72:819–24.
11. Control of the Leishmaniasis. Report of a meeting of the WHO expert committee on the control of Leishmaniases. 2010; Geneva.
12. Pan American Health Organization. Leishmaniasis in the Americas: treatment recommendations. Washington, D.C.: PAHO; 2018; http://iris.paho.org.
13. Sundar S, Chakravarty J. Leishmaniasis: an update of current pharmacotherapy. Expert Opin Pharmacother. 2013;14(1):53–63.
14. Sundar S, Chakravarty J. An update on pharmacotherapy for leishmaniasis. Expert Opin Pharmacother. 2015;16(2):237–52.
15. Chakravarty J, Sundar S. Current and emerging medications for the treatment of leishmaniasis. Expert Opin Pharmacother. 2019;20(10):1251–65.

14 Fungal Infection and Ulceration

Tuhina Banerjee, Swati Sharma, and Priyanka Singh

14.1 Introduction

The evolution of humans over the years has occurred in parallel with the evolution of microorganisms. Hence the association of microbes and disease in humans is constantly evolving. In this relevance, in recent years, fungal infections have been increasingly recognized as an emerging cause of morbidity and mortality. The impact of fungal infection is so severe that globally it affects over 300 million people with nearly 1.6 million deaths each year [1]. The ubiquitous presence of fungal elements in the environment, their commensal status on human body and their opportunistic nature has accounted for increasing recognition of their disease-causing ability. Additionally, changing lifestyle, climatic challenges, urbanization, and comorbidities have also facilitated the spread of fungal infections. Simultaneously, development in diagnostic modalities and a better understanding of several strategies and mechanisms of fungi to survive and persist have helped in their awareness.

When considering fungal infections and ulcerations in wounds, it must be acknowledged that it becomes doubly challenging to timely diagnose, treat, and ensure healing sets in. Some interesting facts on this aspect have been recently revealed through in-depth research, though limited studies on mycobiome component of microbiome on skin and in ulcer or wounds have shown the coevolution of fungi and bacteria in a symbiotic manner benefitting from each other's existence. This renewed interest has put forward several answers and challenges towards fungal infections in wounds and skin ulceration. Presently, when several approaches are being made to study the entire microbial environment in the form of microbiome

T. Banerjee (✉) · S. Sharma · P. Singh
Department of Microbiology, Institute of Medical Sciences, Banaras Hindu University, Varanasi, India
e-mail: drtuhina105@bhu.ac.in

A. K. Khanna, S. K. Tiwary (eds.), *Uncommon Ulcers of the Extremities*,
https://doi.org/10.1007/978-981-99-1782-2_14

in different anatomical sites, the "wound" bed serves as an excellent environment to constitute or support microorganisms.

In this chapter, we have reviewed the concepts of the mycobiome in relation to the microbiome, the reported fungal infections in wounds, the developments in diagnostic modalities, and a standard protocol for their management and prevention.

14.2 The Wound Microbiome

With the recent developments in our understanding of the wound environment, the role of the entire microbiota in the wound rather than the culturable ones is being emphasized. It is now evident that the microbial load along with the diversity in microflora and the role of this flora as pathogens matter in the response towards treatment. It is interesting that wound microbiomes are heterogenous. This heterogeneity is influenced by ulcer depth, duration, and other host-related factors [2]. Findings from studies mostly on diabetic foot ulcer (DFU) microbiome have revealed that certain genera of bacteria are in abundance in the wound microbiome namely: *Anaerococcus*, *Staphylococcus*, *Corynebacterium*, *Porphyromonas*, *Streptococcus*, *Peptoniphilus*, *Pseudomonas,* etc. [3].

Large-sized chronic wounds are colonized by polymicrobial communities, because of which persistent inflammation and impaired wound healing occur. The common hypothesis is once colonized, the communities within the wound form a biofilm and disrupt the healing process. The skin niche in case of the invasion or injury can influence the composition and activity of the wound microflora [4]. The commensals bacteria and fungi not only coexist at anatomical sites, but also interact for their existence, which sometimes is detrimental to the host. There are several reasons for evolutions of these cooperative strategies between the bacteria and fungi as summarized in Fig. 14.1.

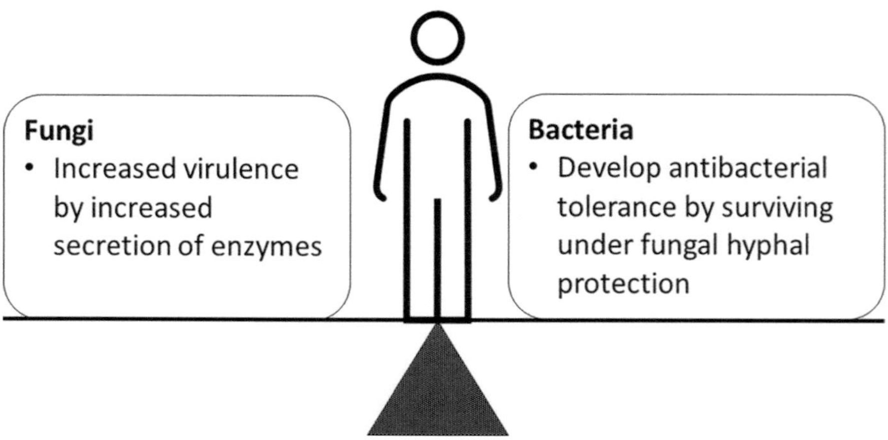

Fig. 14.1 Coevolution strategies of bacteria and fungi in human anatomical sites

The wound microbiome therefore is not limited to bacterial flora but includes complex interactions of microbial communities resulting in the formation of inter-kingdom mixed species biofilms [5, 6]. The understanding of these niches on the wound surface is imperative for the management of infected wounds.

14.2.1 Mycobiome

Our understanding of wound microbiome has heavily relied on improved methods of detection of microbes based on their genomic data. In this way, the study of 16S rRNA gene of bacteria by sequencing has helped in the identification of genetic diversity. However, the 16S rRNA gene amplification method is "bacteriocentric." The fungal counterpart in the microbiome is often overlooked [7]. Therefore, the mycobiome component of the "microbiome" is often lacking, though both bacteria and fungi constitute the commensal population in the skin.

Unlike previous research which has mainly focused on the bacterial flora in wounds and infections, there is emerging evidence that many human commensal fungi are also members of this microflora community. It is interesting to note that while sufficient number of research publications has targeted bacterial profiling of wounds, a negligible number of studies have focused on fungal profiling. Studies have suggested that over 25% of all DFUs consists of fungal flora that are missed by the routine diagnostic procedures [7]. One study had determined the changes in the DFU mycobiome [4]. In this study, it was found that the two most abundant species were *Cladosporium herbarum* and *Candida albicans* (*C. albicans*) both belonging to the phylum Ascomycota. A total of 17 phylotypes were identified, 10 belonged to Ascomycota filamentous fungi, which are ubiquitous in the environment and others were opportunistic pathogens like *Trichosporon* and *Rhodosporidium*. This study has also revealed that highly heterogenous mycobiome exists varying with different patients at different times. This mycobiome was more diverse in patients with systemic administration of antibiotics that selectively kill bacterial counterpart of the wound microbiome facilitating fungal growth.

Multispecies biofilm with bacteria was seen in the DFU microbiome in this study. Interestingly, the co-cultures revealed close relation between the bacterial and yeasts cells wherein the yeast cells were the "core" of the biofilm with the bacterial cells at the periphery. The hyphae of varying thickness of the yeast cells were directed outside the colony. The interactions were, however, not competitive. Additionally, *C. albicans* has been previously correlated with *Alcaligenes*. It was also reported that these hyphae help in adhesion to the surface thus providing substrate for binding for the bacteria. In this regard, the association of *C. albicans* with *Staphylococcus aureus* (*S. aureus*) whereby *S. aureus* coats itself with the secreted polysaccharides of the yeast often enhances resistance to penetration of antimicrobial agents. Similarly, *Citrobacter freundii* and *Candida* have been related for providing attachment or scaffolding [7]. The arrangement of the bacterial and fungal communities in mixed biofilms on wound surface can be visualized in Fig. 14.2.

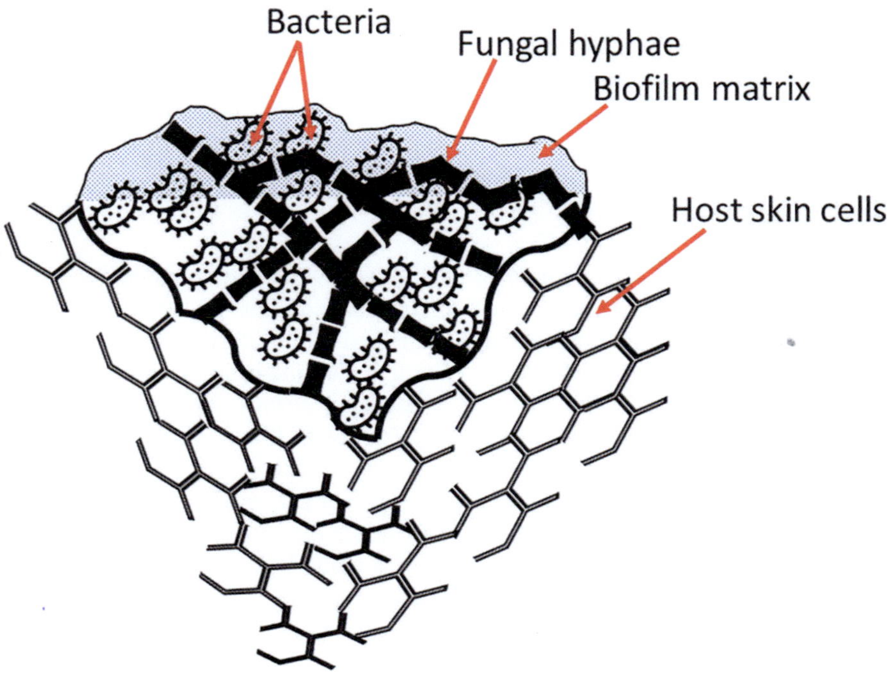

Fig. 14.2 Arrangement of the bacterial and fungal communities in mixed biofilms

When DFU mycobiome was categorized as "pathogens" and "allergens" owing to the fact that many skin commensal filamentous fungi are opportunistic pathogens or allergens, it was seen that both these groups clustered separately. Pathogens were higher in non-healing wounds. In reference to necrosis, the level of pathogens was significantly higher in ulcers with more than 75% necrotic tissues [4].

However, elucidating wound mycobiomes is challenging. In the process of molecular DNA sequencing, band analyzing, the problem is that even in reference database, adequate representation of fungal data may not be adequate for full characterization of the microbiome. In this regard, the available fungal database represents only 1.5% of the total fungal diversity [4, 7].

14.3 Fungal Infections and Ulcerations

Chronic ulcerations in the leg often represent an important health problem with most of these ulcers being related to peripheral vascular disease. *Candida* species is an otherwise harmless commensal, which if gets opportunity in form of host immunocompromised status due to malignancy, long term antibiotic therapy, use of intravenous devices and invasive traumatic injuries, causes infection [8]. *C. albicans* has been reported in 10% of cases of chronic DFU, second only to *Pseudomonas* as monomicrobial cause of infection [9]. Often *Candida* infections are the preliminary signs of prediabetic stage or stage of developing diabetes [7].

Burn wounds are often colonized with commensal yeast which later finds an opportunity to infect the wound. This colonization is usually seen after the third and fourth week. Regarding fungi, translocation from gut flora does not seem to be the source of infection. Instead, skin flora modified with the application and administration of topical and systemic agents facilitate fungal colonization. Consequently, such wounds are infected with *Candida* species in normal circumstances [10].

However, fungal wound infections (FWIs) have been an independent predictor of morbidity as revealed by multivariate analysis. Geographical locations of the injury are important in terms of etiology because the reservoir of most of the fungi is soil. Therefore, contamination of wounds with fungi like *Fusarium* species and *Apophysomyces* is likely. *Aspergillus* has been noted to be the most common cause of fatal FWIs. Infection with Mucorales takes a more aggressive course [11]. Fungi implicated in deep infections are mycetoma, sporotrichosis, chromoblastomycosis, blastomycosis, histoplasmosis, and lobomycosis [12].

Most of the wound infections following trauma due to molds have been reported from penetrating wounds in soldiers or post natural disasters, where soil contamination of wounds by molds is a pre-requisite for colonization to proceed to infection [13, 14].

Pathogens like *Candida* species, *Trichosporon*, and *Rhodotorula* have been associated with poor wound healing often leading to chronicity in wounds. Delayed wound healing is encountered with these pathogens. However, allergens like *Cladosporium*, *Aspergillus*, *Penicillium*, *Alternaria*, and *Fusarium* are also detected in abundance in wounds [7]. An extensive study from India on fungal causes of deep tissue infections in diabetic foot ulcers had revealed prevalence rates of *C. parapsilosis* (25.5%), *C. tropicalis* (22.7%), *Trichosporon asahii* (12.8%), *C. albicans* (10.6%), and *Aspergillus* species (5.0%) with considerable resistance to the azoles [15]. Clinical acumen and signs of infection help to decide the true pathogen implicated and the management regime. *Trichophyton,* which is a common cause of tinea capitis, has been reported as a rare cause of post-surgical scalp infection [16].

List of fungi that have been reportedly isolated from invasive fungal infections has been provided in Table 14.1.

Table 14.1 List of common fungal agents isolated from invasive fungal wounds

Fungal group	Agents
Mucorales	*Actinomucor* spp.
	Apophysomyces spp.
	Cunninghamella spp.
	Lichtheimia spp.
	Mucor spp.
	Rhizomucor spp.
	Rhizopus spp.
	Saksenaea spp.
	Syncephalastrum spp.
Aspergillus	*A. flavus*
	A. fumigatus
Candida spp.	*C. albicans*
	C. tropicalis
Others	*Fusarium* spp.
	Scedosporium spp.
	Alternaria
	Penicillium
	Paecilomyces
	Bipolaris

14.4 Diagnosis of Fungal Infections

For any infection, cause of infection, and ulceration in wounds, the role of prompt diagnosis in predicting the cause of the infection cannot be overemphasized. Unfortunately, in case of fungal infections, diagnostic modalities are not only limited to advanced centers, but the etiological agents are much overshadowed by their bacterial counterpart. Recently, with the emergence of fungal causes of infections, the diagnostic possibilities have also been developed. Nevertheless, the usual cause of diagnosis of FWI is non-responsive to conventional antibacterial therapy. Classical laboratory diagnosis approach is microscopy of wound culture/histopathological examination (HPE). However, suboptimal sensitivity for each method is often seen. For example, positive HPE but false negative on culture can range from 17 to 56%, whereas 11% of HPE negative samples can be culture positive [13]. Rapid assays like serum galactomannan and Beta-D-glucan can help in disseminated cases. Polymerase chain reaction (PCR) and Matrix-Assisted Laser Desorption/Ionization-Time of Flight (MALDI-ToF) can be used for exact identification [17]. However, with the latest methods, the problem of limited fungal data in the respective databases as mentioned above is the major hinderance. Diagnosis can be elaborated in the following steps:

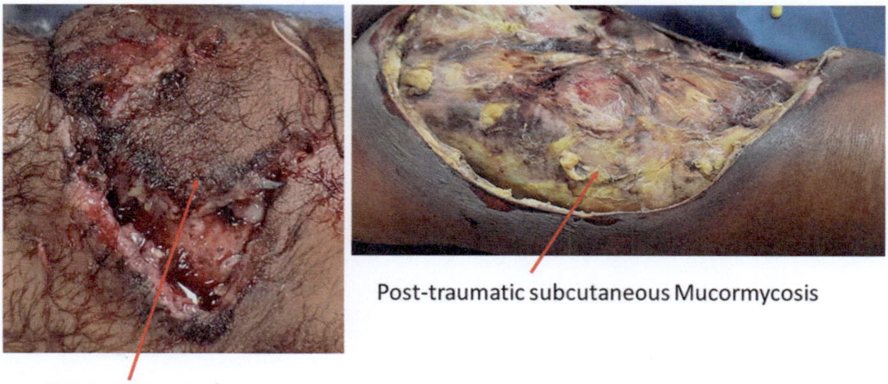

Fig. 14.3 Wounds showing blackening and non-viable tissue

14.4.1 Sample Collection

On physical examination, color changes in wound with the appearance of white clusters for *Aspergillus* or blackening (Mucor) or increase in non-viable tissue hint towards fungal infection as shown in Fig. 14.3. Relevant serial sampling might be required to elucidate the dynamic microbial flora in case of chronic wound. Patients' history including the use of empirical antifungal treatment should also be included.

14.4.2 Microscopy

Direct microscopy of wound tissue exudate can aid in early identification of fungal infection provided sample has been properly collected. The microscopic findings have been shown in Fig. 14.4. HPE of relevant tissue samples can also aid in early detection of FWIs.

14.4.3 Conventional Culture

Diagnostic culture is largely biased as only culturable microbes are presumed to be the cause of infection. This often leads to empirical use of antimicrobials and cause delay in wound healing by promoting drug-resistant strains. However, in resource limited settings, fungal culture is limited to few centers and there who performs it can provide species level identification and antifungal susceptibility testing. Culture-based methods are severely plagued with delay in diagnosis and difficulty in delineation of colonizers or contaminants from true pathogens.

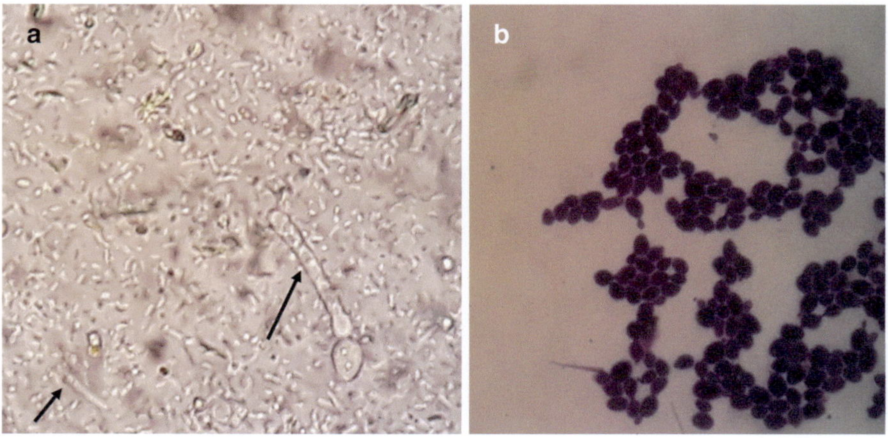

Fig. 14.4 Direct microscopy (**a**) showing fungal elements like yeast cells and pseudohyphae (40X); (**b**) budding yeast cells in gram stain (100X)

14.4.4 Nonculture-Based Techniques

14.4.4.1 Estimation of Markers

Estimation of certain cell wall fungal components like beta-D-glucan in invasive fungal infections or galactomannan in case of invasive *Aspergillosis* is often performed. These modalities lack the exact identification of the fungal agent but aid in the diagnosis of probable fungal infections.

14.4.4.2 Polymerase Chain Reaction

Molecular detection of the internal transcribe spacer (ITS) region (ITS-1 and ITS-2) of 18S rRNA by PCR can help in rapid and accurate diagnosis and is recently being used in most of the developed centers.

14.4.4.3 Metagenomics Sequencing

To study the entire mycobiome, use of whole genome shotgun sequencing provides a superior, unbiased assessment of the entire fungal flora of the wound. However, the procedure dose not delineate colonizers and pathogens. An overview of these approaches has been provided in Fig. 14.5 and Table 14.2.

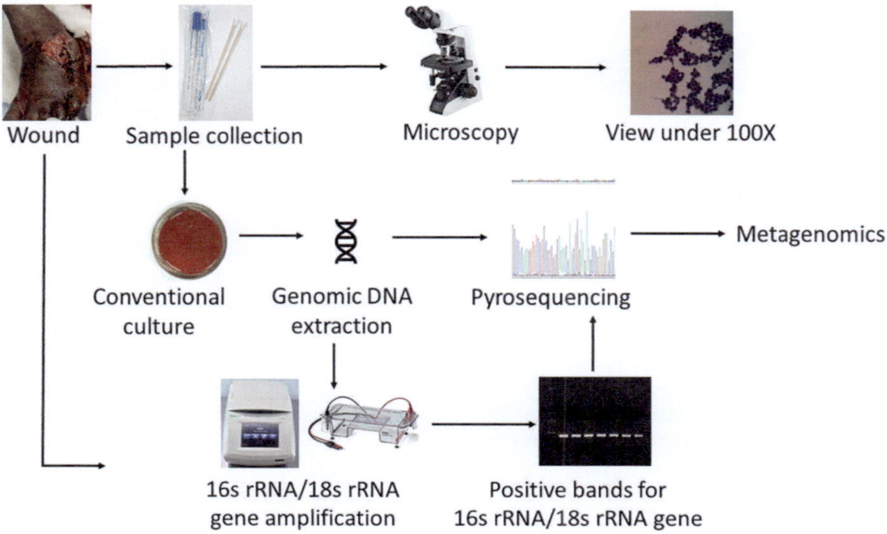

Fig. 14.5 Overview of diagnostic approaches for fungal infections

Table 14.2 Salient features of various diagnostic modalities for fungal infections

Diagnostic method	Advantages	Disadvantages
Microscopy	• Allows presumptive identification and empirical therapy	• Exact fungal identification not possible
Histology	• Allows diagnosis of invasive infections • Detects angioinvasion • Detects necrosis	• Exact fungal identification not possible
Culture	• Allows exact identification of the fungi • Allows antifungal susceptibility testing	• Poor yield in contaminated wounds • Need resources
Non-culture-based molecular methods	• Allows exact identification • Advanced methods predict entire microbiome	• Expensive • Labor intensive • Does not differentiate pathogens from colonizers

14.5 Management

Once diagnosis is achieved, prompt management is the key to successfully treating fungal infection in wounds. Management encompasses both non-medical measurements and administration of antifungal agents [14, 18, 19].

Table 14.3 Antifungal agents commonly used in fungal infections and ulcerations

Antifungal agent	Dosage	Antifungal spectrum
Amphotericin B (liposomal)	5–10 mg/kg/day intravenous	*Mucorales*, *Aspergillus*, *Fusarium* First-line therapy in mold-associated traumatic injuries
Voriconazole	Loading dose: 6 mg/kg every 12 h (first 24 h) Maintenance dose: 4 mg/kg twice daily (after 24 h) intravenous	*Aspergillus* (including *Aspergillus terreus*), *Fusarium*, and *Scedosporium* Often used in combination empirically for invasive fungal infections Not active against *Mucorales*
Posaconazole	Loading dose: 300 mg twice daily (first 24 h) Maintenance dose: 300 mg daily (after 24 h) intravenous	*Mucorales*, *Aspergillus* (including *Aspergillus terreus*), *Fusarium,* and *Scedosporium*
Isavuconazole	Loading dose: 200 mg thrice daily (first 48 h) Maintenance dose: 200 mg daily (12–24 h after the last loading dose) intravenous	*Mucorales*, *Aspergillus* (including *Aspergillus terreus*), *Fusarium,* and *Scedosporium*

14.5.1 Non-Medical Measures and Local Therapies

- Repeated and aggressive surgical debridement of necrotic materials.
- Dakin's solution: 0.025% sodium hypochlorite solution.
- Vacuum-assisted closure (VAC) therapy.
- Application of ointments Nystatin and Amphotericin B locally.

14.5.2 Medical Management

The use of antifungal agents based on the fungal etiology has been summarized in Table 14.3.

14.6 Prevention

Fungal infections and ulceration can be prevented in several ways. However, owing to their ubiquitous presence both in indoor and outdoor settings, prevention of exposure is quite challenging. Fungal elements in indoor air depend on the composition in outdoor air which is affected by geographical location as well as environmental factors like temperature, humidity, level of pollution, etc. Besides, infected pets or plants, leaking plumbing systems and heating, ventilation and air conditioning systems (HVAC) also affect the fungal composition of indoor air [16]. Strict vigilance and avoidance of exposure to these sources can prevent fungal ulcerations. Another important factor is damp living conditions, the moisture content helping in survival and persistence of fungal spores. Fungi like *Alternaria*, *Aspergillus*, *Cladosporium*, and *Rhodotorula* have been reported in moist places. In this context, "sick building syndrome" is an entity wherein contaminated building surfaces with fungal spores often lead to symptoms among the building occupants. Consequently, source tracking by swabbing probable surface reservoirs can detect potential reservoir of infection. Building materials that minimize fungal colonization should be studied and used. Lastly, prompt diagnosis, preferably prior to the transition from colonization to pathogenic state, can help in early management and prevention. The use of metagenomics to completely understand the fungal counterpart in the microbiota both in humans and in the environment can be helpful under these circumstances [20].

14.7 Conclusion and Future Directions

There have been sufficient "bacteriocentric" microbiome studies due to improved techniques of bacterial 16S rRNA gene sequencing. Similar methodologies should be applied for the fungal counterpart through extensive research. A better understanding of several interactions of the microbial communities in wounds could help in better and early management. Antifungal stewardship and the development of new antifungal agents should be targeted to prevent undue drug resistance. The future of wound management largely lies on restoring "healthy mycobiome" as early as possible based on improved understanding of resident mycobiomes and their interactions with host factors.

References

1. Stop neglecting fungi. Nat Microbiol. 2017;2:17120.
2. Gardner SE, Hillis SL, Heilmann K, Segre JA, Grice EA. The neuropathic diabetic foot ulcer microbiome is associated with clinical factors. Diabetes. 2013;62(3):923–30. https://doi.org/10.2337/db12-0771.
3. Misic AM, Gardner SE, Grice EA. The wound microbiome: modern approaches to examining the role of microorganisms in impaired chronic wound healing. Adv Wound Care (New Rochelle). 2014;3(7):502–10. https://doi.org/10.1089/wound.2012.0397.
4. Kalan L, Loesche M, Hodkinson BP, Heilmann K, Ruthel G, Gardner SE, Grice EA. Redefining the chronic-wound microbiome: fungal communities are prevalent, dynamic, and associated with delayed healing. MBio. 2016;7(5):e01058–16. https://doi.org/10.1128/mBio.01058-16.
5. Ghannoum M. Cooperative evolutionary strategy between the bacteriome and mycobiome. MBio. 2016;7(5):e01951–16. https://doi.org/10.1128/mBio.01951-16.
6. Hoarau G, Mukherjee PK, Gower-Rousseau C, Hager C, Chandra J, Retuerto MA, Neut C, Vermeire S, Clemente J, Colombel JF, Fujioka H, Poulain D, Sendid B, Ghannoum MA. Bacteriome and mycobiome interactions underscore microbial dysbiosis in familial Crohn's disease. mBio. 2016;7:e01250–16. https://doi.org/10.1128/mBio.01250-16.
7. Kalan L, Grice EA. Fungi in the wound microbiome. Adv Wound Care (New Rochelle). 2018;7(7):247–55. https://doi.org/10.1089/wound.2017.0756.
8. Jud P, Valentin T, Regauer S, Gary T, Hackl G, Rief P, Brodmann M, Hafner F. Invasive *Candida krusei* infection and Candida vasculitis of a leg ulcer in an immunocompetent patient: a case report. Int J Infect Dis. 2017;55:96–8. https://doi.org/10.1016/j.ijid.2017.01.010.

9. Banerjee T, Das A, Singh A, Bansal R, Basu S. The microflora of chronic diabetic foot ulcers based on culture and molecular examination: a descriptive study. Wound Manag Prev. 2019;65(5):16–23. https://doi.org/10.25270/wmp.2019.5.1623.
10. de Macedo JL, Santos JB. Bacterial and fungal colonization of burn wounds. Mem Inst Oswaldo Cruz. 2005;100(5):535–9. https://doi.org/10.1590/s0074-02762005000500014.
11. Pruskowski KA, Mitchell TA, Kiley JL, Wellington T, Britton GW, Cancio LC. Diagnosis and management of invasive fungal wound infections in burn patients. Eur Burn J. 2021;2:168–83. https://doi.org/10.3390/ebj2040013.
12. Sehgal VN. Leg ulcers caused by deep mycotic infection. Clin Dermatol. 1990;8(3–4):157–65.
13. Giacobbe DR, Riccardi N, Vena A, et al. Mould infections of traumatic wounds: a brief narrative review. Infect Dis Ther. 2020;9:1–15. https://doi.org/10.1007/s40121-020-00284-8.
14. Kronen R, Liang SY, Bochicchio G, Bochicchio K, Powderly WG, Spec A. Invasive fungal infections secondary to traumatic injury. Int J Infect Dis. 2017;62:102–11. https://doi.org/10.1016/j.ijid.2017.07.002.
15. Chellan G, Shivaprakash S, Karimassery Ramaiyar S, Varma AK, Varma N, Thekkeparambil Sukumaran M, Rohinivilasam Vasukutty J, Bal A, Kumar H. Spectrum and prevalence of fungi infecting deep tissues of lower-limb wounds in patients with type 2 diabetes. J Clin Microbiol. 2010;48(6):2097–102. https://doi.org/10.1128/JCM.02035-09.
16. Gaffar S, Birknes JK, Cunnion KM. Trichophyton as a rare cause of postoperative wound infection resistant to standard empiric antimicrobial therapy. Case Rep Pediatr. 2018;2018:3483685. https://doi.org/10.1155/2018/3483685.
17. Tiew PY, Mac Aogain M, Ali NABM, et al. The Mycobiome in health and disease: emerging concepts, methodologies and challenges. Mycopathologia. 2020;185:207–31. https://doi.org/10.1007/s11046-019-00413-z.
18. Lat A, Thompson GR 3rd. Update on the optimal use of voriconazole for invasive fungal infections. Infect Drug Resist. 2011;4:43–53. https://doi.org/10.2147/IDR.S12714.
19. Revankar SG. Antifungal drugs—infectious diseases—MSD manuals. https://www.msdmanuals.com/en-in/professional/infectious-diseases/fungi/antifungal-drugs#. Accessed 24 Dec 2021.
20. Johnson TR, Gómez BI, McIntyre MK, Dubick MA, Christy RJ, Nicholson SE, Burmeister DM. The cutaneous microbiome and wounds: new molecular targets to promote wound healing. Int J Mol Sci. 2018;19(9):2699. https://doi.org/10.3390/ijms19092699.

15 Covid and Ulceration

Rohit Kumar Singh and Puneet Kumar

Although the SARS-Cov-2 Corona virus primarily affects the respiratory system, causing the acute respiratory distress syndrome and pneumonia, but it can involve the other organs also including skin. COVID-19 induced illness has been coupled with various dermatologic manifestations, including rash, urticaria, retiform purpura, and vasculitis. Numerous dermal manifestations of COVID-19 occur, like lymphocytic vasculitis presenting with lesions on the toes, feet, heals, and hands occurs in COVID-19 patients. Vasculitis is a type of leukocytoclastic vasculitis with deposition of immunocomplexes. Commonly involving the children and adolescents. But none of the mechanism can explain the mechanism of ulcer formation among the COVID-19 infected patients. Moreover, pressure ulcers are a wearisome comorbidity for patients admitted with COVID-19 due to impaired perfusion and reduced mobility in patients with compromised respiratory function.

15.1 Introductions

In the year 2020, when the World Health Organization confirmed that corona virus disease 2019 to be pandemic disease. By that time most of the cities around the world had become the epicentre of the COVID-19. In the beginning of year 2020, novel corona virus named SARS-CoV-2 was recognized in Wuhan city of China. Corona virus spread very rapidly to the different geographical regions of globe,

R. Kumar Singh · P. Kumar (✉)
Department of Surgery, Institute of Medical Sciences, Banaras Hindu University, Varanasi, India

A. K. Khanna, S. K. Tiwary (eds.), *Uncommon Ulcers of the Extremities*, https://doi.org/10.1007/978-981-99-1782-2_15

causing a worldwide pandemic [1, 2]. Although the virus primarily affects the respiratory system, causing the acute respiratory distress syndrome and pneumonia, but it can involve the other organs also including skin [3, 4]. It was rapidly accepted that SARS-CoV-2 is but one of a big pool of pre-pandemic SARS-like bat corona viruses which reproduce in primary human airway epithelial cells, using human Angiotensin Converting Enzyme (ACE)2 entry receptors patients [5, 6].

Chronic ulcer wounds are not uncommon it occurs in 1–2 per 100,000 population in the western countries. Chronic wounds are usually associated with the similar comorbidities that augment the threat for mortality from Corona virus disease 2019 (COVID-19) [7]. Transmission of infection with severe acute respiratory syndrome corona virus 2 (SARS-CoV-2) is extremely contagious and its transmission among humans is extremely quick. It has a long incubation period of average 6 days during this period asymptomatic carriers can infect others. Hence, throughout the care of patients with ulcers, following appropriate safety measures is vital to lessen the risk in this susceptible population. The duty of caring both high-risk patients and health care providers by minimizing contact to SARS-CoV-2 is necessary [8, 9]. During this pandemic health care sectors have suffered a major setback, leading to major interruptions in the health care services together with the care of patients with wounds. Unavoidably the delivery of wound care and all others essential medical services have been shifted [10]. In addition, until pre-covid era device-related pressure ulcers (DRPUs) and actions to avoid them have been concerned with the consequence of device on patients. But in the COVID-19 era, stuffs have changed, and it is now the medical professionals who need help in preventing skin damage and DRPUs. A huge amount of focus has been shifted towards the effects of DRPUs during the COVID-19. By such a substantial worldwide rise in the numbers of patients requiring intensive care and the augmented use of prone positioning to manage acute respiratory distress syndrome (ARDS), the occurrence of DRPU is anticipated to increase [7, 10]. Besides, a novel and common type of DRPU coupled with the pandemic appeared within medical personnel is that of facial injuries caused by personal protective equipment (PPE). These injuries are first and foremost caused by medical face masks and goggles, even though reports are now up-and-coming of PPE-induced dermal injure in other areas together with the armpit, groin, and extremities [7].

In addition, this COVID-19 induced illness has been coupled with various dermatologic manifestations, including rash, urticaria, retiform purpura, and vasculitis. Numerous dermal manifestations of COVID-19 occur, like lymphocytic vasculitis presenting with lesions on the toes, feet, heals, and hands occurs in COVID-19 patients [11]. Vasculitis is a type of leukocytoclastic vasculitis with deposition of immunocomplexes. Commonly involving the children and adolescents. But none of the mechanism can explain the mechanism of ulcer formation among the COVID-19 infected patients. Moreover, pressure ulcers are a wearisome comorbidity for patients admitted with COVID-19 due to impaired perfusion and reduced mobility in patients with compromised respiratory function [12–14].

15.2 Risk Factors

The most important risk factors directly attributed to severe COVID-19 include immobility, hypoperfusion, and systemic coagulopathy which are also the features of critical ill COVID-19 patients [15, 16]. Among indirect risk factors that have been seen variably displayed comprise of immobility and recumbency for prolonged periods, mechanical ventilation, intensive care unit (ICU) stay, fever, incontinence poor nutrition, and faecal contamination/irritation [17]. Unlike usual condition, COVID-19 is highly contagious, especially among medical staff.

An ulcerative wound is a break of the normal constitution of the skin, likely extending further deeply, and considered as acute or chronic. Risk factors for COVID-19 in patients with chronic wounds. A nonhealing ulcerative wound is frequently a pinnacle of various underlying medical problems. Majority of the patients with ulcers have several comorbidities, for example, diabetes mellitus, hypertension, and chronic renal disease [18, 19]. These same above-mentioned risk factors place a lot of patients with chronic ulcer wounds in a high-risk group for advancing severe consequences if they get infected with COVID-19. According to the research review and the meta-analysis the most common comorbid conditions associated with the hospitalized COVID-19 patients were diabetes mellitus, hypertension, cardiovascular diseases, smoking, chronic obstructive pulmonary disease (COPD), malignancy, and chronic kidney disease [20]. Patients with these above-mentioned comorbid conditions result in poorer outcomes, so attention should be given to decrease exposure of the virus among these patients with chronic wounds. Beside the conventional risk factors for developing wounds, SARS-CoV-2 is allied with physiologic changes that may influence normal healing. If these changes encourage de novo wound growth or supplement impair healing of chronic ulcer wounds in patients having COVID-19 infection is unknown.

For patients with stage II or above pressure ulcers, the costs of medical resource increase significantly in many hospitals. Meanwhile, patients on mechanical ventilation are difficult to turn, and the risk of medical care exposure infection increases. In addition, diarrhoea is one of the common (2–49.5%) symptoms of COVID-19 and could also contribute to the occurrence of sacral pressure ulcer in ICU patients [20, 21]. The sacral pressure ulcer is also very susceptible to contamination by faeces. Unfortunately, faecal excretion persisted after sputum excretion in 23–82% patients for 1–11 days, suggesting that the faeces of COVID-19 patients are potentially infectious [22, 23]. Sacral/buttocks ulcerations in COVID-19 patients can serve as portals of entry for bacteria, leading to bacteraemia or sepsis. Thus, even if patients are successfully treated for COVID-19-associated ARDS, these ulcers can lead to additional problems prolonging hospitalization, leading to hospital readmission or even death.

Although, these changes may add to the so far augmented risk for pressure-induced skin and soft tissue ulcerative wound in patients with COVID-19 who need extended hospital admissions. Prone positioning and face masks have been associated with pressure-induced injuries among both COVID-19 patients and health care personals, respectively. During the COVID-19 pandemic across the globe sectional reported the prevalence of dermal injuries begins with the PPE use in medical workers, it was found that there are mainly three types of skin injuries [23, 24]. These were device-related pressure ulcers (DRPU, now known as pressure injuries), moisture-associated skin damage, and skin tears.

Multi-level analysis of risk factors coupled with PPE-induced skin injuries revealed higher prevalence among those with daily wearing times greater than 4 h. Various other studies carried out across the globe mentioned the adverse skin reactions among the N95 mask users, the most common of which being nasal bridge scarring followed by facial itching and skin damage. Around more than 50% of health care personnel reported dermal complications due to latex gloves. Aetiology of PPE-induced DRPUs is considered to be very comparable to aetiology of DRPUs from continuous positive airway pressure masks, used for sleep apnoea [25].

15.3 Pathophysiology

Pathophysiology of COVID-19-associated ulcer is unclear but may possibly comprise immune dysregulation, vasculitis, vessel thrombosis, or neoangiogenesis. Severe COVID-19 may define a type of microvascular injury syndrome mediated by the activation of complement pathways and an associated procoagulant state [26, 27]. Complement pathways activation and related procoagulant state has been seen in severe COVID-19 which characterize a type of microvascular injury syndrome. SARS-CoV-2 infection causes downregulation of angiotensin-converting enzyme 2 due to which cumulation of angiotensin II occurs, leading to vasoconstriction and increased vascular permeability [28, 29]. However, direct thrombogenic effects can also produce tissue ischemia. While few of the authors have reported the association of ulcerative wounds with disseminated intravascular coagulation (DIC) among the COVID-19 patients [30]. Histopathological samples taken from the skin and lung tissue from the COVID-19 infected patients revealed considerable deposits of the terminal complement components C5b-9 (membrane attack complex), C4d, and mannose binding lectin (MBL)-associated serine protease (MASP) 2 in the microvasculature along with systemic activation of the alternative and lectin-based complement pathways [31–34]. Studies over several patients have established increased risk for pulmonary embolism, high incidence of thrombosis involving multiple organs, and amputations secondary to arterial thrombosis among COVID-19 patients which support that COVID-19 is a hypercoagulable state [35].

A few studies and case reports have also mentioned the unusual clinical course of coronavirus disease 2019. Some researchers have proposed that acute limb ischemia be supposed to recognized as an unusual complication related with COVID-19.

The exact pathogenesis behind this hypercoagulable state is not entirely understood, few researchers believes that main culprit is variation in prothrombic factors, such as elevated levels of factor VIII and fibrinogen while other believes the reason behind the hypercoagulable state is the inflammatory response and cytokine storm associated with the disease [36–38]. Among several studies it is noted that some of the risk factors associated with the risk of thrombosis are of D-dimer, C-reactive protein, and co-morbidity such as hypertension. Various studies have point out towards the thrombotic complications among the COVID-19, especially venous thromboembolic events such as pulmonary emboli and deep vein thromboses [39].

However, rare but some of the studies and few case reports have mentioned the acute limb ischemia in patients with COVID-19. A study conducted in Italy on the 20 patients with acute limb ischemia with special attention on the incidence and the outcome. They found that the incidence of acute limb ischemia to be higher in the months of 2020 compared with 2019, and they credited this elevated incidence to the augmentation in the cases caused by thromboembolic disease associated with COVID-19. In conclusion, acute limb ischemia must be approved as an unusual complication coupled with COVID-19. It is essential to increase knowledge of arterial thrombosis as a potential complication of the hypercoagulable state caused by SARS-CoV-2 since timely identification is crucial for early diagnosis and treatment [40, 41].

SARS-CoV-2 is a novel enveloped, positive-sense, single-stranded RNA virus that comes under the genus Betacoronavirus. For SARS-CoV-2 virus the only receptors which is present is Angiotensin-converting enzyme 2 (ACE2) which help this virus to invade and cause infection in human. This virus mainly involves the respiratory tract, ACE2 gene expression has been seen in various human tissues, including gastrointestinal and cutaneous tissue. In recent studies on 31 Genotype-Tissue Expression human tissue, have recognized that among all organs, small intestine, testis, kidneys, heart, thyroid, and adipose tissue found to have the upmost ACE2 gene expression levels, at the same time blood, spleen, bone marrow, brain, blood vessels, and muscle found to have the lowest levels [42, 43]. Organs other than mentioned above such as lungs, colon, liver, bladder, and adrenal glands have intermediate gene expression of ACE2 in the human body. Researchers looked over the existed data sets available for (GEPIA2 and ARCHS4) to search ACE2 mRNA expression and ACE2-positive cell constitution in skin tissue. The study established that the genetic expression of ACE2 was much higher in keratinocytes than other cellular compartments in skin tissues, such as fibroblasts and melanocytes. This extensive expression of ACE2 advocate that this virus might be accountable for infecting other human tissues beside the lungs and could possibly result in further clinical manifestations. The exact pathophysiologic mechanisms involved in COVID-19 and its skin manifestations (ulcers) are unexplored still, many assumptions have been considered. Some of the studies advocated the cause to be due to an adverse reaction to pharmaceutical COVID-19 drugs or excess production of cytokines triggered by hyperinflammation. While others believe that there may be other possible molecular mechanisms like "immune dysregulation", vasculitis, vessel thrombosis, or neoangiogensis, pauci-inflammatory thrombogenic vasculopathy with extensive deposition of complement components C5b-9 and C4d within the cutaneous microvasculature [8, 44]. Other aetiology of these skin lesions could be adverse dermatological side effects to medications used for COVID-19, DIC, and macrothromboses. In less severe COVID-19 infections, these lesions are understood to be a result of microthrombi formation created by inflammatory cytokines or

ACE2 entry into cells or from "cytokine storm" due to hyperactivity of the immune system [45, 46].

In the beginning pathology studies of COVID-19 patients established diffuse alveolar damage (DAD) with oedema, hyaline membranes, and inflammation, accompanied by type II pneumocyte hyperplasia, features characteristic of typical ARDS [47, 48]. However, some patients with COVID-19 associated severe respiratory distress have a delayed onset of respiratory distress, then evident comparatively well-preserved lung mechanics, despite of the severity of hypoxemia, characterized by high respiratory compliance and high shunt fraction, and extended requisite for ventilation. Thus, major aspects of the pathology of COVID-19 may be estimated to differ from classic ARDS [27, 49, 50].

Vasculitis is an illustrative word for a broad variety of conditions marked by inflammation of the blood vessels that happens as a primary process or secondary to a fundamental disease. Occlusive vasculopathy is a separate clinical entity described by skin changes and ulceration of the lower extremities (Fig. 15.1) as a consequence of thrombosis of the small vessels of the dermis and is generally related with pre-thrombotic conditions [51].

Various microbial agents, counting bacteria, viruses, protozoa, and fungi have been marked out in association with vasculitis. The diagnosis of vasculitis is, hence, wide-ranging and aims to exclude other potential aetiologies of malignancy, autoimmune diseases, and other infections [52, 53]. Vasculopathy is related with risk factors predisposing to thrombosis. Coronaviridae are reported to be associated with thrombotic events.

Some of the authors have reported vasculitis among the corona virus positive patients. The patient has gone through wide-ranging radiological and laboratory investigations that were negative apart from positive coronavirus OC43. Even biopsy of the tissue was performed. In view of the clinical presentation and the investigations performed, the diagnosis of small vessel vasculopathy following coronavirus OC43 has been recommended by the authors [54, 55].

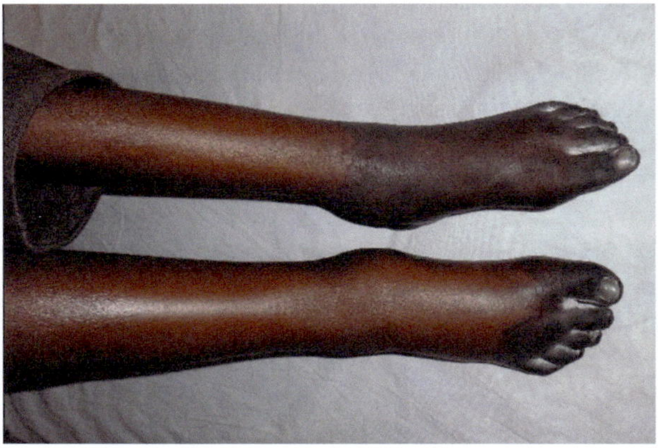

Fig. 15.1 Image of skin changes and ulceration of the lower extremities because of vasculitis in COVID-19 positive patients

Several recent studies demonstrate potential association of coronavirus OC43 with vascular pathology that the authors believe is post-immune inflammation, but the diagnosis of vasculopathy has been also suggested by experienced clinicians. Corona virus mainly involves the respiratory tract; however, there is facts relating them to systemic disease [56]. COVID-19 infection has been involved in the pathogenesis of Kawasaki disease. HCoV-OC43 and HCoV-229E were detected more often among the multiple sclerosis patients from their brain samples when compared with healthy individuals. The current COVID-19 pandemic has discovered vasculopathic activity of some coronaviruses and there is well-established evidence of COVID-19-associated vasculitis. Various viruses have well-built connection with vasculitis such as HCV, HBV, and HIV, has also been look over. However, it is difficult to say whether that rash was linked with a coronavirus OC43 infection or was related to another pathology. Two theories have been advocated for the explanation of the pathogenesis of dermal manifestations among the –COVID-19. The main pathogenesis behind dermal lesions in Covid 19, appears to be triggering of coagulative cascade pathways and the complement activation pathways with a cross link among the two [56, 57]. Unfortunately, consensus is deficient within the authors as to the pathology and pathogenesis of the skin lesions of COVID-19. Though researchers do not have diagnostic histology of vasculitis, but they believe this to be a case of small vessel vasculitis caused by coronavirus OC43 infection. Supplementary research is required to offer more strong evidence for this potential association [58]. Histological and immunohistochemistry studies delineate a blueprint of cutaneous and pulmonary pathology involving microvascular injury and thrombosis, steady with activation of the alternative pathway (AP) and lectin pathway (LP) of complement (Fig. 15.2). Co-localization of SARS-CoV-2-specific spike glycoproteins with complement components in the lung and skin was also recognized [60].

Among various dermal worries caused by PPE, DRPU/pressure injuries are the most worth mentioning. Pressure ulcer/injury is defined by the National Pressure Injury Advisory Panel (NPIAP) as “localized damage to the skin and underlying soft tissue usually over a bony prominence or related to a medical or other device” [61]. Prior to the COVID-19 pandemic, DRPU were chiefly seen in patients who were significantly ill; but this virulent disease has introduced DRPU as a novel complication resulting in facial injuries (ulcers) within health care workers wearing PPE. The PPE devices worn amongst medical personnel inducing DRPU were N95 respirators, goggles, and protective masks. In medical personnel’s PPE-induced DRPU had an, in general, prevalence of nearly 30%, the maximum among PPE-induced skin injuries. In 2019 a review study was carried out in which prevalence of non-PPE-acquired DRPU in adult patients was found to be only 11%, which is much low when compared to DRPU in medical personnel during COVID-19. The majority of PPE-induced DRPU were located on the nasal bridge and cheeks; lesser-known locations included the auricle, forehead, zygoma, mandible, and eyebrow arch. Non-PPE-acquired DRPU locations included head, face, ears, feet, neck, sacrum, and buttocks. Around more than 95% of DRPU reported in the medical staff belonged to Stage 1 and Stage 2 of pressure ulcer categories [61, 62] (Fig. 15.3).

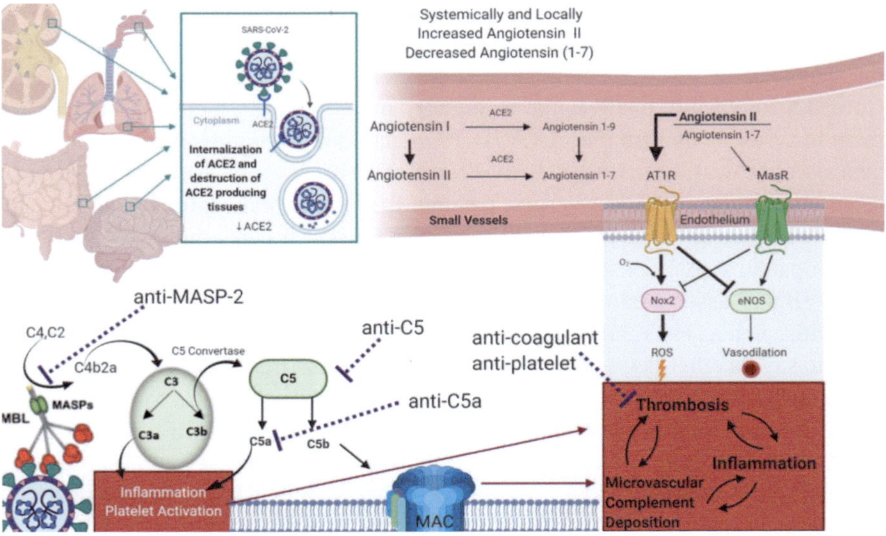

Fig. 15.2 Model for AP and LP complement activation by SARS-CoV2, and its interaction with coagulation cascades "This figure is reprinted with permission from source, Magro et al., 2020 [59]"

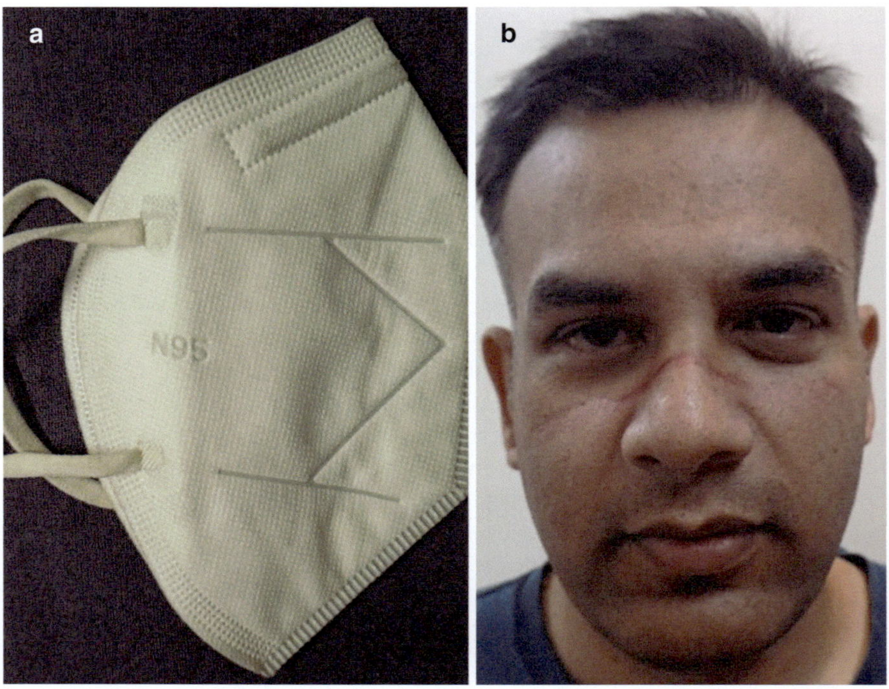

Fig. 15.3 PPE-induced pressure ulcers seen during the COVID-19 pandemic. (**a**) N95 respirator mask worn by health care professionals. (**b**) Pressure sore, secondary to N95 mask, located on the nasal bridge

15.4 Clinical Features

COVID-19's cutaneous symptoms become evident in patients of each and every age group with differing levels of severity. At present, the value of these symptoms remains comparatively unidentified by many health care personnel due to a scarcity of literature reviews [8, 12]. COVID-19 is extremely communicable, mostly due to its spread through respiratory droplets. Following an incubation period of 1–14 days, common clinical symptoms such as "fever cough, fatigue, sputum production, shortness of breath, sore throat, and headache" begin to show. In addition to these symptoms, novel symptoms like a variety of dermal manifestations have been reported worldwide. During the first wave of COVID-19 few of the studies across the globe documented dermal manifestations in the established cases of COVID-19 positive patients to be less than 1%, on the other hand, data from various other studies later on shown a much higher percentage with dermal manifestations [63, 64]. Even though disparity in prevalence, reports of dermal lesions have turn out to be even more in various age groups, collectively with children who were previously considered to be asymptomatic to the infection.

Various studies evaluated pressure ulcers in patients with COVID-19 and found that these cutaneous lesions were coupled with obesity, immobility in the setting of critical illness, incontinence, and malnutrition [65] (Fig. 15.4).

Even though some patients in these studies developed thrombotic complications of COVID-19 such as pulmonary embolism, deep vein thrombosis, and cerebrovascular accident, dermal biopsies of dependent purpura and ulcers were in favour of pressure injury rather than thrombotic vasculopathy. Even though our knowledge of the skin manifestations of COVID-19 and their primary pathophysiology is still in progress, this chapter contributes to the insufficient literature on ulcers in patients with COVID-19 [66, 67]. Although, purpuric pressure necrosis lacking thrombotic vasculopathy seems to be a common complication of COVID-19-related hospital admission.

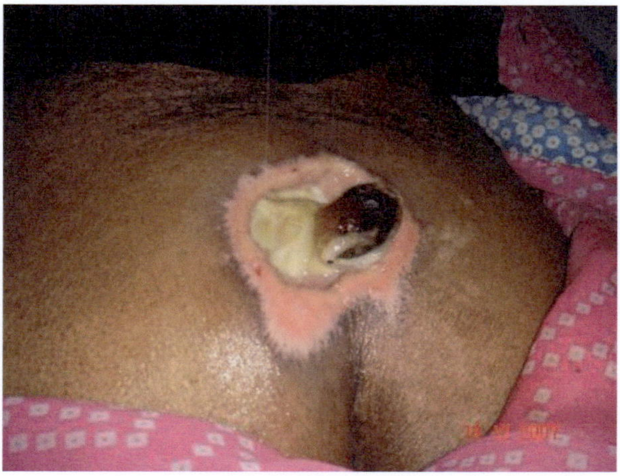

Fig. 15.4 Pressure ulcers in patient with COVID-19

Several dermatological manifestations have been coupled with COVID-19 including purpuric skin lesions such as pernio-like changes of the fingers/toes, macular purpuric rashes on the extremities, palpable purpura, and retiform purpura [11, 68]. Among the various dermatological finding Retiform purpura is common in patients with coronavirus disease 2019 (COVID-19). But recently some of the studies have reported that Retiform purpura on the buttocks can be a presenting sign of COVID-19 [69]. It has been observed that occurrence of retiform purpura, including purpuric patches on the buttocks, is mainly associated with very serious COVID-19 patients, supporting it is a poor prognostic indicator. Histopathology studies propose that thrombotic vasculopathy that causes the retiform purpura involves complement activation and platelet aggregation resistant to standard anticoagulation. Few authors also advocate that COVID-19-associated vasculopathy seems to be associated with a minimal type-I interferon immunologic response, excessive viral replication, and extensive complement activation [3, 8]. Even though complement activation has been a central reason for the vasculopathy, there is ample evidence that platelet dysfunction also acts in COVID-19 coagulopathy. Results from the key histopathological work up reveals that the biopsy specimens from pressure ulcers do not correlate with features seen in patients with retiform purpura biopsies, however, it is not clear whether histopathologic evaluation of lesional biopsy specimens can distinguish between COVID-19-associated vasculopathy and pressure-induced injury [70, 71] (Fig. 15.5).

In summary, few studies have reported the development of sacral/buttock retiform purpura on the buttocks as an ominous presenting sign of severe COVID-19. Clinicians should be extremely suspicious of COVID-19 if this cutaneous abnormality is observed among the patients. Recognition of sacral/buttocks retiform purpura and its likely connection with severe COVID-19 course may allow aggressive early treatment that minimizes end-organ damage and death. Moreover, research is required to establish the role of pressure-induced injury in sacral/buttocks (Fig. 15.6) purpura that arises after COVID-19 diagnosis and a prolonged bedbound state [72].

Additional research is necessary to establish efficient strategies for prevention and management of pressure-related injury in patients with COVID-19.

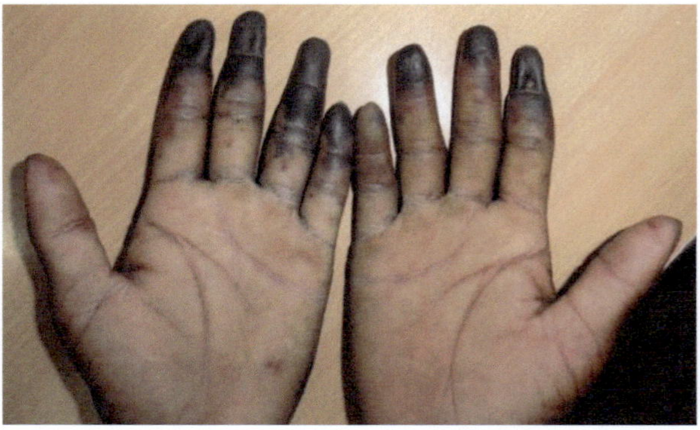

Fig. 15.5 Thrombotic ulcer in COVID-19 patient in upper limb

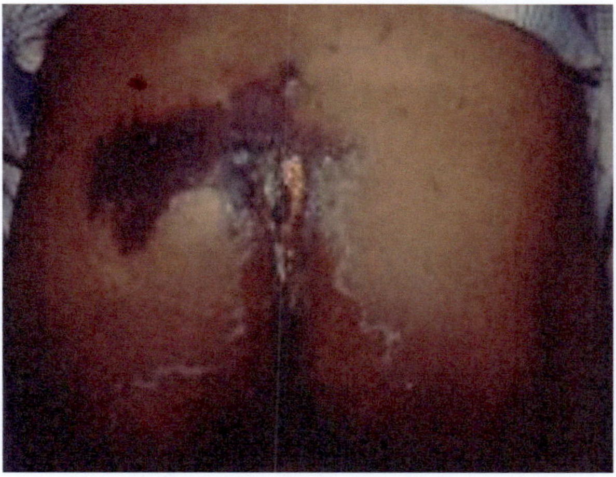

Fig. 15.6 Pressure-induced injury in sacral/buttocks of patient with COVID-19 infection

15.5 Treatment

Treatment policies differ among studies because of low number of cases reported. Some of the case series where health care workers presenting with nasal bridge pressure ulcers associated with N95 respirators, in all these cases which were, categorized as grade 1 pressure ulcers and treated with hydrocolloid dressings, while those with grade 3 pressure ulcer and treated with BETAplast [73]. Thin hydrocolloid dressing was also used as treatment in patients presenting with a grade 2 pressure ulcer on the nasal bridge. One of the groups proposed an enhanced treatment choice for health care personnel adding up of a benzalkonium chloride patch to the pressure ulcer prior to using hydrocolloid dressing and applying the N95 mask [74]. Logic following this way incorporated protection of the existing pressure ulcer, at the same time as preventing further severity of the ulcer when the patch was removed.

Other treatment recommendations for PPE-induced ulcers incorporated wet dressing to encourage wound convergence, silver ion dressings to avoid infection and secondary damage by regular dressing replacements, and epidermal growth [75].

15.6 Management

Look up fundamental contributing factors, such as antishock treatment to improve skin perfusion [69, 76–90].

- Offer pressure redistribution with correct positioning and appropriate use of pressure-reducing devices.
- Improve mobility (such as augmented physical therapy and discourage use of sedatives), avoiding excess moisture, and enhancing the nutrition.

- Reinforce the preventive education of pressure sores for medical personnel.
- Vigilant routine monitoring of the pressure ulcer, the dressing, the adjacent skin, and any potential complications.
- For stage 1, action should focus on preventive measures and wound protection. For stage 2, dressings are required to maintain a moist wound environment. For stages 3 and 4, treatment consists of available wound infection, debridement of necrotic tissue, and proper dressings.
- Medical insurance may cover partial extra payments when patients with COVID-19 in ICU develop stage 3 or 4 during the pandemic.

15.7 Complication

Potential complications arising from PPE-induced ulcers may well involve a beginning to new infections and a breach of PPE protocol leading to increased contamination. Interestingly, the introduction of viral infections other than COVID-19 or bacterial infections could lead to cutaneous manifestations of their own, mimicking those associated with COVID-19. Due to these complications, prevention of PPE-induced pressure ulcers is paramount [91]. One of the preventative methods discussed include proper PPE training; this could reinforce the proper use of an N95 respirator and discuss problems associated with extremely tight N95 mask securement. Other preventative measures include the relief of pressure build-up in N95 masks every 2 hr and the addition of prophylactic barrier creams at least 30 min before applying the respirator mask. Finally, wearing a properly fitted mask, correct goggle use, the application of moistures/gels, and management of skin indentations could help protect one from a pressure injury [62, 91].

15.8 Summary and Recommendations

- Ulcers are not uncommon and are usually associated to the similar comorbidities (e.g., diabetes mellitus, hypertension, obesity, and chronic renal disease) that augment the chances of mortality if the patient gets infected with severe acute respiratory syndrome coronavirus 2 (SARS-CoV-2). While providing the care to the patients with ulcers, it is extremely essential to supervise the proper safety measures in order to reduce the risk in this vulnerable group. The chances of spread are likely less in the home care surroundings with proper safety measures, compared with other health care settings.
- SARS-CoV-2 is allied with some physiologic changes that might influence healing process. It is not very sure if these changes encourage de novo wound development or in addition impair healing of chronic ulcers in patients infected with COVID-19. COVID-19 infected patients may present with ulcerative skin lesions as a consequence of microvascular injury. Thrombotic events (arterial thrombosis) have higher chance to occur in COVID-19 hospitalized patients.

- Timely wound care is important to prevent complications and reduce the time to healing. In order to prevent complications and short down the time to healing it is very essential that appropriate wound care should be provided to the patients at the right time. Various modifications in the delivery of wound care have happened during this COVID-19 pandemic because of disruption of wound care paradigms. Major endeavour for wound management all through the COVID-19 pandemic is to guarantee a better level of wound care at the same time restricting unnecessary in-person visits to reduce contact to the virus for both patients and health care staffs.
- Throughout the COVID-19 pandemic one of the ways to diminish the risk of COVID-19 transmission is to deliver the wound care in the home setting is promoted irrespective of the type of wound.
- Superior patients' satisfaction along with better wound care through Telehealth visits have been pointed in several studies. Many countries across the globeopted telehealth as an option to provide cost-effective and minimal resource-demanding medical care. The form of wound care adopted throughout the pandemic, which places importance on distant care, can facilitate to deal with patients in the future. Throughout this pandemic Telehealth appears to be the most supportive in evaluating the wound of the patients.

References

1. Coronavirus resource center. https://coronavirus.jhu.edu/. Accessed 28 May 2020.
2. Coronavirus disease (COVID-19) outbreak situation. World Health Organization. www.who.int/emergencies/diseases/novel-coronavirus-2019. Accessed 11 Apr 2020.
3. Freeman EE, McMahon DE, Lipoff JB, et al. The spectrum of COVID-19-associated dermatologic manifestations: an international registry of 716 patients from 31 countries. J Am Acad Dermatol. 2020;83(4):1118–29.
4. Tang J, Li B, Gong J, Li W, Yang J. Challenges in the management of critical ill COVID -19 patients with pressure ulcer. Int Wound J. 2020;17(5):1523–4.
5. Li L, Li R, Wu Z, et al. Therapeutic strategies for critically ill patients with COVID-19. Ann Intensive Care. 2020;10(1):45.
6. Girard R, Baboi L, Ayzac L, Richard JC, Guerin C, Proseva Trial Group. The impact of patient positioning on pressure ulcers in patients with severe ARDS: results from a multicentre randomised controlled trial on prone positioning. Intensive Care Med. 2014;40(3):397–403.
7. Mervis JS, Phillips TJ. Pressure ulcers: pathophysiology, epidemiology, risk factors, and presentation. J Am Acad Dermatol. 2019;81(4):881–90.
8. Magro C, Mulvey JJ, Berlin D, et al. Complement associated microvascular injury and thrombosis in the pathogenesis of severe COVID-19 infection: a report of five cases. Transl Res. 2020;220:1–13.
9. WHO Timeline-COVID-19. https://www.who.int/news-room/detail/27-04-2020-who-timeline%2D%2D-covid-19. Accessed 28 May 2020.
10. Coronavirus resource center. https://coronavirus.jhu.edu/map.html. Accessed 28 May 2020.
11. Bosch-Amate X, Giavedoni P, Podlipnik S. Retiform purpura as a dermatological sign of coronavirus disease 2019 (COVID-19) coagulopathy. J Eur Acad Dermatol Venereol. 2020;34(10):e548–9.

12. Zhao Q, Fang X, Pang Z, Zhang B, Liu H, Zhang F. COVID-19 and cutaneous manifestations: a systematic review. J Eur Acad Dermatol Venereol. 2020;34(11):2505–10.
13. Martinengo L, Olsson M, Bajpai R, et al. Prevalence of chronic wounds in the general population: systematic review and meta-analysis of observational studies. Ann Epidemiol. 2019;29:8.
14. Nussbaum SR, Carter MJ, Fife CE, et al. An economic evaluation of the impact, cost, and medicare policy implications of chronic nonhealing wounds. Value Health. 2018;21:27.
15. Galván Casas C, Català A, Carretero Hernández G, et al. Classificationof the cutaneous manifestations of COVID-19: a rapidprospective nationwide consensus study in Spain with 375cases. Br J Dermatol. 2020;183(1):71–7. https://doi.org/10.1111/bjd.19163.
16. Manalo IF, Smith MK, Cheeley J, Jacobs R. A dermatologic manifestation of COVID-19: transient livedo reticularis. J Am Acad Dermatol. 2020;83(2):700. https://doi.org/10.1016/j.jaad.2020.04.018.
17. Zhang Y, Cao W, Xiao M, et al. Clinical and coagulation characteristicsof 7 patients with critical COVID-2019 pneumoniaand acro-ischemia. Zhonghua Xue Ye Xue Za Zhi. 2020;41:E006. https://doi.org/10.3760/cma.j.issn.0253-2727.2020.0006.
18. Hicks CW, Selvarajah S, Mathioudakis N, et al. Burden of infected diabetic foot ulcers on hospital admissions and costs. Ann Vasc Surg. 2016;33:149.
19. Llamas-Velasco M, Muñoz-Hernández P, Lázaro-González J, et al. Thrombotic occlusive vasculopathy in skin biopsy from alivedoid lesion of a COVID-19 patient. Br J Dermatol. 2020;183:591. https://doi.org/10.1111/bjd.19222.
20. Magro C, Mulvey JJ, Berlin D, et al. Complement associatedmicrovascular injury and thrombosis in the pathogenesis ofsevere COVID-19 infection: a report of 5 cases. Transl Res. 2020;220:1–13.
21. Rondinelli J, Zuniga S, Kipnis P, et al. Hospital-acquired pressure injury: risk-adjusted comparisons in an integrated healthcare delivery system. Nurs Res. 2018;67(1):16–25. https://doi.org/10.1097/NNR.0000000000000258.
22. Tang J, Li B, Gong J, Li W, Yang J. Challenges in the managementof critically ill COVID-19 patients with pressure ulcer. Int Wound J. 2020;17:1523. https://doi.org/10.1111/iwj.13399.
23. Connors JM, Levy JH. COVID-19 and its implications for thrombosis and anticoagulation. Blood. 2020;135(23):2033–40. https://doi.org/10.1182/blood.2020006000.
24. Helms J, Tacquard C, Severac F, et al. High risk of thrombosisin patients with severe SARS-CoV-2 infection: a multicenter prospective cohort study. Intensive Care Med. 2020;46(6):1089–98. https://doi.org/10.1007/s00134-020-06062-x.
25. Paranjpe I, Fuster V, Lala A, et al. Association of treatment dose Anticoagulation with in-hospital survival among hospitalized patients with COVID-19. J Am Coll Cardiol. 2020;76(1):122–4. https://doi.org/10.1016/j.jacc.2020.05.001. pii: S0735–1097(20)35218–9. [Epub ahead of print].
26. Chaturvedi S, Braunstein EM, Yuan X, et al. Complement activity and complement regulatory gene mutations are associated with thrombosis in APS and CAPS. Blood. 2020;135:239. https://doi.org/10.1182/blood.2019003863.
27. Magro CM, Poe JC, Kim C, et al. Degos disease: a C5b-9/interferon-a-mediated endotheliopathy syndrome. Am J Clin Pathol. 2011;135:599–610. https://doi.org/10.1309/AJCP66QIMFARLZKI.
28. Ruffatti A, Calligaro A, Lacognata CS, et al. Insights into thepathogenesis of catastrophic antiphospholipid syndrome. A casereport of relapsing catastrophic antiphospholipid syndrome andreview of the literature on ischemic colitis. Clin Rheumatol. 2019;39:1347. https://doi.org/10.1007/s10067-019-04888-5.
29. Vaduganathan M, Vardeny O, Michel T, et al. Renin-angiotensin-aldosterone system inhibitors in patients with Covid-19. N Engl J Med. 2020;382:1653.
30. Manrique-Caballero CL, Peerapornratana S, Formeck C, DelRio-Pertuz G, Gomez Danies H, Kellum JA. Typical and atypicalhemolytic uremic syndrome in the critically ill. Crit Care Clin. 2020;36:333. https://doi.org/10.1016/j.ccc.2019.11.004.
31. Zhu N, Zhang D, Wang W, et al. A novel coronavirus from patients with pneumonia in China. N Engl J Med. 2019;382:727. https://doi.org/10.1056/NEJMoa2001017.

32. Cucinotta D, Vanelli M. WHO declares COVID-19 a pandemic. Acta Biomed. 2020;91(1):157–60. https://doi.org/10.23750/abm.v91i1.93973.
33. cdc.gov/coronavirus/2019.ncov.
34. Wang D, Hu B, Hu C, et al. Clinical characteristics of 138 hospitalized patients with 2019 Novel coronavirus-infected pneumonia in Wuhan, China. JAMA. 2020;23:1061. https://doi.org/10.1001/jama.2020.1585.
35. Tang N, Li D, Wang X, Sun Z. Abnormal coagulation parameters are associated with poor prognosis in patients with novel coronavirus pneumonia. J Thromb Haemost. 2020;18:844. https://doi.org/10.1111/jth.14768.
36. World Health Organization (WHO). WHO coronavirus disease (COVID-19) dashboard. Geneva: WHO. https://covid19.who.int/.
37. Baj J, Karakuła-Juchnowicz H, Teresiński G, et al. COVID-19: specific and non-specific clinical manifestations and symptoms: the current state of knowledge. J Clin Med. 2020;9(6):1753.
38. Cuker A, Peyvandi F. Coronavirus disease 2019 (COVID-19): hypercoagulability. Waltham, MA: UpToDate; 2020. https://www.uptodate.com/contents/coronavirus-disease-2019-covid-19-hypercoagulability.
39. Phan T. Novel coronavirus: from discovery to clinical diagnostics. Infect Genet Evol. 2020;79:104211. https://doi.org/10.1016/j.meegid.2020.104211.
40. Gralinski LE, Sheahan TP, Morrison TE, et al. Complement activation contributes to severe acute respiratory syndrome coronavirus pathogenesis. MBio. 2018;9:e01753–18.
41. Xu Z, Shi L, Wang Y, et al. Pathologic findings of COVID-19associated with acute respiratory distress syndrome. Lancet Respir Med. 2020;8:420–2.
42. Zhang H, Zhou P, Wei Y, et al. Histopathologic changes andSARS-Cov-2 immunostaining in the lung of a patient withCOVID-19. Ann Intern Med. 2020;173:324. https://doi.org/10.7326/M20-0533.
43. Zhou F, Yu T, Du R, et al. Clinical course and risk factors for mortality of adult inpatients with COVID-19 in Wuhan, China: a retrospective cohort study. Lancet. 2020;395:1054–62.
44. Magro CM, Momtahen S, Mulvey JJ, Yassin AH, Kaplan RB, Laurence JC. The role of the skin biopsy in the diagnosis of a typical hemolytic uremic syndrome. Am J Dermatopathol. 2015;37:349–59.
45. Magro CM, Pope Harman A, Klinger D, et al. Use of C4d as adiagnostic adjunct in lung allograft biopsies. Am J Transplant. 2003;3:1143–54.
46. Magro CM, Deng A, Pope-Harman A, et al. Humorally mediated post transplantation septal capillary injury syndrome as a commonform of pulmonary allograft rejection: a hypothesis. Transplantation. 2002;74:1273–80.
47. Yao XH, Li TY, He ZC, et al. A pathological report of threeCOVID-19 cases by minimally invasive autopsies. Zhonghua Bing Li Xue Za Zhi. 2020;49(5):411–7. https://doi.org/10.3760/cma.j.cn112151-20200312-00193.
48. Gattinoni L, Coppola S, Cressoni M, Busana M, Chiumello D. Covid-19 does not lead to a "typical" acute respiratory distress syndrome. Am J Respir Crit Care Med. 2020;201:1299.
49. 10.1164/rccm.202003-0817LE.
50. Chen J, Wang X, Zhang S. Findings of acute pulmonary embolism in COVID-19 patients. Lanc Infect Dis. 2020.
51. Haq SA, Pagnoux C. Infection-associated vasculitides. Int J Rheum Dis. 2019;22:109–15.
52. Teng GG, Chatham WW. Vasculitis related to viral and other microbial agents. Best Pract Res Clin Rheumatol. 2015;29:226–43.
53. Jennette JC, Falk RJ, Bacon PA, et al. 2012 revised international chapel hill consensus conference nomenclature of vasculitides. Arthritis Rheum. 2013;65:1–11.
54. Connors JM, Levy JH. Thromboinflammation and the hypercoagulability of COVID-19. J Thromb Haemost. 2020;18:1559–61.
55. Zhang Y, Xiao M, Zhang S, et al. Coagulopathy and antiphospholipid antibodies in patients with Covid-19. N Engl J Med. 2020;382:e38.

56. Ackerman AB, Boer A, Bennin B, Gottlieb G. Vasculitis: basic patterns and analysis of them in histologic diagnosis of inflammatory skin diseases. In: An algorithmic method based on pattern analysis. 3rd ed. New York: Ardor Scribendi; 2005. p. 278–88.
57. Jennette JC, Falk RJ, Bacon PA, Basu N, Cid MC, Ferrario F, et al. Revised international chapel hill consensus conference nomenclature of vasculitides. Arthritis Rheum. 2013;65:1–11.
58. Drerup C, Metze D, Ehrchen J, et al. Evidence for immunoglobulin-mediated vasculitis caused by monoclonal gammopathy in monoclonal gammopathy of unclear significance prompting oncologic treatment. JAAD Case Rep. 2019;5:288–91.
59. Magro C, Mulvey JJ, Berlin D, Nuovo G, Salvatore S, Harp J, et al. Complement associated microvascular injury and thrombosis in the pathogenesis of severe COVID-19 infection: a report of five cases. Transl Res. 2020;220:1–13. https://doi.org/10.1016/j.trsl.2020.04.007.
60. Zhu N, Zhang D, Wang W, et al. A novel coronavirus from patients with pneumonia in China, 2019. N Engl J Med. 2020;382:727–33.
61. Hu K, Fan J, Li X, Gou X, Li X, Zhou X. The adverse skin reactions of health care workers using personal protective equipment for COVID-19. Medicine (Baltimore). 2020;99:e20603.
62. Gefen A, Ousey K. Update to device-related pressure ulcers: SECURE prevention. COVID-19, face masks and skin damage. J Wound Care. 2020;29:245–59.
63. Zhou F, Yu T, Du R, et al. Clinical course and risk factors for mortality of adult inpatients with COVID-19 in Wuhan, China: a retrospective cohort study. Lancet. 2020;395:1054.
64. Lu R, Zhao X, Li J, et al. Genomic characterisation and epidemiology of 2019 novel coronavirus: implications for virus origins and receptor binding. Lancet. 2020;395:565.
65. Qian GQ, Yang NB, Ding F, et al. Epidemiologic and clinical characteristics of 91 hospitalized patients with COVID-19 in Zhejiang, China: a retrospective, multi-centre case series. QJM. 2020;113:474.
66. Bouaziz JD, Duong TA, Jachiet M, et al. Vascular skin symptoms in COVID-19: a French observational study. J Eur Acad Dermatol Venereol. 2020;34:e451.
67. Wollina U, Karadağ AS, Rowland-Payne C, et al. Cutaneous signs in COVID-19 patients: a review. Dermatol Ther. 2020;33:e13549.
68. Zhang Y, Cao W, Xiao M, et al. Clinical and coagulation characteristics of 7 patients with critical COVID-2019 pneumonia and acro-ischemia. Zhonghua Xue Ye Xue Za Zhi. 2020;41:E006.
69. Tang J, Li B, Gong J, et al. Challenges in the management of critical ill COVID-19 patients with pressure ulcer. Int Wound J. 2020;17:1523.
70. Galvan Casas C, Catala A, Carretero Hernandez G, et al. Classification of the cutaneous manifestations of COVID-19: a rapid prospective nationwide consensus study in Spain with 375 cases. Br J Dermatol. 2020;183(1):71–7.
71. Magro C, Mulvey JJ, Laurence J, et al. The differing pathophysiologiest hat underlie COVID-19 associated perniosis and thrombotic retiform purpura: a case series. Br J Dermatol. 2021;184(1):141–50.
72. Garrido Ruiz MC, Santos-Briz A, Santos-Briz A, et al. Spectrum of clinicopathologic findings in COVID-19-induced skin lesions: demonstration of direct viral infection of the endothelial cells. Am J Surg Pathol. 2021;45(3):293–303.
73. Zhou N-Y, Yang L, Dong L-Y, et al. Prevention and treatment of skin damage caused by personal protective equipment: experience of the first-line clinicians treating 2019-nCoV infection. Int J Dermatol Venereol. [Epub ahead of print]. https://doi.org/10.1097/JD9.0000000000000085.
74. Jiang Q, Song S, Zhou J, et al. The prevalence, characteristics, and prevention status of skin injury caused by personal protective equipment among medical staff in fighting COVID-19: a multicenter, cross-sectional study. Adv Wound Care (New Rochelle). 2020;9:357–64.
75. Gefen A, Ousey K. Prevention of skin damage caused by the protective equipment used to mitigate COVID-19. J Wound Care. 2020;29:311.
76. Cichowitz A, Pan WR, Ashton M. The heel: anatomy, bloodsupply, and the pathophysiology of pressure ulcers. Ann Plast Surg. 2009;62:423–9.
77. Brown KL, Phillips TJ. Nutrition and wound healing. Clin Dermatol. 2010;28:432–9.
78. Ma S, Yuan Z, Peng Y, Chen J, Li H, Luo Q, et al. Experience andsuggestion of medical practices for burns during the outbreakof COVID-19. Burns. 2020;46:749–55.

79. Hahnel E, El Genedy M, Tomova-Simitchieva T, Hauß A, Stroux A, Lechner A, et al. The effectiveness of two silicone dressingsfor sacral and heel pressure ulcer prevention comparedwith no dressings in high-risk intensive care unit patients: arandomized controlled parallel-group trial. Br J Dermatol. 2020;183:256–64.
80. Apirag C, Peerasak C, Jupaporn K. Cost-effectiveness analysisin comparing alginate silver dressing with silver zinc sulfadiazinecream in the treatment of pressure ulcers. Arch Plast Surg. 2013;40:589–96.
81. Mataro I, Lanza A, Di Franco S, Di Franco L, Sangiuolo M, Notaro M, et al. Releasing burn-ınduced compartment syndromeby enzymatic escharotomy-debridement: a case study. J Burn Care Res. 2020;41:1097–103.
82. Batra RK, Aseeja V. VAC therapy in large ınfected sacral pressureulcer grade ıv can be an alternative to flap reconstruction? Indian J Surg. 2014;76:162–4.
83. Forrester JD, Nassar AK, Maggio PM, Hawn MT. Precautions for operating room team members during the COVID-19 pandemic. J Am Coll Surg. 2020;230:1098–101.
84. Surajit B, Mishra K. Pressure ulcers: current understanding andnewer modalities of treatment. Indian J Plast Surg. 2015;48:4–16.
85. Dincer M, Doger C, Tas SS, Karakaya D. An analysis of patientsin palliative care with pressure injuries. Niger J Clin Pract. 2018;21:484–91.
86. Cox J, Schallom M. Pressure injuries in critical care: a survey ofcritical care nurses. Crit Care Nurse. 2017;37:46–55.
87. Wall BM, Mangold T, Huch KM, Corbett C, Cooke CR. Bacteremiain the chronic spinal cord injury population: risk factors for mortality. J Spinal Cord Med. 2003;26:248–53.
88. Ferrell BA, Josephson K, Norvid P, Alcorn H. Pressure ulcersamong patients admitted to home care. J Am Geriatr Soc. 2000;48:1042–7.
89. Rogers LC, Armstrong DG, Capotorto J, et al. Wound center without walls: the new model of providing care during the COVID-19 pandemic. Wounds. 2020;32:178.
90. Prachand VN, Milner R, Angelos P, et al. Medically necessary, time-sensitive procedures: scoring system to ethically and efficiently manage resource scarcity and provider risk during the COVID-19 pandemic. J Am Coll Surg. 2020;231:281.
91. Zingarelli EM, Ghiglione M, Pesce M, et al. Facial pressure ulcers in a COVID-19 50-year-old female intubated patient. Indian J Plast Surg. 2020;53:144.

16 Neuropathic Ulcers

P. Harnarayan, D. Harnanan, and V. Naraynsingh

16.1 Introduction

Neuropathic ulcers occur in areas which are subjected to increased pressures due to stress and repetitive injuries. They are seen in a foot that is typically warm, well perfused with bounding pulses in the areas of high pressure such as the plantar surface of the metatarsal heads and the heel of the foot. These ulcers arise in patients who have a neurologic deficit, typically a loss of peripheral sensation, as seen in peripheral neuropathy. The term neuropathic encompasses a broad meaning to include a lack of sensation, reduced movement, autonomic dysfunction and reduced feedback [1]. It is of necessity for clinicians to recognize the predictive conditions for neuropathic ulcer formation, allowing them to reduce or eliminate ulcers in susceptible patients. It is also important to recognize and diagnose these ulcers early and institute the appropriate treatment, since neuropathic ulcers can lead to acute infection, chronic osteomyelitis with the risk of major amputation [2].

16.2 Epidemiology

Neuropathic ulcers are most commonly found in diabetic patients and can be classified as neuro-ischaemic, ischaemic or neuropathic in nature. The lifetime risk of an ulcer in diabetes is 15% [3] with the annual population-based incidence having a range of 1.0–4.1% [4]. The prevalence has a range of 4–10%, but up to 25% patients may present with an ulcer during their lifetime [5, 6]. Over the age of 60, 7% of diabetics have foot ulceration, and in the 15–50 age group, 45–60% are neuropathic, 25–45% neuro-ischaemic and only 10% purely ischemic [7].

P. Harnarayan · D. Harnanan · V. Naraynsingh (✉)
Department of Clinical Surgical Sciences, University of the West Indies, Republic of Trinidad and Tobago

A. K. Khanna, S. K. Tiwary (eds.), *Uncommon Ulcers of the Extremities*, https://doi.org/10.1007/978-981-99-1782-2_16

Although many studies have looked at neuropathic ulcers in the diabetic foot, information in the non-diabetic neuropathic population is limited. One Australian study looked at non-diabetic foot ulcers and found that one-third of patients had a neuropathy as one of their comorbidities. The mean age of non-diabetic patients with foot ulcers was found to be higher than in diabetics. The study also found that the main aetiology of these non-diabetic neuropathic ulcers was end stage renal disease (ESRD), vitamin B12 deficiency, rheumatoid arthritis, scleroderma, gout and cerebral palsy [8].

Another Australian study confirmed the lack of information on non-diabetic foot ulcer populations generally but found that only 15% of patients in their study were non-diabetic. Foot ulcers were found to be neuropathic in 51.6% cases, neuro-ischaemic in 17.8%, ischaemic in 7.2%, postsurgical in 6.6% and 16.8% were described as "other." The most common sites were the digits of the foot (52%), the heel (25%), the plantar surface of foot (12%) and the dorsal aspect of the foot (11%) [9].

Peripheral neuropathy is the pre-existing condition that leads to neuropathic ulceration. This has a prevalence of up to 50% of diabetic patients during their lifetime [1, 10]. The incidence amongst Type 1 diabetics is 30–34% and Type II diabetes ranges from 6% to 51% (average 35–45%). As expected, it is seen at younger ages in Type I diabetes than Type II, with the incidence increasing with age [11, 12]. In terms of gender distribution, even though peripheral neuropathy is seen in both men and women, it is more common in male patients [13]. Diabetic polyneuropathy is seen more commonly in the elderly and those with long standing Type I and II diabetes [14] and appears to be less common in those of South Asian descent than in Europeans and Afro-Caribbeans [15]. However, South Asians suffer more painful diabetic neuropathy than the other population sub-types [15].

16.3 Aetiology

Systemic derangements that contribute to peripheral neuropathy include deficiencies seen in Vitamin B_1, B_6 and B_{12} together with toxins such as heavy metal poisoning, and organophosphate exposure. Excessive alcohol consumption and drugs (chemotherapeutic agents, antimicrobials and cardiovascular) have also been associated with peripheral neuropathy [16]. Endocrine and metabolic causes of peripheral neuropathy include diabetes mellitus, thyroid, renal and chronic liver diseases. Infectious diseases such as HIV, leprosy and syphilis as well as autoimmune diseases like Sjögren's syndrome have also been implicated. There are also less common causes such as the neurologic disorders Charcot-Marie-Tooth syndrome, syringomyelia and demyelinating polyneuropathy [16]. Anatomical abnormalities such as sciatic nerve compression, nerve entrapments (e.g., tarsal tunnel syndrome) and spinal cord trauma are also included. Spina bifida and meningomyelocele are the commonest causes in the childhood population.

16.4 Pathophysiology

The development of a neuropathic ulcer is a complex process [17] involving many factors but the initiating factor is a lack of the protective sensation of the plantar foot surface. Patients with deformities of the foot and those with reduced joint movements are prone to such ulcers [18]. Limited joint mobility is also thought to contribute to ulcer formation in a susceptible neuropathic foot [19]. It is thought that non-enzymatic glycosylation of the soft tissues around the joints creates a hard non-yielding surface. This predisposes to increased friction at the prominent areas of the foot during ambulation, in an area which has reduced or no sensation due to the neuropathy. The lack of ability to appreciate sensation, feel pain and then withdraw foot from a painful source, allows mechanical forces to breach the epidermal layer allowing initiation of the process of ulcer formation.

When these forces are applied to an area for long periods, a combination of local inflammation, tissue ischemia, epidermal destruction and then ulceration occur [20]. It has been shown that ulcerative areas correspond to those areas with the highest plantar pressure [21]. The combination of walking, repetitive forces and neuropathy expose the foot to high pressures and stressful forces [22]. High foot pressures and neuropathy were found to be independent risk factors for ulceration in a diabetic population [23]. In one study, peak plantar pressures were significantly higher in feet with ulcers (83.1+/−24.7 N/cm^2, range:10–125) than in control patients (62.7+/−24.4 N/cm^2, range 7.3–113.0, $p < 0.001$) [24].

In patients with peripheral neuropathy, sensory nerve injury progresses to a loss of protective sensation whilst motor nerve injury leads to deformities of the foot. Repetitive stress at high-pressure areas then cause a breach in the epidermis and dermis of the skin, causing skin ulceration which allows passage of microorganisms into the soft tissue and ultimately the bone. This gives rise to soft tissue infections, abscess formation and osteomyelitis.

16.5 Assessing Patients

16.5.1 History

The importance of the patient's medical history includes many of the facts we consider to be routine but which become critically significant when treatment is considered. The length of time they have had the ulcer, the presence of causative or contributory diseases, investigations done and treatment offered are important. Clinicians sometimes neglect to ask about the level of control of comorbidities, medicinal compliance as well as previous documented admissions to hospital or health care facility. Past surgical history including debridement, minor or major surgery are needed and any recent blood investigations should be included. A history of metabolic, endocrine, haematological or autoimmune disorders which can be linked to foot ulcer formation should be sought. Personal insight from the patient about their own observations, such as the slipping of the patient's slipper from their foot whilst walking (the Slipping slipper sign) is relevant. This is a previously undocumented marker of peripheral neuropathy [25].

16.5.2 Physical Examination

Clinical examination should include an examination of the neurological, musculo-skeletal and vascular systems. A thorough neurological examination involves the entire peripheral nerve supply including motor, sensory and autonomic nerve evaluation, since each component can ultimately give rise to deficits, which may initiate or perpetuate ulcer formation. Two-point discrimination and monofilament pinpoint testing are the basic tools required but nerve conduction studies are also useful. In specialized neuropathic foot clinics, the diagnosis depends on the finding of an inability to appreciate a 5.07 Semmes-Weinstein hair (which applies 10 g of pressure) areflexia and impaired vibration sense [26]. This is measured by an instrument termed a biothesiometer (Xilas Medical, San Antonio, Texas, USA), a hand-held device for measuring the threshold of perception of vibration sense, in neuropathies.

Modified neuropathy disability scoring, in which a structured interview and clinical examination are done by one observer, can be utilized [27]. Neuropathic signs can also be assessed using a screening tool (e.g., The Michigan Neuropathy Screening Instrument, MNSI) which visualizes a structured assessment of the patient's feet to identify various abnormalities. These include deformities, calluses, dry skin, fissures, ulcers and the presence of infection. It also includes an examination of reflexes at the ankle, and vibratory sense of the great toe. The neurological assessment is then added to nerve conduction studies to produce a score used to confirm or exclude a neuropathy [28].

The musculo-skeletal system is examined taking special note of abnormality in gait, structural deformities, the type of foot arches, presence of muscle wasting and pressure points, during a full mechanical examination. Foot pressure measurements, including peak plantar pressures, should also be recorded at this time.

Although pure ischemic ulcers are uncommon, a thorough vascular examination is carried out to exclude a neuro-ischaemic aetiology, since these are the second most common type of ulcers seen in the foot. All pulses should be palpated, compared with the contralateral side and a hand-held Doppler (HHD) should be used to auscultate the dorsalis pedis, posterior tibial and perforating peroneal arteries as an objective assessment. The ankle –brachial index (ABI) should be obtained for all three vessels, since this gives a quantitative assessment of the vascular supply, to determine if patients require further investigation by way of angiography.

16.5.3 Clinical Evaluation

The purpose of the clinical evaluation is to diagnose and confirm and the presence of a neuropathy. Laboratory investigations are essential, and those commonly requested are the full blood count, electrolytes, renal function tests, fasting glucose and haemoglobin A_1C. The special tests are the erythrocyte sedimentation rate (ESR), thyroid function tests, vitamin B_{12} levels and the specific tests for autoimmune diseases. Wound swabs and tissue sampling should also be done to confirm or exclude an infection.

The physical examination is then used in conjunction with these biochemical plasma markers and electromyoneurographic (EMG) studies. The electromyogram and nerve conduction testing (NCT) give objective evidence on muscle contractility and the speed of conduction of impulses along the peripheral nerves. Although these are commonly used in the investigation of peripheral neuropathies they are seldom, if at all, used in neuropathic ulcers [1].

16.5.4 Tissue Sampling

The specific probe to bone test allows the clinician to feel the bone in an ulcer and sometimes a loose fragment can be acquired for laboratory analysis. This was at one time considered the "gold-standard test", retrieving bone and sending for both pathological and microbiological evaluation. Recent debates have shown that the quality of reporting of both the sensitivity and specificity varies tremendously and are surprisingly, very clinician dependent. However, tissue culture remains a mainstay of diagnosis for infection in an ulcer, and this supersedes the value of wound swabs.

A punch biopsy of the skin around the ulcer, or at its edge, can be used to calculate the epidermal nerve fibre density, a test which allows diagnosis of small-fibre peripheral neuropathy objectively. The number of intra-epidermal nerves per unit area (the epidermal nerve density) remains constant through our lifetime, so a reduction is therefore clinically significant. These small fibres may give rise to small-fibre neuropathy which can occur with persistent vibratory forces (e.g., use of a jackhammer) or in chronic alcohol abuse, some types of vasculitis, amyloidosis and also patients with HIV infection.

16.5.5 Radiological Imaging

The relative value of conventional radiography, magnetic resonance imaging (MRI), computerized tomography (CT) and radio nucleotide bone scans, must be understood when evaluating a neuropathic ulcer which may not be infected. Radiographs are very useful and are the initial first line of imaging in the neuropathic foot. They show the stature of the foot, identifying areas of suspected stress points due to flexion or extension deformities. They also give views of bone demineralization with or without cortical destruction and periosteal reaction, which may be either thickening or elevation. Fat stripping and muscle atrophy which contribute to bony prominences, in addition to features of osteomyelitis are readily visualized by radiography (Fig.16.1).

Fig. 16.1 Osteomyelitis

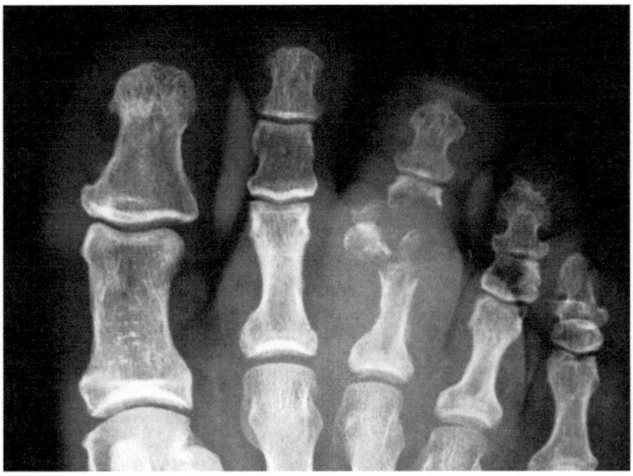

Osteomyelitis proximal phalanx -3rd toe

Computerized tomography (CT) and magnetic resonance imaging (MRI) are other imaging modalities available in evaluating neuropathic ulceration. CT scans have more sensitivity when dealing with bone, since the resolution is better than both conventional radiography and MRI. CT is especially good in detecting erosions of the cortex, periosteal reaction and small sequestra formation. However, the ability to give useful information on the state of the soft tissue is lacking.

MRI is based on showing morphologic features giving mainly structural information about the neuropathic foot. It has evolved, now using contrast agents in different phases to give much more quantitative information. Since MRI is a non-ionizing radiation, it is useful for repeat investigations in the younger population and can be used to detect soft tissue infections easily. MRI is the imaging of choice in detecting osteomyelitis (OM) and soft tissue complications of neuropathies [29, 30], and has a sensitivity of 90% and a specificity of 83% in detection of OM [31, 32].

Radionuclide scans, useful in both the diabetic foot and non-diabetic neuropathic feet, find much more use in the former. The Technetium ^{99m}Tc- MDP bone scan and the $^{111-}$Indium labelled WBC scan are quite useful in detecting infections in these ulcers. When combined, they have a sensitivity of 93% and a specificity of 83% and will show if infection in a neuropathic ulcer is localized and limited to soft tissue only or if it involves bone. This dual scan shows site and extent of OM in the neuropathic foot [26].

16.5.6 The Charcot Foot

Charcot's foot is a neuropathic arthropathy with severe bone and joint changes that accompany a peripheral neuropathy, primarily due to a loss of sensation. It is an inflammatory condition due in part to the insensate foot, leading to dislocation of joints, fracture of bones, osseous subluxation and bone remodelling.

Radiologically, there is destruction of the articular surfaces with joint debris, deformity and bony dislocation observed. Osteolysis of the distal metatarsals and phalanges can occur and it can present as ulceration of mid-foot or hind-foot.

Even though the Charcot foot is seen primarily in diabetics, it can also be seen in a variety of clinical conditions which have a sensory or autonomic neuropathy. These causes may be infective (syphilis, leprosy, HIV) neurologic (Parkinson's Disease, syringomyelia) or in patients with chronic alcoholism, those on renal dialysis or those with spinal cord injury.

16.6 Management of Neuropathic Ulcers

The management of neuropathic ulcers can be conceptualized under three main headings:

Prevention, Ulcer Healing with Maintenance and Surgery.

16.6.1 Prevention

Guidelines have recommended that persons at very low risk for ulceration be screened annually, for loss of protective sensation and peripheral artery disease and persons at higher risk would require more frequent follow-up with more aggressive surveillance. For preventing a foot ulcer, educate the at-risk patient about appropriate foot self-care and treat any pre-ulcerative sign on the foot. Instruct moderate-to-high risk patients to wear accommodative, properly fitting therapeutic footwear. Prescribe therapeutic footwear that has a demonstrated plantar pressure-relieving effect during walking, to prevent plantar foot ulcer recurrence. In patients that fail non-surgical treatment for an active or imminent ulcer, consider surgical intervention. Provide integrated foot care for high-risk patients, to prevent ulcer recurrence [33].

16.6.2 Ulcer Healing

Neuropathic ulcers require a detailed evaluation and staging of the ulcers, so as to determine how aggressive should be the management strategy. Understanding the biomechanical evaluation behind the structures at risk, help inform clinical practice guidelines, including orthotic prescriptions and modifications. This includes possible surgical intervention and reconstruction of underlying deformities to decrease plantar loading [34]. Up to 25% of patients with diabetes mellitus will develop foot ulcers in their lifetime and when these patients present, a detailed clinical evaluation would enable categorization into two main groups. Those with only neuropathic features–with or without infection and those with neuro-ischaemic features—with or without infection. Whilst neuropathic ulcers are twice as common to that of neuro-ischaemic ulcers there is a trend towards increasing vasculopathy in these patients, and as such neuro-ischaemic wounds will also require revascularization in order to achieve wound healing [35].

The depth and extent of tissue loss in addition to features of sepsis would allow for a tailored approach to achieving wound healing. Wound debridement remains the mainstay of management of wounds complicated by necrotic tissue and ascending infection. Neuropathic ulcers invariably are located over pressure points and bone prominences and as such osteomyelitis is usually one of the major features resulting in minor/major amputations. Wound debridement is performed to change the environment of chronic non-healing or septic wounds to an environment which encourages wound healing. This is done by removing abnormal tissues such as hyperkeratotic epidermis, necrotic dermal tissue, septic and nonviable connective tissue including tendons, muscle and bone. Debridement converts a stagnant non-healing wound into an active healing wound by encouraging the release of platelet derived growth factor, inhibiting proteinases and limits the action of the bacterial biofilm [36]. There are various modalities of performing wound debridement which include surgical, mechanical, enzymatic and biological. Because these wounds are neuropathic, surgical debridement can be performed with minimal discomfort (Fig. 16.2).

Once an underlying soft tissue infection is suspected, culture and sensitivity directed antibiotic therapy as well as proper wound care techniques would be required. Once osteomyelitis is suspected, the gold-standard approach for evaluation is bone biopsy with both pathology and microbiology analysis [36]. Standard techniques of encouraging wound healing by maintaining a moist wound, free of

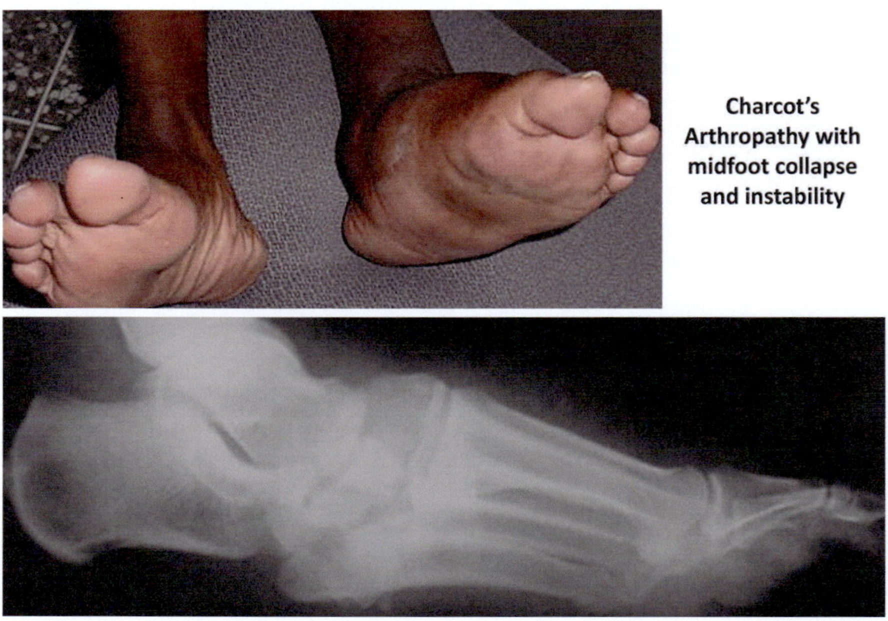

Fig. 16.2 Charcot's arthropathy

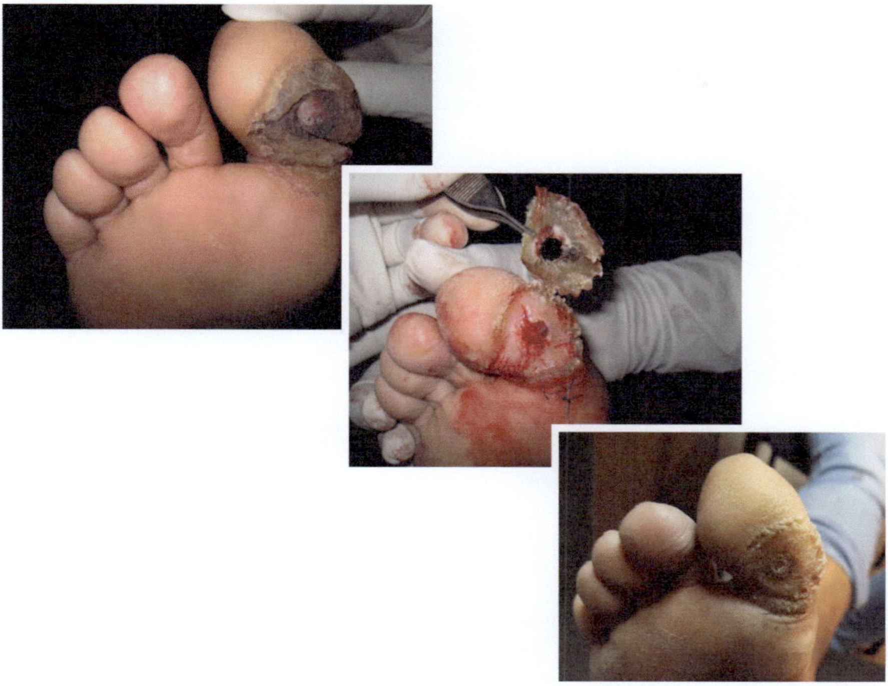

Fig. 16.3 Surgical Debridement

sepsis with a stable pH, allows time for closure of wounds. However, wounds that fail to progress as expected and do not meet the target of 50% reduction in size by 6 weeks, or non-healing by 3 months, may require advanced wound care manoeuvres. These include negative pressure wound therapy, hyperbaric oxygen therapy and ultrasonic wound debridement (Fig. 16.3).

16.6.3 Maintenance

All ulcerations should be offloaded to decrease the pressure and redistribute forces to the surrounding tissues and thus facilitate all phases of wound healing. The likelihood of wound healing is synonymous with the effectiveness of offloading and patient compliance. This has been evaluated in many studies and shown to help prevent recurrence of neuropathic ulcers, as well as promote healing in current ulcerations. Offloading treatment comes in many forms and includes total contact casting, controlled ankle motion (CAM) boot therapy, forefoot casting and wedge shoes. These are extremely important in patients with plantar wounds [37, 38]. There is strong evidence supporting non-removable devices that extend up to near-knee level, as being the primary therapy for offloading, in both forefoot and midfoot ulcerations [39]. The International Working Group on the Diabetic Foot (IWGDF) updated guidelines, for offloading the foot in patients with neuropathic ulcers,

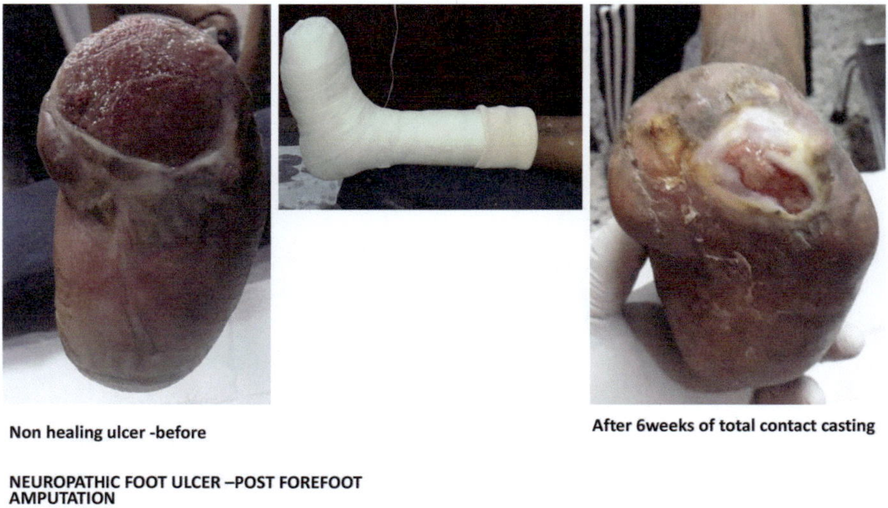

Fig. 16.4 Total Contact Casting

recommends non-removable, knee-high devices, as first-line therapy for offloading. Removable knee-high devices are considered second-line, removable ankle-high offloading are the third line, with felted foam or custom footwear, as the fourth line for offloading ulcerations [40]. Once healing has been achieved, it is crucial that a structured surveillance plan is instituted. This must include custom-made orthotics, prescription foot wear and foot hygiene, in order to prevent re-ulceration. Patients who have significant tissue loss and foot deformity, may require custom-made ankle-foot-orthoses (AFO) in order to achieve adequate long-term offloading [41] Fig. 16.4.

16.6.4 Surgery

Surgical offloading for recalcitrant plantar neuropathic ulcers is another very useful option. These are ideally suited for plantar ulcers that are located over the metatarsal heads or tips of hammer toes or in the cases of Charcot's deformities with ulcers over bony prominences. Surgical offloading can be bony offloading or tendon lengthening procedure. Bony offloading includes metatarsal osteotomy, resection arthroplasty and metatarsal head resection. Tendon lengthening procedures include Achilles tendon lengthening, gastrocnemius recession, tibialis anterior lengthening and flexor tenotomies. Whilst surgical offloading techniques have been mainly utilized for recalcitrant or recurrent neuropathic ulcers, recent data suggests that early surgical intervention results in earlier and more sustainable wound healing [42] (Figs. 16.5, 16.6 and 16.7).

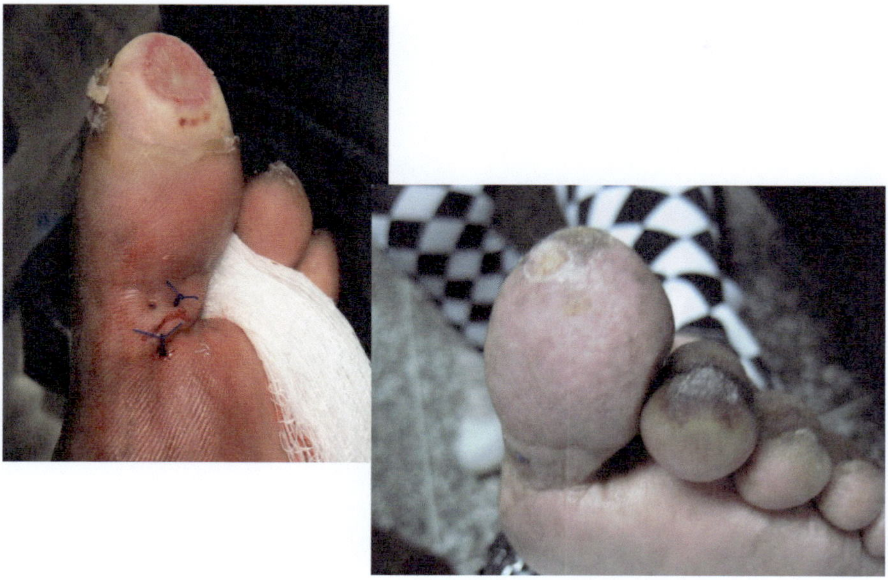

Fig. 16.5 Flexor Tenotomy

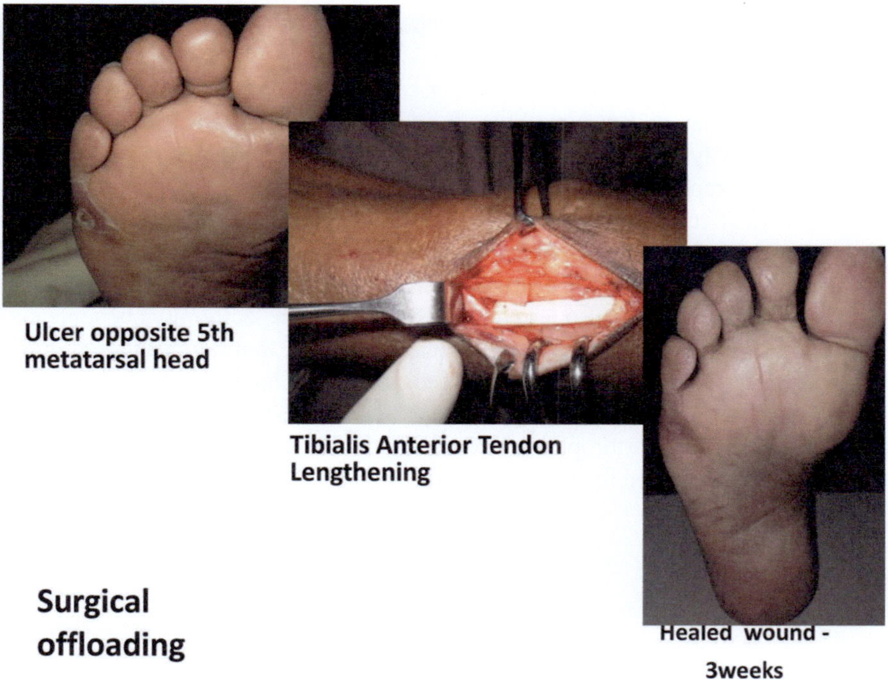

Fig. 16.6 Tibialis Anterior Lengthening

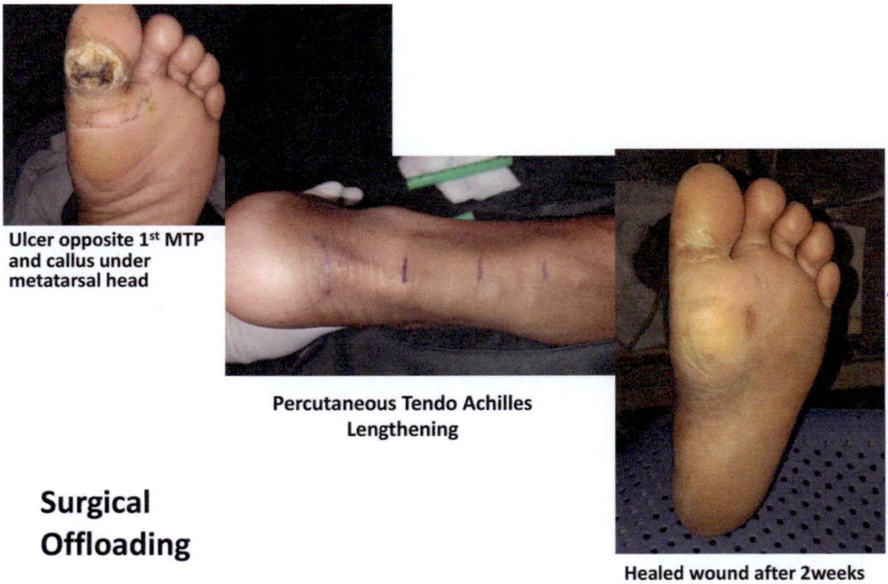

Fig. 16.7 Tendo-Achilles Lengthening

16.6.5 Treatment of Charcot's Neuroarthropathy

Charcot neuroarthropathy is a devastating complication of peripheral neuropathy especially seen in diabetes mellitus. It is synonymous with progressive, non-infectious, osteolysis-induced bone and joint destruction and is seen in patients who have sustained repeated trauma to the foot and ankle. When the ankle, mid-foot and hind-foot are affected, the talo-calcaneo-navicular complex is destroyed, leading to significant ankle instability. In its later stages, there can be complete subluxation of the ankle mortis with weight bearing diverted onto the malleoli. Collapse of the midfoot and foot arch can also lead to the "Rocker bottom" deformity phenomenon, ultimately resulting in plantar ulceration and eventually, midfoot instability. Initial management revolves around custom-made orthoses and braces, to prevent progression of the disease. However, whilst arthrodesis is the most commonly used surgical procedure, resectional arthroplasty, internal fixation, external fixation or a combination of both, can be used for treatment [43] (Fig. 16.8).

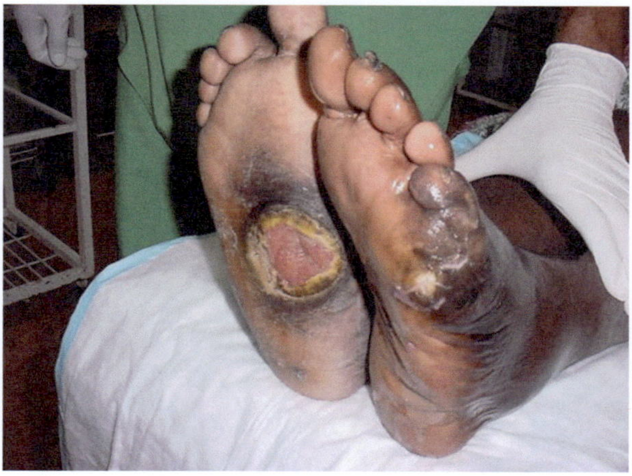

Fig. 16.8 Midfoot Plantar Ulcer due to mid-foot collapse –"Rocker bottom" foot deformity

16.7 Conclusion

In a multicentre prospective study, it was found that 17.4% of patients with diabetic foot ulcers die within 14 years, compared to 3.1% in patients without a pedal ulcer. In the diabetic foot ulcer group, the 5-year mortality rate was 22%, and the 10-year mortality rate was 71%, and about 29% of all patients underwent some form of limb amputation. Twenty-five percent of diabetic patients will develop a foot ulcer in their lifetime, and many would have either minor or major amputation. Neuropathic ulcers are twice as common as neuro-ischaemic ulcers and whilst there are other causes for neuropathic ulcers, peripheral neuropathy secondary to diabetes mellitus is by far the most common [44]. In order to prevent major limb amputation, early and aggressive management must be instituted, utilizing a multidisciplinary approach. If patients have a history of previous ulceration, peripheral vascular disease or a history of previous minor amputations, an aggressive surveillance strategy should be implemented with regular specialist physician evaluations. If patients have any diagnosis related to peripheral neuropathy, they should be seen at a minimum of once per year by their specialist, with primary care appointments more often for overall medical management. Patients' education about daily pedal examinations, whilst at home, is crucial in ensuring early recognition. The best strategy to decrease the probability of neuropathic ulcerations is vigilance and proper treatment of the underlying causes of neuropathy. Early intervention with proper offloading is the key to decreasing morbidity and mortality associated with neuropathic ulcers [45, 46] (Figs. 16.9, 16.10 and 16.11).

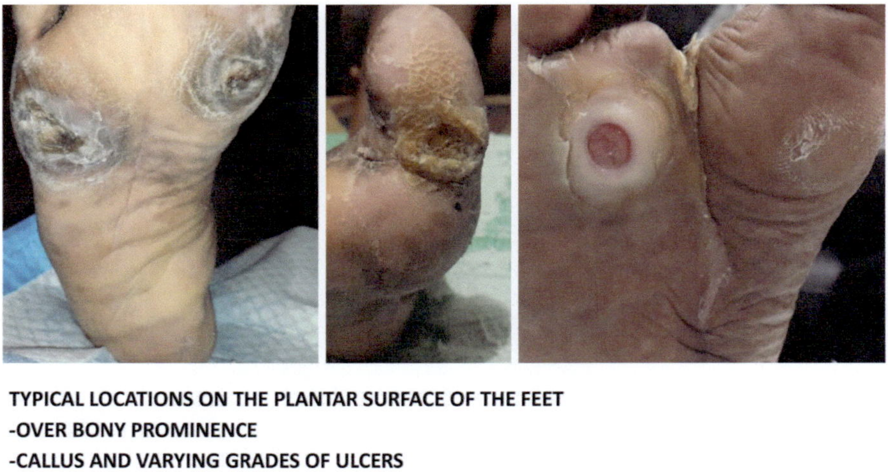

Fig. 16.9 Neuropathic Ulcers

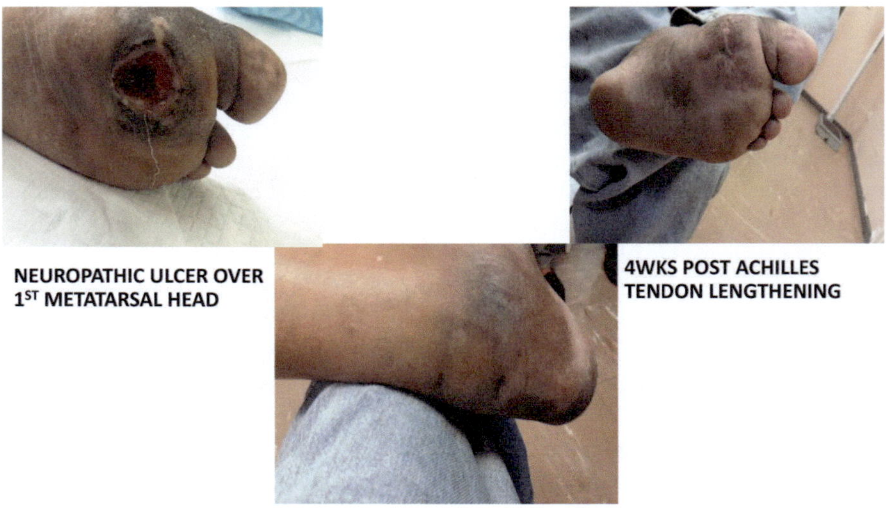

Fig. 16.10 Case of Neuropathic foot ulcer healed by Tendo-Achilles Lengthening

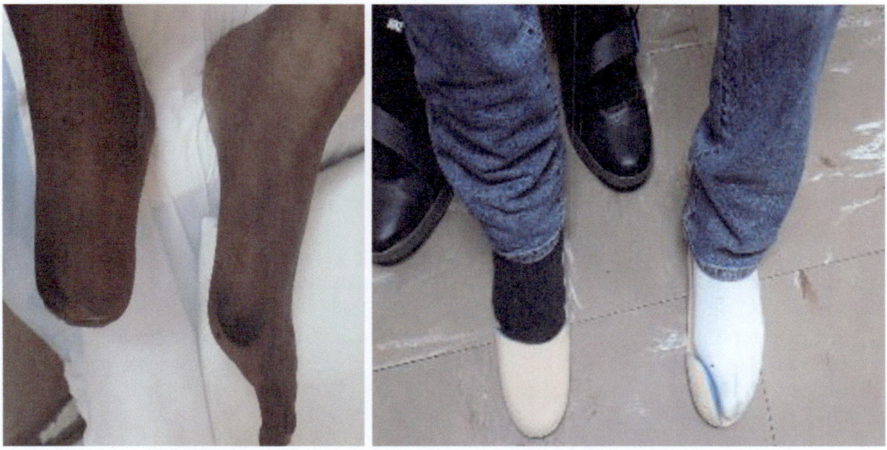

RIGHT FOREFOOT AMPUTATION
LEFT HALLUX AMPUTATION

RIGHT FOREFOOT FILLER INSOLE
LEFT HALLUX FILLER INSOLE

Fig. 16.11 Insoles for prevention of Ulcer recurrence

References

1. Eastman DM, Dreyer MA. Neuropathic ulcer. [updated 2021 Jul 27]. In: Stat Pearls [internet]. Treasure Island, FL: Stat Pearls Publishing; 2021. https://www.ncbi.nlm.nih.gov/books/NBK559214.
2. Singh N, Armstrong DG, Lipsky BA. Preventing foot ulcers in patients with diabetes. JAMA. 2005;293(2):217–28.
3. Reiber GE. The epidemiology of diabetic foot problems. Diabet Med. 1996;13(suppl 1):S6–S11.
4. Reiber GE. Epidemiology of foot ulcers and amputations in the diabetic foot. In: Bowker JH, Pfeifer MA, editors. The diabetic foot. St Louis, Mo: Mosby; 2001. p. 13–32.
5. International Working Group on the Diabetic Foot. Epidemiology of diabetic foot infections in a population-based cohort. Paper presented at: international consensus on the diabetic foot. May 22-24, 2003; Noordwijkerhout, The Netherlands.
6. Lavery LA, Armstrong DG, Wunderlich RP, Tredwell J, Boulton AJ. Diabetic foot syndrome: evaluating the prevalence and incidence of foot pathology in Mexican Americans and non-Hispanic whites from a diabetes disease management cohort. Diabetes Care. 2003;26:1435–8.
7. Harnarayan P, Ramdass M, Maharaj R, Naraynsingh V. Chapter III/3,types of ulcers of lower extremity. In: Khanna AK, Tiwary SK, editors. Ulcers of the lower extremity. Cham: Springer; 2016. https://doi.org/10.10007/978-81-322-2635-2_3.
8. Haji Zaine N, Hitos K, Vicaretti M, et al. Characteristics of non-diabetic foot ulcers in Western Sydney, Australia. J Foot Ankle Res. 2016;9:6.
9. Lazzarini PA, O'Rourke SR, Russell AW, Derhy PH, Kamp MC, d'Emden MC, Kinnear EM. Queensland's high risk foot database: tracking the length and width of Queensland's foot ulcers. J Foot Ankle Res. 2013;6(Suppl 1):O21.
10. Kumar S, Ashe HA, Parnell LN, Fernando DJ, Tsigos C, Young RJ, Ward JD, Boulton AJ. The prevalence of foot ulceration and its correlates in type 2 diabetic patients: a population-based study. Diabet Med. 1994;11(5):480–4.
11. Ismail-Beigi F, Craven T, Banerji MA, Basile J, Calles J, Cohen RM, Cuddihy R, Cushman WC, Genuth S, Grimm RH, Hamilton BP, Hoogwerf B, Karl D, Katz L, Krikorian A, O'Connor

P, Pop-Busui R, Schubart U, Simmons D, Taylor H, Thomas A, Weiss D, Hramiak I, ACCORD trial group. Effect of intensive treatment of hyperglycaemia on microvascular outcomes in type 2 diabetes: an analysis of the ACCORD randomised trial. Lancet. 2010;376(9739):419–30.

12. Duckworth W, Abraira C, Moritz T, Reda D, Emanuele N, Reaven PD, Zieve FJ, Marks J, Davis SN, Hayward R, Warren SR, Goldman S, McCarren M, Vitek ME, Henderson WG, Huang GD, Investigators VADT. Glucose control and vascular complications in veterans with type 2 diabetes. N Engl J Med. 2009;360(2):129–39.
13. Hicks CW, Selvin E. Epidemiology of peripheral neuropathy and lower extremity disease in diabetes. Curr Diab Rep. 2019;19(10):86.
14. Tovi J, Svanborg E, Nilsson BY, Engfeldt P. Diabetic neuropathy in elderly type 2 diabetic patients: effects of insulin treatment. Acta Neurol Scand. 1998;98(5):346–53.
15. Abbott CA, Malik RA, van Ross ER, Kulkarni J, Boulton AJ. Prevalence and characteristics of painful diabetic neuropathy in a large community-based diabetic population in the U.K. Diabetes Care. 2011;34(10):2220–4.
16. Mayans L, Mayans D. Causes of peripheral neuropathy: diabetes and beyond. J Fam Pract. 2015;64(12):774–83.
17. Van Damme H, Limet R. The diabetic foot. Rev Med Liege. 2005;60:516–25.
18. Moretti B, Notarnicola A, Maggio G, et al. The management of neuropathic ulcers of the foot in diabetes by shock wave therapy. BMC Musculoskelet Disord. 2009;10:54.
19. Fernando DJ, Masson EA, Veves A, Boulton AJ. Relationship of limited joint mobility to abnormal foot pressures and diabetic foot ulceration. Diabetes Care. 1991;14(1):8–11.
20. Brand PW. The diabetic foot. In: Ellenberg M, Rifkin H, editors. Diabetes mellitus, theory and practice. New York: Medical Examination Publishing; 1983. p. 803–28.
21. Duckworth T, Betts RP, Franks CI, Burke J. The measurement of pressure under the foot. Foot Ankle. 1982;3:130.
22. Boulton AJM. The importance of abnormal foot pressure and gait in causation of foot ulcers. In: Connor H, Boulton AJM, Ward JD, editors. The foot in diabetes. Chilchester: Wiley; 1987. p. 11–26.
23. Frykberg RG, Lavery LA, Pham H, Harvey C, Harkless L, Veves A. Role of neuropathy and high foot pressures in diabetic foot ulceration. Diabetes Care. 1998;21(10):1714–9.
24. Armstrong DG, Peters EJ, Athanasiou KA, Lavery LA. Is there a critical level of plantar foot pressure to identify patients at risk for neuropathic foot ulceration? J Foot Ankle Surg. 1998;37(4):303–7.
25. Teelucksingh S, Ramdass MJ, Charran A, et al. The slipping slipper sign: a marker of severe peripheral diabetic neuropathy and foot sepsis. Postgrad Med J. 2009;85:288–91.
26. Crerand S, Dolan M, Laing P, Bird M, Smith ML, Klenerman L. Diagnosis of osteomyelitis in neuropathic foot ulcers. J Bone Joint Surg Br. 1996;78(1):51–5.
27. Kumar S, Ashe HA, Parnell LN, Fernando DJ, Tsigos C, Young RJ, Ward JD, Boulton AJ. The prevalence of foot ulceration and its correlates in type 2 diabetic patients: a population-based study. Diabet Med. 1994;11(5):480.
28. Feldman EL, Stevens MJ, Thomas PK, Brown MB, Canal N, Greene DA. A practical two-step quantitative clinical and electrophysiological assessment for the diagnosis and staging of diabetic neuropathy. Diabetes Care. 1994;17:1281–9.
29. Donovan A, Schweitzer ME. Use of MR imaging in diagnosing diabetes-related pedal osteomyelitis. Radiographics. 2010;30:723–36.
30. Tan PL, Teh J. MRI of the diabetic foot: differentiation of infection from neuropathic change. Br J Radiol. 2007;80:939–48.
31. Walker EA, Beaman FD, Wessell DE, Cassidy RC, Czuczman GJ, Demertzis JL, Lenchik L, Motamedi K, Pierce JL, Sharma A, et al. Expert panel on musculoskeletal imaging. ACR appropriateness criteria® suspected osteomyelitis of the foot in patients with diabetes mellitus. J Am Coll Radiol. 2019;16:S440–50.
32. Kapoor A, Page S, Lavalley M, Gale DR, Felson DT. Magnetic resonance imaging for diagnosing foot osteomyelitis: a meta-analysis. Arch Intern Med. 2007;167:125–32.

33. Bus SA, Lavery LA, Monteiro-Soares M, Rasmussen A, Raspovic A, Sacco ICN, van Netten JJ. Guidelines on the prevention of foot ulcers in persons with diabetes (IWGDF 2019 update. International working group on the diabetic foot). Diabetes Metab Res Rev. 2020;36(Suppl 1):e3269.
34. DiLiberto FE, Baumhauer JF, Nawoczenski DA. The prevention of diabetic foot ulceration: how biomechanical research informs clinical practice. Braz J Phys Ther. 2016;20:101–5.
35. Bajaj S, Mahajan A, Grover S, Mahajan V, Goyal P, Gupta VK. Peripheral vascular disease in patients with diabetic foot ulcers. J Assoc Physicians India. 2017;65(5):14–7.
36. Lipsky BA, Berendt AR, Cornia PB, Pile JC, Peters EJ, Armstrong DG, Deery HG, Embil JM, Joseph WS, Karchmer AW, Pinzur MS, Senneville E. Infectious Diseases Society of America clinical practice guideline for the diagnosis and treatment of diabetic foot infections. Clin Infect Dis. 2012;54(12):e132–73.
37. Bus SA. The role of pressure offloading on diabetic foot ulcer healing and prevention of recurrence. Plast Reconstr Surg. 2016;138(3 Suppl):179S–87S.
38. Bus SA, van Deursen RW, Armstrong DG, Lewis JE, Caravaggi CF, Cavanagh PR. Footwear and offloading interventions to prevent and heal foot ulcers and reduce plantar pressure in patients with diabetes: a systematic review. Diabetes Metab Res Rev. 2016;32(Suppl 1):99–118.
39. Lazzarini PA, Jarl G, Gooday C, Viswanathan V, Caravaggi CF, Armstrong DG, Bus SA. Effectiveness of offloading interventions to heal foot ulcers in persons with diabetes: a systematic review. Diabetes Metab Res Rev. 2020;36(Suppl 1(Suppl 1)):e3275.
40. Bus SA, Armstrong DG, Gooday C, Jarl G, Caravaggi C, Viswanathan V, Lazzarini PA. Guidelines on offloading foot ulcers in persons with diabetes (IWGDF 2019 update). Diabetes Metab Res Rev. 2020;36(Suppl 1):e3274.
41. Bus SA, van Deursen RW, Armstrong DG, Lewis JE, Caravaggi CF, Cavanagh PR. Footwear and offloading interventions to prevent and heal foot ulcers and reduce plantar pressure in patients with diabetes: a systematic review. International working group on the diabetic foot. Diabetes Metab Res Rev. 2016;32(Suppl 1):99–118.
42. Yammine K, Assi C. Surgical offloading techniques should be used more often and earlier in treating forefoot diabetic ulcers: an evidence-based review. Int J Low Extrem Wounds. 2020;19(2):112–9.
43. Ogut T, Yontar NS. Surgical treatment options for the diabetic Charcot Hindfoot and ankle deformity. Clin Podiatr Med Surg. 2017;34(1):53–67.
44. Rastogi A, Goyal G, Kesavan R, Bal A, Bhansali A, Kumar H, Mangalanadanam, Kamath P, Jude EB, Armstrong DG. Long term Outcomes after Incident Diabetic Foot Ulcer: multicenter large cohort prospective study (EDI-FOCUS investigators) epidemiology of diabetic foot complications study. Diabetes Res Clin Pract. 2020;162:108113.
45. Andrews KL, Dyck PJ, Kavros SJ, Vella A, Kazamel M, Clark V, Litchy WJ, Dyck PJB, Lodermeier KA, Davies JL, Carter RE, Klein CJ. Plantar ulcers and neuropathic arthropathies: associated diseases, polyneuropathy correlates, and risk covariates. Adv Skin Wound Care. 2019;32(4):168–75.
46. Bartus CL, Margolis DJ. Reducing the incidence of foot ulceration and amputation in diabetes. Curr Diab Rep. 2004;4(6):413–8.

Drug Induced Ulceration of Extremities 17

Upinder Kaur

17.1 Introduction

Medications are a rare and often ignored cause of limb ulcers. It is presumed that around 1.1% of chronic leg ulcers can be caused by drugs [1]. Limb ulcers can be related to the pharmacological action of drugs or can be the manifestation of drug induced vasculitis or immunological alterations. Early suspicion of drug involvement in the induction of ulcers can result in timely intervention and can prevent considerable morbidity and mortality. Cutaneous ulcers can be observed in complicated cases of drug related immunological conditions such as Stevens-Johnson syndrome (SJS) and drug induced bullous eruptions. Though such association is well documented for some antiepileptics such as phenytoin and antimicrobials like sulphonamides, no drug is completely devoid of risk of hypersensitivity reactions. Discussion of such immunological reactions is hence beyond the scope of this chapter. The aim of the present chapter is to provide a comprehensive review on common drugs implicated in limb ulcers, the possible mechanisms of ulcer development, the phenotypic patterns of drug induced extremity ulcers, their management, and outcomes. Description of such drugs is given individually in the section below as well as in Table 17.1.

17.1.1 Hydroxyurea

Hydroxyurea, also known as hydroxycarbamide, is a hydroxylated version of urea and is used in various haematologic conditions such as chronic myeloid leukaemia, essential thrombocytosis, polycythaemia vera, sickle cell anaemia, and refractory

U. Kaur (✉)
Department of Pharmacology, Institute of Medical Sciences, Banaras Hindu University, Varanasi, UP, India

A. K. Khanna, S. K. Tiwary (eds.), *Uncommon Ulcers of the Extremities*, https://doi.org/10.1007/978-981-99-1782-2_17

Table 17.1 Common drugs implicated in limb ulcers, the associated features, HPE findings and possible mechanisms of ulcer generation

Drug	Used for	Time of onset of ulcers	Affected individuals	Location of ulcers	Associated features	HPE	Tentative mechanism / risk factor	Treatment required	Outcomes
Hydroxyurea	CML, PV, ET	5–6 years	Mainly elderly	Lower limbs (peri malleolar> feet, heel, tibia) > forearms	Disproportionate pain, xerosis, hyperpigmentation of skin, nail discoloration	Epidermal necrosis, dermal fibrosis, and perivascular infiltrates. No evidence of vasculitis or vascular thrombosis	DNA damage and direct toxicity of skin cells, megaloblastic erythrocytes impairing blood flow	Drug discontinuation and symptomatic management	Heal over weeks-months
Warfarin	DVT, PE	3–10 days	Mainly middle aged-elderly females	Fatty areas: Buttocks, thigh, breast, abdomen>distal limbs, toes	Preceded by ecchymotic patch with bluish black discoloration	Thrombosis of dermal venules. No evidence of vasculitis	High starting dose of warfarin without heparin cover. Underlying protein C deficiency/anti thrombin III deficiency/ factor V Leiden mutation precipitates thrombosis by warfarin	Drug discontinuation and alternative anticoagulants such as heparin or NOAC. Surgical debridement is often required for large ulcers	Heal over weeks-months

Heparin	DVT, PE, ACS	5–10 days	–	Injection site: Thigh, abdomen, arms Non injection site: Venous thrombosis of lower limbs	Thrombocytopenia, serum positivity for anti-heparin-PF-4 antibody	Thrombosis of dermal venules, epidermal necrosis or a type III hypersensitivity reaction in the form of vasculitis	Anti-heparin-PF-4 antibody causes platelet aggregation and thrombosis	Drug discontinuation and alternative anticoagulants such as anti-Xa agents or DTI	Heal over weeks-months
Methotrexate	Psoriasis, RA	Days-weeks in psoriasis, 3–10 years in RA	Middle aged-elderly	Lower limbs, hands, elbows, psoriatic skin	Pancytopenia and oral ulcers	–	Inhibition of DNA replication resulting in direct cytotoxicity of epidermal cells. Concomitant use of NSAIDs or steroids hastens the risk.	Drug discontinuation and symptomatic management	Heal over weeks
Propylthiouracil (PTU)	Hyperthyroidism	3–5 years	Mainly adult females	Lower limbs, upper limbs, trunk, and face	Preceded by fever, arthralgia and palpable purpura, p-ANCA and ANA positive, renal involvement common	Vasculitis and perivascular inflammatory infiltrates	Immune mediated small vessel vasculitis secondary to anti-MPO-PTU antibody	Drug discontinuation and symptomatic management. Steroids and immunomodulators such as cyclophosphamide may be required. Surgical debridement is required for large ulcers	Heal over weeks-months

(continued)

Table 17.1 (continued)

Drug	Used for	Time of onset of ulcers	Affected individuals	Location of ulcers	Associated features	HPE	Tentative mechanism / risk factor	Treatment required	Outcomes
Hydralazine	Hypertension, heart failure, PIH	3 years	Elderly females>males	Legs, feet, fingers	Vesiculopustular to ulcerative lesions. Dyspnoea, weight loss, polyarthralgia, GIT and renal involvement. P-ANCA and ANA positive, other antibodies such as anti-histone, anti-dsDNA may also be positive	Leukocytoclastic vasculitis and deposition of IgM, fibrin, and complement protein C3 in the cutaneous blood vessels	Immune mediated small vessel vasculitis secondary to anti-MPO-drug antibody	Drug discontinuation and symptomatic management. Steroids and immunomodulators such as cyclophosphamide may be required.	Heal over weeks-months
Nicorandil	Stable angina	2–4 years	Mainly elderly males	Mainly lower limbs	History of surgery or mild physical trauma may be present. Oral and perianal ulcers	–	Vascular steal phenomenon and accumulation of nicotinic acid metabolites in skin cells	Drug discontinuation and symptomatic management	Heal over weeks-months

Ergotamine	Migraine	Years	Adults	Mainly lower limbs	Claudication and paraesthesia in lower limbs, decreased to absent pulses	–	Constriction of iliac and femoral blood vessels. Cigarette smoking and adrenergic agonists hasten the risk	Drug discontinuation, vasodilators such as nifedipine, prazosin and antiplatelet drugs	Heal over weeks-months

ACS acute coronary syndrome, *ANA* antinuclear antibody, *CML* chronic myeloid leukaemia, *DNA* deoxyribonucleic acid, *DTI* direct thrombin inhibitors, *DVT* deep venous thrombosis, *ET* essential thrombocytosis, *GIT* gastrointestinal tract, *HPE* histopathologic examination, *MPO* myeloperoxidase, *NOAC* novel oral anticoagulants, *NSAIDs* non-steroidal anti-inflammatory drugs, *p-ANCA* perinuclear-anti neutrophil cytoplasmic antibody, *PE* pulmonary embolism, *PF-4* platelet factor-4, *PIH* pregnancy induced hypertension, *PV* polycythaemia vera, *RA* rheumatoid arthritis hyper eosinophilia. Given at the therapeutic dose of 500–1000 mg twice a day, the drug is known to cause mucocutaneous adverse effects (AEs) such as xerosis, hyperpigmentation of skin, discolouration of nails, and cutaneous ulcers. Numerous case reports and a large case series ($n = 41$) of hydroxyurea associated limb ulcers exist in literature [2–6]. Around 12% patients on hydroxyurea therapy may develop cutaneous ulcers [7]. Ulcers occur after years of therapy (mean time of onset ≈ 5 years) and have been reported as early as after 6 months of drug intake. Elderly are commonly affected, with no sex wise differences. Ulcers can be single or multiple and are typically located on the peri malleolar area, lower half of the anterior aspect of tibia, feet, and heel (Fig. 17.1). In rare cases, the forearm can also be involved [8]. Well demarcated margins of ulcers with surrounding erythema, cutaneous atrophy, and associated hyperpigmentation of skin are the presenting features. Severe pain out of proportion to the ulcer is another typical complaint. Ulcers can be preceded by trivial trauma such as a minor scratch and are often refractory to conservative treatment unless the drug is discontinued. Secondary bacterial infections and cellulitis may develop in undiagnosed cases [2, 3]. Histopathologic examination (HPE) of ulcer shows epidermal necrosis, dermal oedema and fibrosis, hyalinization of vessels and perivascular inflammatory infiltrates, with no evidence of vasculitis [3, 7]. Ulcers heal over a period of weeks–months with drug discontinuation and symptomatic management. Though the mechanism behind the ulcerogenic state is not fully clear, the drug is known to impair DNA synthesis thereby causing cell cycle arrest of rapidly proliferating cells such as the keratinocytes. The drug also causes megaloblastic changes in erythrocytes leading to their poor deformability, impairing cutaneous blood flow.

17.1.2 Anagrelide

Anagrelide is another drug used in the treatment of myeloproliferative disorders and thrombocythemia. The drug acts by inhibiting phosphodiesterase (PDE) and increasing c-AMP inside platelets and vascular smooth muscle cells. It interferes

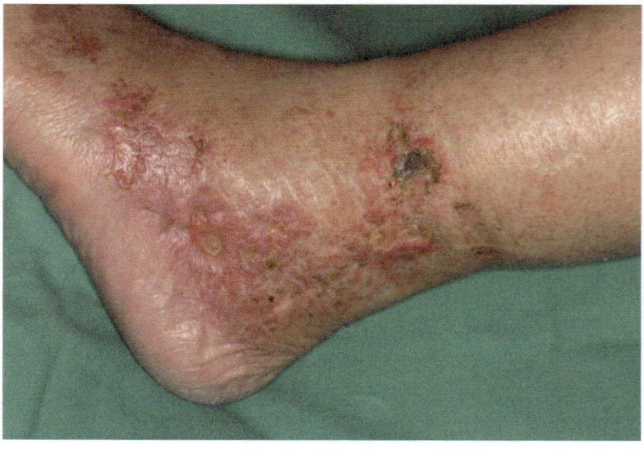

Fig. 17.1 Hydroxyurea induced lower limb ulceration

with maturation of megakaryocytes to platelets and thus decreases platelet count. Common AEs of anagrelide are related to the pharmacological action and include headache, hypotension, and tachycardia. The drug can also cause mucocutaneous AEs such as xerosis and hyperpigmentation and in rare cases, cutaneous ulcers. Ulcers are generally located on lower limbs, mainly around the lateral malleolar area and are painful [9, 10]. Time of onset varies from 6 weeks to 1 year. Ulcers are refractory to symptomatic therapy including surgical debridement and heal only following drug discontinuation. Whether pathogenesis of ulcer development is related to the thrombotic milieu of underlying disorders or is solely related to drug, needs further understanding [9, 10].

17.1.3 Warfarin

Warfarin is an oral anticoagulant used for the prevention and treatment of thromboembolic states such as deep venous thrombosis and pulmonary embolism and in the prophylaxis against stroke in patients of atrial fibrillation. Bleeding is the most common AE of the drug. Rarely, the drug can cause cutaneous disturbances in the form of dermatitis, urticaria, maculopapular lesions, and skin necrosis. The exact incidence of warfarin induced skin necrosis (WISN) is not known due to rarity of the event but is thought to affect 0.01–0.1% of drug users [11]. The condition starts within 3–10 days of warfarin intake and is common in middle aged–elderly, obese women. Individuals with deficiency of protein C, protein S, factor V Leiden mutation, antithrombin III deficiency and those with anti-phospholipid antibodies are particularly vulnerable to this disabling condition [12, 13]. Loading with high dose of warfarin without pre-treatment with heparin is another potential risk factor. Classically affected areas are the fatty regions such as of breast, abdomen, thighs, and buttocks. Penile involvement may occur in men. Uncommonly, distal parts of lower limbs and toes can be affected. WISN may start as paresthesias in the affected area followed by appearance of erythema and ecchymotic patch (Fig. 17.2). The lesion is purplish to begin with, is followed by a blue-black discolouration and often, is misdiagnosed as haematoma. Appearance of haemorrhagic bullae often leads to permanent full thickness damage of the skin and exposure of underlying muscles and tendons. HPE of lesion shows thrombosis of venules and fibrin deposits in the cutaneous vessels. Vasculitis and inflammatory infiltrates are less common. Treatment requires warfarin discontinuation and administration of systemic anticoagulants such as heparin or novel oral anticoagulants like dabigatran along with optimal wound care. Purified protein C concentrates can be given but their availability and high cost are the limiting factors. Small lesions may heal with this conservative approach, but surgical debridement and grafting is usually required for large lesions. Since benefits of drug overweigh the risk of WISN, resumption of drug at low dose may be tried in future if no alternatives are available. This should always be preceded by adequate heparin coverage [11].

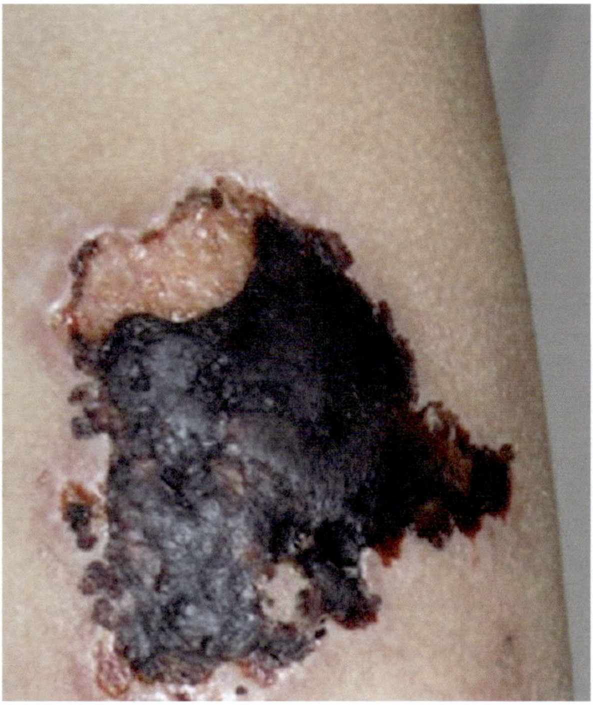

Fig. 17.2 Warfarin induced skin erythema, necrosis, and ulceration

17.1.4 Heparin

Unfractionated heparin (UFH) and low molecular weight heparin (LMWH) are systemic anticoagulants used in the prevention and treatment of venous thrombosis, in the immediate management of acute coronary syndromes and to prevent coagulation in extracorporeal circuit in patients undergoing dialysis. Bleeding is their most common AE. The drugs in rare cases can cause thrombocytopenia also known as heparin induced thrombocytopenia (HIT). Around 0.5–1% patients on UFH may be complicated by HIT and the incidence rate is further low (0.2–0.3%) with LMWH. Major morbidity in HIT is not because of thrombocytopenia but is rather accounted by thrombosis, defined better as heparin induced thrombocytopenia and thrombosis (HITT). Thrombocytopenia is usually not severe, and platelet fall below 20,000/μL is uncommon. IgG antibodies induced by heparin-platelet factor-4 (PF-4) complex activate the platelets and lead to the hypercoagulable state. Thrombosis classically develops within 5–10 days of heparin use, is common in post-surgery period and predominantly involves veins than arteries. Local skin sites such as of abdomen, thigh, and arms are usually affected. Lesions can be erythematous to begin with and can be necrotizing to non-necrotizing. Involvement of distant sites is not uncommon. Fatalities due to stroke and myocardial infarction can occur in missed cases. Bilateral deep venous thrombosis developing during heparin therapy is a strong clue towards the development of HITT and if undiagnosed leads to potential sequelae in the form of venous gangrenes. Splanchnic, cerebral, and adrenal veins are some other atypical sites involved in HITT. Diagnosis of HITT is mainly clinical and supported by four Ts (Thrombocytopenia, thrombosis, timing, and other causes ruled out). Anti-heparin-PF-4 antibody is present in majority of cases. In the event of suspicion of HITT, heparin should be discontinued, and alternative anticoagulants should be initiated for the treatment of thrombus and prevention of its progression. Direct thrombin inhibitors such as bivalirudin and dabigatran, and anti-Xa agents such as fondaparinux are preferred in this setting. Other emerging therapies include oral factor Xa inhibitors such as rivaroxaban and apixaban. Warfarin can also be given but its use should be preceded by direct thrombin inhibitors as possible aggravation of skin necrosis can occur in undiagnosed protein C deficiency states. HPE of skin lesions may show epidermal necrosis, thrombosis of dermal vessels or features of type III hypersensitivity reaction such as vasculitis, induced by heparin-PF4-antibody immune complexes. In the event of occurrence of HITT, reinstitution of heparin in future can be allowed for short term such as to cover the peri-operative need, if platelet activating antibodies are undetectable in serum. This should be followed by careful clinical monitoring as well as monitoring of platelet count for at least 10 days post-last dose of heparin as possibility of occurrence of delayed HITT exists [14–16].

17.1.5 Ergot Compounds

Ergot compounds such as ergotamine and ergotoxine are used in the treatment of migraine attacks. The compounds act as partial agonist at adrenergic α and serotonergic receptors resulting in vasoconstriction. Claviceps purpurea, a fungus growing on grains such as rye is the source of natural ergot compounds. Attacks of ergot poisoning or "ergotism" in the form of limb gangrenes and convulsions were witnessed in the Middle Ages with some reports occurring in the nineteenth century and few in 1950s in France. Following the association of fungus with these symptoms, cases of ergotism have declined. Rare cases of ergot compound toxicity in the form of limb ischaemia and ulcers over the lower limbs are reported with ergotamine intake [17]. Chronic consumption of ergotamine over years for migraine attacks is a consistent feature in these reports. In sensitive individuals, however, dose as low as 2 mg can provoke significant ischaemia [17–19]. Constriction of iliac and femoral blood vessels is evident in early phases, followed by more severe involvement of distal blood vessels. Cases resolve with discontinuation of ergot preparation and administration of vasodilators such as prazosin and nifedipine, and antiplatelet drugs such as aspirin.

17.1.6 Methotrexate

Methotrexate associated skin ulcers were described initially in patients of psoriasis. Ulcers can involve the psoriatic skin or can arise de novo over the uninvolved skin. The dose of methotrexate has varied from 7.5 mg–25 mg/week in reported cases.

When involving the psoriatic skin, ulcers arise usually within days-weeks of start of therapy while the time of onset is variable when non psoriatic skin is involved. Ulcers heal successfully within weeks of drug discontinuation [20].

Cutaneous ulcers with methotrexate have also been reported in nonpsoriatic conditions such as rheumatoid arthritis (RA) particularly in old age patients. The onset of ulcers is often delayed, varying from 3–10 years of therapy [21, 22]. Lower limbs, hand, and elbows are the typical sites involved. Patients may have concomitant oral ulcers and pancytopenia and may have other contributory conditions such as diabetes, cardiovascular diseases, renal insufficiency, and haematological malignancies. The development of ulcers is hastened with concomitant intake of steroids, biologicals, and non-steroidal anti-inflammatory drugs (NSAIDs) [21]. Foot ulcers as early as within days have been reported with a low 5 mg dose of methotrexate consumed erroneously on daily basis [23]. Treatment requires drug discontinuation and symptomatic management, and significant healing occurs over weeks. The mechanism of ulcer induction by methotrexate has been hypothesized to be related to the pharmacological inhibition of folate synthesis and DNA replication. Rapidly proliferating cells such as of skin are consequently affected resulting in cutaneous atrophy and ulceration.

17.1.7 Leflunomide

Leflunomide is another dug with disease modifying roles in immune conditions such as RA and psoriasis. Diarrhoea and liver toxicity are its common AEs. Mucocutaneous adverse effects such as rashes and alopecia are also not uncommon. Cutaneous ulcers on lower limbs and forearms have been reported mainly in elderly females after months of therapy with leflunomide. The drug inhibits dihydroorotate dehydrogenase enzyme involved in pyrimidine synthesis as well as blunts the action of growth factors such as epidermal derived growth factor (EDGF). Both mechanisms can explain the ulcerogenic potential of drug. HPE done in limited cases has shown evidence of inflammation in dermis and subcutaneous tissue with necrosis of collagen fibres and presence of granulation tissue. Granulomas with giant cells may also be seen. Following drug discontinuation, healing starts, albeit slowly and full healing may require a span of 8–18 months. Leflunomide has active metabolite with a long t-half of 1–4 weeks. The drug activity may last for months, explaining the delayed healing process [24, 25].

17.1.8 Sedative Use and Limb Ulcers

Sedatives such as members of barbiturate class, benzodiazepines, Z- compounds like zolpidem, antihistaminics like diphenhydramine, and other drugs with sedative action such as opioids, all have been linked with ulcers on the lower limbs. Ulcers are generally of pressure ulcer type and located on the lower back or interior aspects of knees. In one study, nearly 45% elderly patients with pressure ulcers were using sedative drugs. Furthermore, the risk of severe ulceration was observed to be five times higher in patients using sedatives versus those not using sedatives [26].

Opioid abuse: Opioids such as pentazocine have been linked with cutaneous ulcers [27, 28]. Ankles, tibial sites, and cubital fossa are the typical sites involved and the time of onset can vary from 10 days to years of drug abuse. Ulcers start with bullous lesion and upon rupture expose deeper tissues such as muscles. Ulcers have a necrotic base, hyperpigmented margins, and surrounded by indurated skin. Thrombophlebitis, multiple scars, and venous sclerosis may also be evident. Other associated features include non-pitting oedema of hands and feet, typically known as the puffy hand syndrome and muscle contractures. HPE findings include epidermal necrosis, perivascular infiltrates of neutrophils and lymphocytes in dermis, vasculitis, and neutrophilic abscesses. Typical location of ulcers at easily accessible sites, difficulty in accessing the peripheral veins, presence of hand oedema and muscle contractures are some of the potential clues of pentazocine abuse leading to ulcers. Urinary pentazocine screening should be done but can be negative if patient has not taken the drug recently. Though conservative management has been tried successfully by some, excision followed by grafting is required in majority of the cases [27]. Drug discontinuation should be done cautiously with vigilance for withdrawal features. Psychiatry referral should be done for counselling and de-addiction therapies.

17.1.9 Propylthiouracil

Propylthiouracil is used in the management of hyperthyroidism. Common AEs of this drug include hepatitis and cutaneous reactions. A characteristic but uncommon AE is agranulocytosis. In rare cases (<1/10000), the drug is known to cause vasculitis [29]. Case reports of pyoderma gangrenosum also exist with PTU [30]. Vasculitis occurs predominantly in females (F/M: 8/1) and after years of therapy (median duration of therapy≈ 42 months). Systemic symptoms such as fever, rash, and arthralgia are the initial manifestations. Rash starts as palpable purpura and patchy lesions (Fig. 17.3). Gradually, full thickness of skin is involved, lesions become necrotic and widespread. Common sites are lower limbs and upper limbs. Trunk and face may also be affected. Patients usually test positive for perinuclear-anti neutrophilic cytoplasmic antibodies (p-ANCA) and antinuclear antibodies (ANA). Concomitant renal involvement is seen in more than 50% of cases. HPE of ulcers shows evidence of vasculitis and perivascular inflammatory infiltrates. Significant recovery occurs with drug discontinuation and administration of steroids with or without immunomodulators. Large ulcers may necessitate surgical debridement and grafting. Nearly 8–9% patients may succumb to the disease because of renal involvement and sepsis [29]. A high index of suspicion for vasculitis should be kept in patients on PTU developing early signs of cutaneous involvement. In the event of vasculitis, the drug should never be reintroduced.

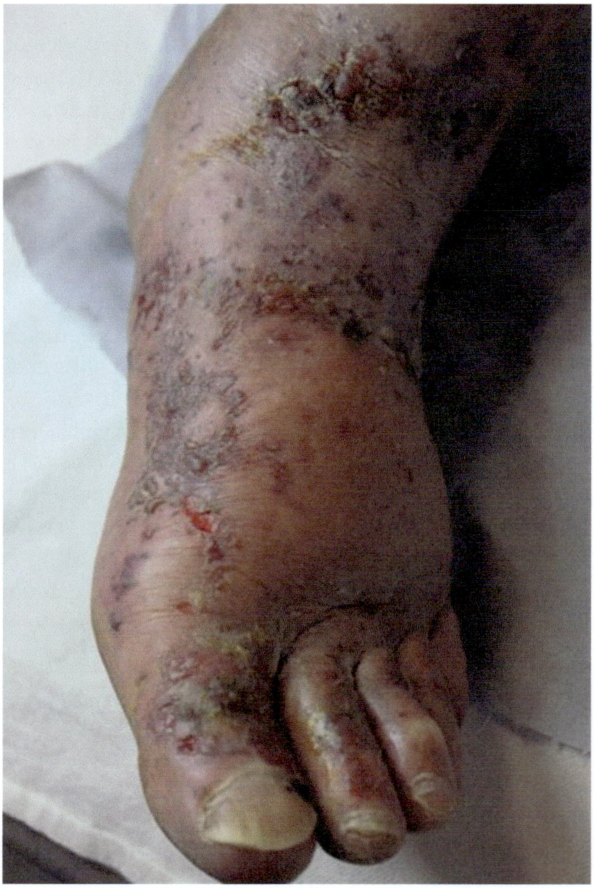

Fig. 17.3 Propylthiouracil associated vasculitis and patchy skin lesions

17.1.10 Hydralazine

Hydralazine is an arteriolar vasodilator used in the treatment of hypertension, pregnancy induced hypertension, and congestive heart failure. Hypotension, tachycardia, and headache are its common AEs. Uncommonly and after years of therapy, the drug is implicated in immunological conditions such as drug induced lupus and ANCA positive vasculitis. Females, older age, and increased dose of hydralazine are the traditional risk factors of these disorders. Vasculitis manifests as dyspnoea, weight loss, rash, and polyarthralgia. Rash is vesiculopustular to ulcerative and commonly involves legs, feet, and fingers. Among other systemic features, mucosal involvement of airways and gastrointestinal tract and rapidly progressive renal involvement are characteristic of hydralazine associated vasculitis. Fatalities can occur in missed cases. In nearly all cases, patients test positive for p-ANCA and ANA in serum. Not uncommon is the presence of anti-ds-DNA, anti-histone, and anti-cardiolipin antibodies. HPE of ulcer site shows evidence of leukocytoclastic vasculitis and deposition of IgM, fibrin, and complement protein C3 in the cutaneous blood vessels. Discontinuation of drug and symptomatic management form the mainstay of therapy. Steroids and immunomodulators such as cyclophosphamide may be required in some cases. Larger ulcers may need surgical debridement. Occurrence of vasculitis is an absolute contraindication of re-use of hydralazine [31, 32].

17.1.11 Levamisole

Levamisole is an anthelminthic and immunomodulator drug. The drug is used off label in nephrotic syndrome, gastrointestinal malignancies, and rheumatoid arthritis. Because of serious AEs like agranulocytosis, the drug was withdrawn from the USA. Having similarity with cocaine in taste and appearance and a euphoria supplementing action, the drug is mixed with cocaine unscrupulously. Following the use of levamisole adulterated cocaine, reports of vasculitis and cutaneous ulcerations have been reported in cocaine users. The entity is now named as cocaine-levamisole-induced vasculopathy syndrome (CLIVS). Lesions start as painful purpura on pinna, lower limbs, and upper limbs with gradual progression to full thickness skin lesions and ulcerations. HPE of lesions shows leukocytoclastic vasculitis and thrombosis of dermal blood vessels. Because of rarity of events, the exact pathogenesis needs to be delineated. Affected individuals show neutropenia and serum positivity for p-ANCA and c-ANCA. Urinary examination shows the presence of cocaine and levamisole. Treatment requires discontinuation of both offending drugs, symptomatic care and counselling. Corticosteroids may be required in systemic involvement [33].

17.1.12 Nicorandil

Nicorandil is used as adjuvant therapy in patients of stable angina. By opening the ATP sensitive K+ channels on vascular smooth muscles, the drug acts as a vasodilator and relieves the anginal pain. The common AEs include headache, hypotension, and tachycardia. It was in the late 1990s that the drug began to be associated with new onset mucosal ulcers in the oral cavity and perianal area. This was soon followed by reports of gastrointestinal ulcers involving the ileum, parastomal ulcers, and ulcers in the genital region. First case of pure cutaneous ulceration was reported with nicorandil in 2011 [34]. In a pharmacovigilance-based study of spontaneous reports of ulcerations with nicorandil, cutaneous involvement was seen in 27% of reported cases. In nearly 22% cases, the history of physical trauma or prior cutaneous lesions may be present. Cutaneous ulcers are generally seen in elderly patients, emerge after 2–4 years of therapy and commonly involve the lower limbs. Because of unawareness, often there is a delay of another 7–8 months in attributing the lesions to nicorandil [35]. In the absence of known predictors, a high index of suspicion should be kept at the very onset of ulcerative lesions and the drug should be stopped, and optimal wound care should be provided. Significant healing occurs over next 2–3 months. Vascular steal phenomenon produced by the drug or accumulation of its toxic nicotinic acid metabolite in skin, are some of the mechanisms attributed to ulcer generation. Possibility of immune mediated reaction also exists.

17.1.13 Other Drugs

Tyrosine kinase inhibitors: Epidermal growth factor receptor (EGFR) inhibitors such as gefitinib and afatinib are known for their AEs on skin such as rashes and acneiform eruptions [36]. Multikinase inhibitors such as sunitinib, soratinib, nilotinib, and cabozantinib have been associated with hand and foot reaction and palmoplantar erythrodysesthesias [37]. Case reports of extremity ulcers including pyoderma gangrenosum exist with these inhibitors. Ulcers resolve following discontinuation of the culprit drug and symptomatic management [38–40].

Erythropoietin, Diltiazem, and Nifedipine: Case reports of cutaneous ulceration on lower limbs exist with recombinant erythropoietin (r EPO), diltiazem, and nifedipine [41–43]. Dermal vessel thrombosis leading to ulceration has been reported with r EPO in an elderly male with underlying small vessel disease, diabetes, hypertension, and renal insufficiency [41]. Nifedipine is known to cause dependant oedema in lower limbs that in rare cases can complicate to ulcers [42].

Cutaneous vasculitis and ulcers on lower limbs have been reported with diltiazem. However, patients being on multiple drugs, uncertainty exists with respect to association and mechanism of vasculitis with diltiazem [43].

17.2 Conclusion

Drugs constitute an important cause of new onset cutaneous ulcers. Direct toxicity on epidermal and dermal cells, vascular thrombosis, and vasculitis are the main mechanisms through which medications can produce ulcers over extremities. Ample evidence of extremity ulcers exists for drugs such as hydroxyurea, methotrexate, propylthiouracil, hydralazine, and anticoagulants. The pharmacologically characteristic ergotism is rare nowadays due to decline in the use of ergot compounds. Some drugs such as nicorandil have been characteristically linked with mucosal ulcers. The last decade, however, witnessed many reports of lower limb ulcers with nicorandil. With increase in the use of target-based therapy, evidence on cutaneous lesions and extremity ulcers is piling up for tyrosine kinase inhibitors. Since the field of pharmacologic evaluation is still underdeveloped in many countries, a significant delay occurs in attributing an ulcer developing in response to a drug. Timely involvement of a pharmacologist or performing an intensive drug review can expedite the diagnosis and prevent physical and psychological morbidity.

References

1. Körber A, Klode J, Al-Benna S, Wax C, Schadendorf D, Steinstraesser L, et al. Etiology of chronic leg ulcers in 31,619 patients in Germany analyzed by an expert survey. J Dtsch Dermatol Ges. 2011;9(2):116–21.
2. Dissemond J. Medications A rare cause for leg ulcers. Der Hautarzt. 2011;62(7):516–23.
3. Sirieix M-E, Debure C, Baudot N, Dubertret L, Roux M-E, Morel P, et al. Leg ulcers and hydroxyurea. Arch Dermatol. 1999;135(7):818.
4. Duron D, Blaise S, Cracowski J-L, Roustit M, Khouri C. Drug-induced skin ulcers: A disproportionality analysis from the WHO pharmacovigilance database. J Am Acad Dermatol. 2021;85(1):229–32.
5. Ammad Ud Din M, Hussain SA, Jamshed S. Leg ulcer with long-term hydroxyurea use. Clin Case Rep. 2021;9(4):2487–8.
6. Bryant JR, Andrade P, Hajjar RT, Lumley CR, Chaiyasate K. Malleolar ulceration induced by hydroxyurea therapy for chronic eosinophila. J Am Coll Clin Wound Spec. 2016;8(1–3):47–50.
7. Best PJ, Daoud MS, Pittelkow MR, Petitt RM. Hydroxyurea-induced leg ulceration in 14 patients. Ann Intern Med. 1998;128(1):29–32.
8. de França ER, Teixeira MAG, de Matias KF, Antunes DECM, de Braz RA, CEF S. Efeitos colaterais cutâneos após uso prolongado de hidroxiuréia na Policitemia Vera. An Bras Dermatol. 2011;86(4):751–4.
9. Rappoport L, Körber A, Grabbe S, Dissemond J. Auftreten von Ulcera crurum in Zusammenhang mit der Einnahme von Anagrelid. Dtsch Med Wochenschr. 2007 Feb;132(7):319–21.
10. Oskay T, Özen M. Anagrelide associated with leg ulcers in a case of essential thrombocythaemia. Turk J Hematol. 2021.
11. Chan YC, Valenti D, Mansfield AO, Stansby G. Warfarin induced skin necrosis. Br J Surg. 2002;87(3):266–72.
12. Stewart AJ, Penman ID, Cook MK, Ludlam CA. Warfarin-induced skin necrosis. Postgrad Med J. 1999;75(882):233–5.
13. Kakagia DD, Papanas N, Karadimas E, Polychronidis A. Warfarin-induced skin necrosis. Ann Dermatol. 2014;26(1):96.
14. Handschin AE, Trentz O, Kock HJ, Wanner GA. Low molecular weight heparin-induced skin necrosis—a systematic review. Langenbeck's Arch Surg. 2005;390(3):249–54.
15. Warkentin TE. Clinical picture of heparin-induced thrombocytopenia (HIT) and its differentiation from non-HIT thrombocytopenia. Thromb Haemost. 2016;116(11):813–22.
16. Arepally GM, Padmanabhan A. Heparin-induced thrombocytopenia. Arterioscl Throm Vas Biol. 2020.
17. Garcia GD, Goff JM, Hadro NC, O'Donnell SD, Greatorex PS. Chronic ergot toxicity: a rare cause of lower extremity ischemia. J Vasc Surg. 2000;31(6):1245–7.
18. Glazer G, Myers KA, Davies ER. Ergot poisoning. Postgrad Med J. 1966;42(491):562–8.
19. Merhoff CC, Porter JM. Ergot intoxication. Ann Surg. 1974;180(5):773–9.
20. Lawrence CM, Dahl MGC. Two patterns of skin ulceration induced by methotrexate in patients with psoriasis. J Am Acad Dermatol. 1984;11(6):1059–65.
21. Kurian A, Haber R. Methotrexate-induced cutaneous ulcers in a nonpsoriatic patient: case report and review of the literature. J Cutan Med Surg. 2011;15(5):275–9.
22. Tekur V. Methotrexate-induced nonhealing cutaneous ulcers in a nonpsoriatic patient without pancytopenia. Indian Dermatol Online J. 2016;7(5):418.
23. Hocaoglu N, Atilla R, Onen F, Tuncok Y. Early-onset pancytopenia and skin ulcer following low-dose methotrexate therapy. Hum Exp Toxicol. 2008;27(7):585–9.
24. McCoy CM. Leflunomide-associated skin ulceration. Ann Pharmacother. 2002;36(6):1009–11.
25. Jakob A, Porstmann R, Rompel R. Skin ulceration after leflunomide treatment in two patients with rheumatoid arthritis. JDDG. 2006;4(4):324–7.
26. Lindquist LA, Feinglass J, Martin GJ. How sedative medication in older people affects patient risk factors for developing pressure ulcers. J Wound Care. 2003;12(7):272–5.

27. Prasad HRY, Khaitan BK, Ramam M, Sharma VK, Pandhi RK, Agarwal S, et al. Diagnostic clinical features of pentazocine-induced ulcers. Int J Dermatol. 2005;44(11):910–5.
28. Sahu KK, Sawatkar GU, Sahu SA, Mishra AK, Lal A. Pentazocine-induced skin ulcers. Am J Med Sci. 2020;359(3):182–3.
29. Wall AE, Weaver SM, Litt JS, Rae L. Propylthiouracil-associated Leukocytoclastic necrotizing cutaneous Vasculitis. J Burn Care Res. 2017;38(3):e678–85.
30. Seo JW, Son HH, Choi JH, Lee SK. A case of p-ANCA-positive Propylthiouracil-induced pyoderma Gangrenosum. Ann Dermatol. 2010;22(1):48.
31. Levin LE, Magro C, Horowitz J, Harp J. Hydralazine-associated cutaneous vasculitis presenting with aerodigestive tract involvement. Cutis. 2017;99(5):E25–9.
32. Kumar B, Strouse J, Swee M, Lenert P, Suneja M. Hydralazine-associated vasculitis: overlapping features of drug-induced lupus and vasculitis. Semin Arthritis Rheum. 2018;48(2):283–7.
33. Agdamag AC, Gevorgyan O, Lawrenz Co M, Hassan S. Multiple cutaneous and mucosal lesions in a patient with cocaine-levamisole–induced vasculopathy syndrome. Proc (Bay Univ Med Cent). 2019;32(1):93–5.
34. Mikeljevic J, Highet AS. Nicorandil-induced leg ulceration without mucosal involvement. Clin Exp Dermatol. 2011;36(4):372–3.
35. Babic V, Petitpain N, Guy C, Trechot P, Bursztejn AC, Faillie JL, et al. Nicorandil-induced ulcerations: a 10-year observational study of all cases spontaneously reported to the French pharmacovigilance network. Int Wound J. 2018;15(4):508–18.
36. Warthan MM, Jumper CA, Smith JL. Acneiform eruption induced by Iressa (gefitinib) tablets used to treat non-small cell lung cancer. J Drugs Dermatol. 2004;3(5):569–70.
37. Lipworth AD, Robert C, Zhu AX. Hand-foot syndrome (hand-foot skin reaction, palmar-plantar erythrodysesthesia): focus on sorafenib and sunitinib. Oncology. 2009;77(5):257–71.
38. Sathyanarayanan V, Lokesh KN, Channaviriappa LK, Jacob LA. Gefitinib-induced skin ulceration in metastatic adenocarcinoma lung. Indian J Med Paediatr Oncol. 2014;35(1):109–10.
39. Roger A, Sigal M-L, Bagan P, Sin C, Bilan P, Dakhil B, et al. Ulcères des membres inférieurs développés sous inhibiteurs de tyrosine kinase (sunitinib, nilotinib). Ann Dermatol Venereol. 2017;144(1):49–54.
40. Kuntz T, Koushk-Jalali B, Kreuter A. Sunitinib-induced pyoderma gangrenosum-like skin ulcer. Can Med Assoc J. 2020;192(20):E552–2.
41. Gibson A, Gardner J, O'Donnell J. Erythropoietin and painful leg ulcers: thrombosis or vasculitis? Arthritis Rheum. 2005;53(5):792–2.
42. Luca S, Romeo S. Edema and skin ulcers of the lower limbs as a collateral effect of nifedipine. A clinical case report. Minerva Cardioangiol. 1999;47(6):219–22.
43. Carmichael AJ, Paul CJ. Vasculitic leg ulcers associated with diltiazem. BMJ. 1988;297(6647):562–2.

18 Sickle Cell Anemia and Ulcer

Rajniti Prasad and Meenakshi Pandey

18.1 Introduction

Sickle cell hemoglobin (HbS) is a variant of adult hemoglobin due to mutation of beta chain of globin, which leads to substitution of valine amino acid for glutamic acid at sixth position of beta globin (base pair change: thymine for adenine at sixth codon of β-globin gene). Sickle cell disease refers to any condition in which the production of HbS causes pathophysiological consequences as a result of homozygous inheritance of βS-mutation and referred as either SCD SS or SCA. It includes Sickle cell anemia (SCA), which is the most severe form of the disease but also the compound heterozygotes, where one allele includes sickle cell mutation and second allele includes gene mutation other than the sickle cell mutation, such as HbC, beta thalassemia, HbD, and HbO [1, 2]. Homozygous SS patients are the ones most likely associated with ulcerations.

18.2 History and Epidemiology

Sickle cell disease (SCD) affects millions of people throughout the world and is particularly common among those who had ancestors from Africa, South America, Caribbean, Saudi Arabia, India, and Mediterranean countries. It was first described by the American physician James Herrick who reported the presence of "peculiar elongated and sickle shaped red blood corpuscles" in blood film of the patient with history of leg ulcers, breathlessness, and jaundice. Scientific advances in further decades led to description of molecular structure of HbS molecule, molecular basis

R. Prasad (✉) · M. Pandey
Department of Paediatrics, Institute of Medical Sciences, Banaras Hindu University, Varanasi, India

A. K. Khanna, S. K. Tiwary (eds.), *Uncommon Ulcers of the Extremities*, https://doi.org/10.1007/978-981-99-1782-2_18

of the sickling phenomenon, cloning and sequencing of the beta globin gene, development of diagnostic methods and prenatal diagnosis [1].

The βS-mutation is the classical example of natural selection in humans. It has been seen that heterozygotes, whose red blood cells contain both HbA and HbS, are strongly protected from malaria. The global distribution and the frequency of the βS-mutation reflect the historic incidence of death from malaria. Although sickle cell disease originated in the malaria-endemic world but due to population migration during the last few hundreds of years, first through the slave trade and more recently for economic and work-related reasons, now it is common particularly in developed world. Due to non-availability of newborn screening for sickle cell disease in most resource-poor countries, global data regarding the precise numbers of children born with SCD does not exist [2]. However, on the basis of data on carrier frequencies and global birth rates, it has been estimated that around 312,000 children are born each year with SCD SS (Fig.18.1).

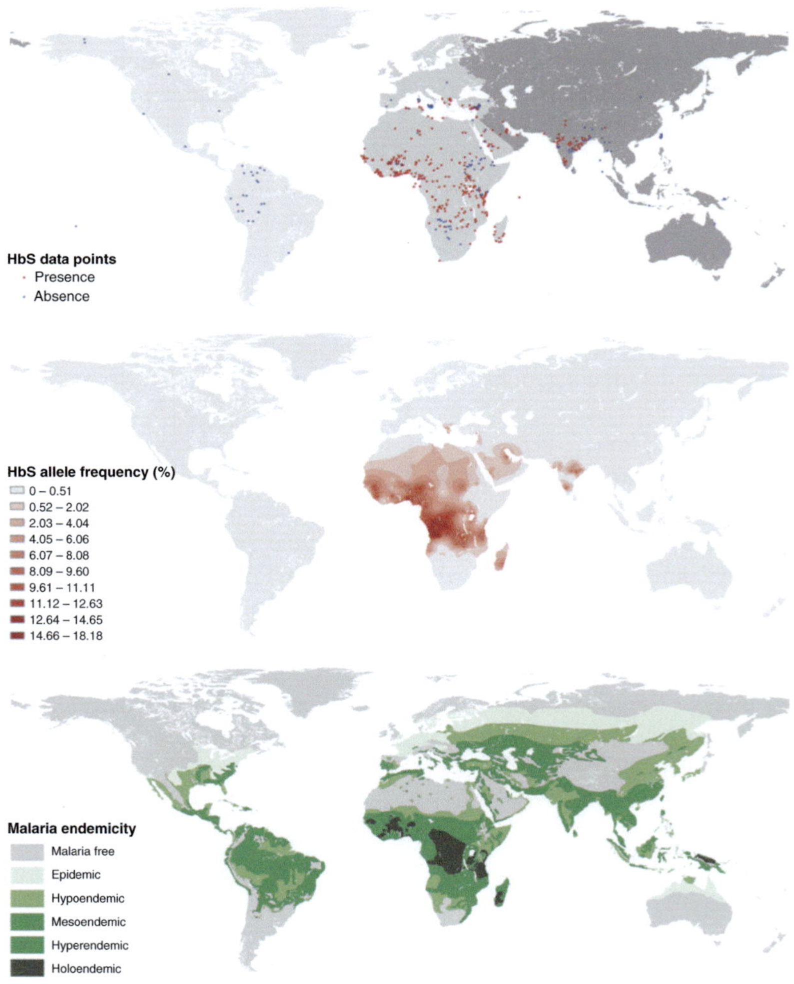

Fig. 18.1 Distribution of HbS allele frequency worldwide with malaria endemicity

18.3 Pathophysiology

Hypoxia, acidosis, and dehydration leads to conformational changes and subsequent polymerization of sickle cell hemoglobin in red blood cells and their characteristics shape, i.e., sickle shape. Sickled red blood cells interact with vascular endothelium and cause microvascular occlusion, ischemia, and reperfusion injury. The increased markers of inflammatory stress, vascular oxidases, inflammatory cytokines, and adhesion molecules suggest it to be an inflammatory disease [3].

Sickle cell ulcer is a frequent complication and its incidence varies from phenotypic and genotypic traits of sickle cell disease. It is rare before 10 years of age and its incidence varies from 3/100 persons per year between 10–19 years and 14.5–19/100 persons per years after 20 years of age inpatients of sickle cell disease. Ulcer is more common in male and genotypes of patients in decreasing order of frequency are homozygous SS sickle cell anemia, compound heterozygous Sβ0 thalassemia, and hemoglobin SCD [4]. The incidence of ulcer has also been correlated with blood level of adult and fetal hemoglobin. Recently vasculopathy (endothelial cell dysfunction, deficiency of nitric oxide, intimal hyperplasia, and vascular smooth cell proliferation) has been correlated with chronic hemolysis in sickle cell disease. Ulcers in sickle cell disease are often associated with high level of lactate dehydrogenase, pulmonary hypertension, and increased risk of death. In mouse model of sickle cell ulcer, deficiency of angiogenesis and chemokines CXCL12 has been reported [5–7].

18.4 Characteristics of Ulcer in Sickle Cell Disease

Most common site of ulceration in sickle cell is lower leg, especially around lateral and medial malleoli and ulcers are often bilateral [4, 8]. Trauma is often the preceding event in causing ulcers. Ulcers usually appear punched out, with well-defined, slightly raised and occasionally rolled margins, and the base is frequently covered with fibrinous material (Fig.18.2). These ulcers last several years. Another type of

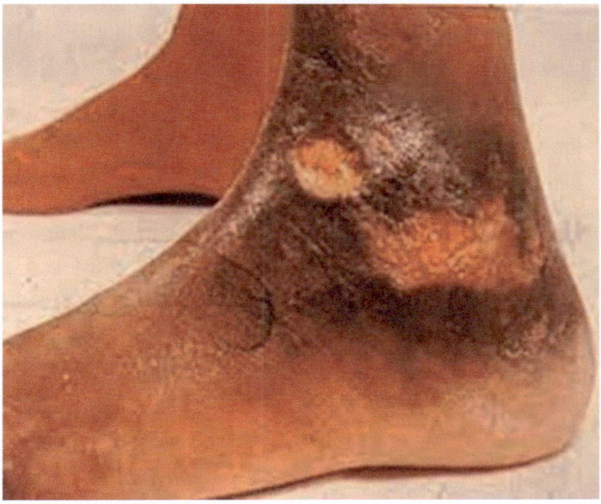

Fig. 18.2 Punched out ulcers over lateral Malleolus in sickle cell disease

ulcer is also seen which develops in the absence of obvious trauma, and progresses through the following stages.

1. Stage of hyperpigmentation.
2. Stage of induration.
3. Stage of dermal necrosis with an intact overlying epidermis, and.
4. Epidermal necrosis, eventuating in a small, deep, and very painful ulcer.

   This type of ulcer, attributed to skin infarction, usually heals relatively quickly (6–9 months). Common complications of these leg ulcers are chronic subcutaneous fibrosis, ulcer osteoma and sometimes acute ankle arthritis/ankyloses [4, 9].

18.5 Deferential Diagnosis

Ulcers in thalassemia are punched out, frequently bilateral, heal slowly, and tend to occur near the malleoli [4, 7].Hereditary spherocytosis, pyruvate kinase deficiency, elliptocytosis, and paroxysmal nocturnal hemoglobinuria are also associated with intractable ulcers of the leg. Cutaneous involvement occurs late in lymphoproliferative disorders and ulceration occurs generally when patient has significant tumor burden or end stage disease. Tumor nodules are found in roughly 7–10% of patients with mycosis fungoides which can later ulcerate and may involve the legs. Ulcerated posterior thigh nodules in granulomatous mycosis fungoides have been reported. In malignant histiocytosis, skin involvement occurs in 10–20% of individuals. Cutaneous ulcer complications seen in polycythemia vera include livedo reticularis with chilblain-like lesions, superficial digital ulcerations, and peripheral gangrene. Disorders of coagulation and fibrinolysis are uncommon causes of cutaneous ulceration, including leg ulceration [1].

18.6 Diagnosis

Clinical findings in the patient may point to the associated hematologic disorder, but the confirmation requires evaluation of red cell indices, blood smear morphology, and other methods such as electrophoresis, HPLC, and genetic testing. Sickle shaped red cells along with target cells on a routine blood smear is diagnostic of Hb S-related disease, but cannot distinguish between Hb SS and HbS-thal states. Hemoglobin electrophoresis studies therefore required for differentiating homozygous from the heterozygous. The former will have high levels of HbSS (80–90%), while carriers have lower values (35–40%). Given the implications of a diagnosis of sickle cell disease versus sickle cell trait with respect to clinical manifestations, evaluating red cell parameters in the parents for genetic counseling cannot be overemphasized (Table 18.1 and Figs.18.3 and 18.4).

In thalassemia major, microcytic, hypochromic anemia with target cells are usual findings on peripheral blood smear. Nucleated red cells, marked

Table 18.1 HPLC pattern of different hemoglobin and their diagnostic significance

Hemoglobin	Disease
Hb A > HbS	Sickle cell trait, sickle α-Thalessaemia
HbS, HbF, and no HbA	Sickle cell anemia, sickle β-Thalassaemia
HbS > HbA and HbF	Sickle β-Thalassaemia
HbA > HbC	HbC trait
HbC, HbF, and no HbA	HbC disease and HbC β-Thalassaemia
HbC > HbA	HbC β-Thalassaemia

[a]*Hb* Hemoglobin

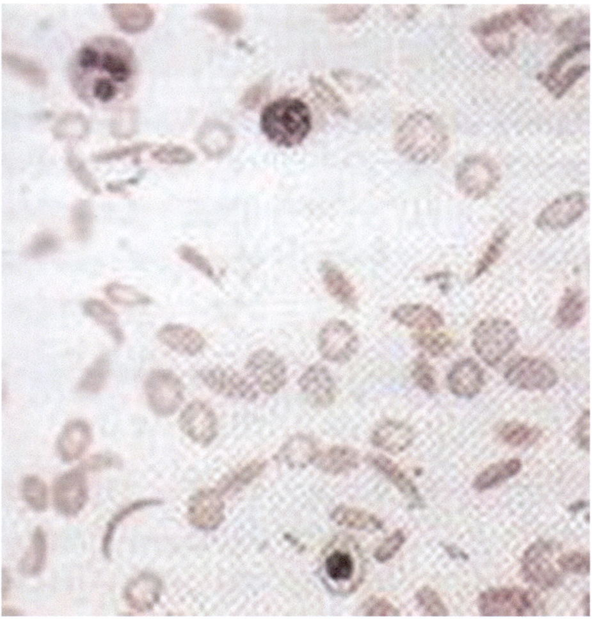

Fig. 18.3 Sickle shaped red cells along with target cells on peripheral blood smear examination

anisopoikilocytosis, and relative reticulocytopenia are typically seen. Hemoglobin electrophoresis can be used for screening purpose, but the mutation analysis, along with testing for common genetic modifiers of the clinical phenotype, is recommended.

When clinical features, cell counts, and peripheral smear are indicative of leukemia then diagnosis is confirmed by bone marrow aspiration and biopsy. In bone marrow examination, more than 25% of cells are lymphoblasts, which is diagnostic for ALL (20% for AML). Immunophenotyping is must while evaluating hematological malignancies. All patients suspected to be having thrombotic disorder should have baseline complete blood count, prothrombin time (PT) and activated partial thromboplastin time (aPTT) to assess coagulation status. It is important to refer to age related normal ranges, when interpreting pediatric coagulation studies.

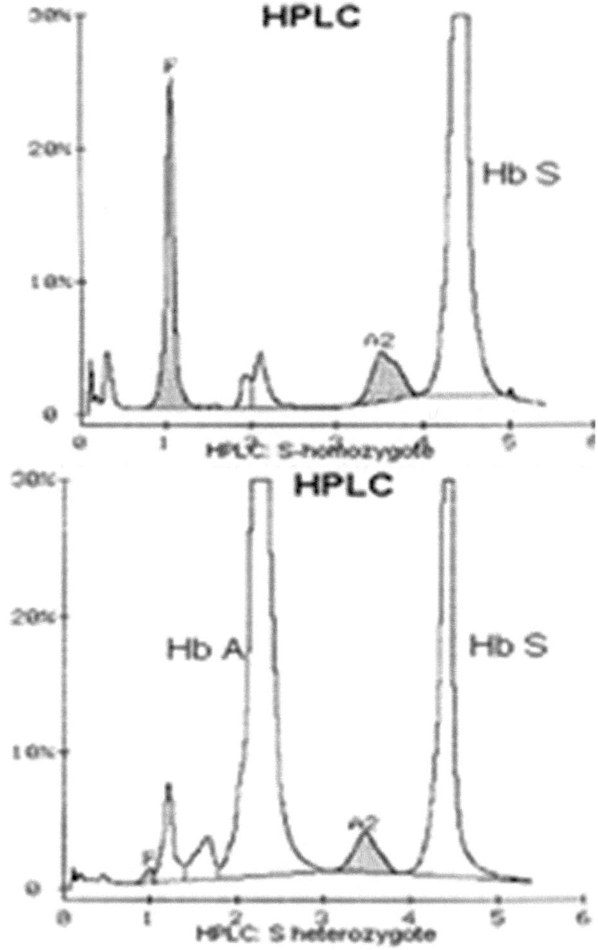

Fig. 18.4 HPLC showing high levels of HbSS (80–90%) in homozygous above, and 35–40% in carriers(lower)

18.7 Treatment and Prevention

First thing required for the management of ulcers in hematological disorders is proper and timely management of the chief hematological disorder. The effective pain management is of paramount importance as vasoconstriction caused by catecholamine release inhibits ulcer healing. NSAIDS are commonly used to relieve pain in SLCUS but topical lidocaine along with opioids is most effective [10]. There is paucity of RCTs in literature regarding the management of sickle cell leg ulcers (SCLUs), so most of the treatment options are based on anecdotal case reports. Management options range from topical medications to systemic therapy and surgical methods.

18.8 Topical Treatment and Dressings

Since SCLUs are extremely painful, heal with difficulty with frequent recurrence, prior local anesthesia is important. Detersive cleaning of fibrin and/ or necrosis is important in care of ulcers. Detersion recommended is first mechanical (with a curette or scalpel) followed by autolytic (hydrogels, alginates or hydrofibers), which should be changed preferably twice in a week. Hydrocolloid dressings are not recommended in SLCUs [11].

Topical application of arginine-glycine-aspartic acid matrix (RGD peptide matrix) shows noticeable benefit in the treatment of SCLUs [12]. This RGD peptide matrix is believed to act as a synthetic extracellular matrix to promote cell migration, keratinocyte layer formation and wound strengthening, thereby promoting healing. Topical application of sodium nitrite has demonstrated a dose-dependent effect on promoting ulcer healing and decreasing pain at the ulcer site [13]. The beneficial effects of solcoseryl (protein free extract of calf blood) ointment, collagen matrix, heparin sulfate and GM-CSF have been reported in some cases and still in experimental phase [14–17].

18.9 Systemic Therapy

Systemic therapies in sickle cell ulcers have not been extensively studied but some trials have shown some benefit of oral zinc [18] and pentoxifylline. Zinc supplements (50 mg/day) reduce the number of vaso-occlusive crisis and decrease the incidence of systemic infections, thus promote faster healing of ulcer. Pentoxifylline improves RBC and leukocyte deformability, thus potentially decreasing blood viscosity and also inhibits platelet aggregation and thrombus formation and decreases plasma fibrinogen levels [19]. These multiple effects ultimately increase microcirculatory flow and tissue oxygen levels and help in SCLU treatment. Blood transfusions are often used in the care of SCD patients. They have also been advocated as a treatment modality for patients with SCLUs as they increase the oxygen delivery to tissues. A variety of transfusion recommendations have been proposed to prevent the recurrence of or to treat existing ulcers [20]. Some authors suggest achieving hemoglobin of 10 g/dL for successful surgical treatment, although a level between 8 and 9 g/dL may be more realistic and adequate for wound healing. Isoxsuprine hydrochloride and levocarnitine have been reported as another treatment modality but their role is unproven in SCLU treatment [21].

Hydroxyurea, a myelosuppressive agent, is the most common drug used in the management of sickle cell anemia. It helps prevent the painful crises, dactylitis, acute chest syndrome (ACS) in sickle cell anemia and also reduces the need of blood transfusion but its role in preventing the occurrence of ulcers is still unproven. The initial dose of hydroxyurea is 15–20 mg/kg given once daily with maximum up to 35 mg/kg/day [22, 23].

18.10 Treatment of Edema

The edema is common with SCLU either due to superficial or deep venous insufficiency (functional venous insufficiency) as observed in Doppler study. Venous compression using multilayered compression bandage to obtain a 30–40 mmHg pressure at ankle is recommended to reduce the edema, pain, and wound healing. After complete healing, compression hosiery should be used to reduce the risk of recurrence [24, 25].

18.11 Surgery and SLCU

Surgical modalities are most frequently used for the treatment of SCLUs but they are associated with high rates of failure and recurrence [26]. Microsurgical free flap transfers are commonly performed but owing to the high rates of failure, numerous recommendations have been made to decrease the incidence of graft failure [27]. The role of endovenous ablation of superficial venous reflux in complete healing of SLCU is debatable but may be useful in associated superficial venous reflux [28]. Perioperative transfusion to decrease HbS levels to less than 30% is recommended, with transfusions beginning 1–2 weeks prior to surgery and continuing for 6 months post-operatively [20]. Use of anticoagulation with heparin and/or aspirin, antibiotics and the rinsing of flaps with warm, heparinized solution prior to attachment also prevents graft failure. Prolonged anticoagulation (heparin or low molecular weight heparin) therapy may be of benefit in such cases where ulcers are associated with thrombotic disorders.

18.12 Cell Based Therapy

Pinch graft currently used in SLCUs appears to be good therapeutic modality in wound healing but their efficacy has not been evaluated in randomized control trial. The spray consisting of human allogenic fibroblasts and keratinocytes, adipocyte-derived stem cells have been found effective in the management of venous ulcers but data on SLCUs are lacking. The efficacy of platelet rich plasma in several randomized trials have been reported as useful modality for treatment of leg ulcers of different origin apart from SCLUs [29–31].

Apligraf, a bilayer epidermis and dermis construct approved by FDA for treatment of venous ulcers has been reported to be beneficial in few patients with SLCUs. Conner et al. had reported reduction in surface area of SLCUs after application of autologous platelet gel at the end of the first week. The postulated hypothesis is probably increase in production of platelet derived growth factor, TGF-β and vascular endothelial growth factor [32].

18.13 Physical Treatment

Topically applied energy-based modalities have also been used for managing sickle cell ulcers. Low-frequency non-contact ultrasound causes effective removal of bacteria and biofilm and the reduction of chronic inflammation [33]. Low-level laser therapy modulates wound healing by increasing mitotic activity, fibroblast production, collagen synthesis, and angiogenesis to help wound healing. There are some case reports about the role of negative pressure wound therapy (NPWT) in the management of SCLUs to obtain granulation tissue in ulcer bed before pinch graft to accelerate inflammatory stage of healing. It also increases release of nitric oxide and growth factor by stimulating angiogenesis and vasodilation [34].

Malnutrition or undernutrition has been observed to be commonly associated with SLCU but supplementation of protein in faster healing of SLCU has not been reported. The administration of vitamin D and folic have been observed to have some beneficial effects in healing of venous ulcer but not in SLCU.

Beyond medications and surgery, bed rest has long been recommended as a useful treatment modality for promoting healing of ulcers in hematological disorders. It reduces venous backpressure and edema around the ulcers. Prevention of any trauma is a useful preventive measure to reduce the occurrence of ulcers, because regardless of all existing treatment modalities, these ulcers are non-healing most of the times with high rate of recurrence.

18.14 Conclusion

The only cure for sickle cell anemia is transplantation with HLA matched hematopoietic stem cells from a sibling or unrelated donor. Most common indications for transplant are recurrent ACS, stroke, and abnormal transcranial Doppler. Genetic counseling and testing should be offered to the family and parents should be done to identify various complications of the disease.

References

1. Rees DC, Williams TN, Gladwin MT. Sickle cell disease. Lancet. 2010;376:2018–31.
2. Powars DR, Chan LS, Hiti A, Ramicone E, Johnson C. Outcome of sickle cell anemia: a 4-decade observational study of 1056 patients. Medicine (Baltimore). 2005;84:363–76.
3. Parent F, Bachir D, Inamo J, et al. A hemodynamic study of pulmonary hypertension in sickle cell disease. N Engl J Med. 2011;365:44–53.
4. Minniti CP, Eckman J, Sebastiani P, Steinberg MH, Ballas SK. Leg ulcers in sickle cell disease. Am J Hematol. 2010;85:831–3.
5. Nouraie M, Lee JS, Yingze ZY. The relationship between the severity of hemolysis, clinical manifestations and risk of death in 415 patients with sickle cell anemia in the US and Europe. Haematologica. 2013;98:464–72.
6. Bunn HF, Nathan DG, Dover GJ, et al. Pulmonary hypertension and nitric oxide depletion in sickle cell disease. Blood. 2010;116:687e92.

7. Nguyen VT, Nassar D, Batteux F, et al. Delayed healing of sickle cell ulcers is due to impaired angiogenesis and CXCL12 secretion in skin wounds. J Invest Dermatol. 2016;136:497–506.
8. Monfort JB, Senet P. Leg ulcers in sickle-cell disease: treatment update. Adv Wound Care. 2020;9(6):348–56.
9. Serjeant GR. Leg ulceration in sickle cell anemia. Arch Int Med. 1974;133:690–4.
10. Altman IA, Kleinfelder RE, Quigley JG, Ennis WJ, Minniti CP. A treatment algorithm to identify therapeutic approaches for leg ulcers in patients with sickle cell disease. Int Wound J. 2016;13:1315–24.
11. Stevens DM, Shupack JL, Javid J, Silber R. Ulcers of the leg in thalassemia. Arch Dermatol. 1977;113:1558–60.
12. Wethers DL, Ramirez GM, Koshy M, Steinberg MH, Phillips G, Siegel RS, et al. Accelerated healing of chronic sickle-cell leg ulcers treated with RGD peptide matrix. RGD Study Group. Blood. 1994;84:1775–9.
13. Minniti CP, Gorbach AM, Xu D, Hon YY, Delaney KM, Seidel M, et al. Topical sodium nitrite for chronic leg ulcers in patients with sickle cell anaemia: a phase 1 dose-finding safety and tolerability trial. Lancet Haematol. 2014;1:e95–103.
14. La Grenade L, Thomas PW, Serjeant GR. A randomized controlled trial of solcoseryl and duoderm in chronic sickle-cell ulcers. West Indian Med J. 1993;42:121–3.
15. Garwood CS, Kim PJ, Matai V, et al. The use of bovine collagen-glycosaminoglycan matrix for atypical lower extremity ulcers. Wounds. 2016;28:298–305.
16. Reindorf CA, Walker-Jones D, Adekile AD, Lawal O, Oluwole SF. Rapid healing of sickle cell leg ulcers treated with collagen dressing. J Natl Med Assoc. 1989;81:866–8.
17. Alikhan MA, Carter G, Mehta P. Topical GM-CSF hastens healing of leg ulcers in sickle cell disease. Am J Hematol. 2004;76:192.
18. Serjeant GR, Galloway RE, Gueri MC. Oral zinc sulphate in sickle-cell ulcers. Lancet. 1970;2:891–2.
19. Frost ML, Treadwell P. Treatment of sickle cell leg ulcers with pentoxifylline. Int J Dermatol. 1990;29:375–6.
20. Eckman JR. Leg ulcers in sickle cell disease. Hematol Oncol Clin North Am. 1996;10:1333–44.
21. Serjeant GR, Howard C. Isoxsuprine hydrochloride in the therapy of sickle cell leg ulceration. West Indian Med J. 1977;26:164–6.
22. Voskaridou E, Christoulas D, Bilalis A, et al. The effect of prolonged administration of hydroxyurea on morbidity and mortality in adult patients with sickle cell syndromes: results of a 17-year, single-center trial (LaSHS). Blood. 2010;115:2354–63.
23. Lanzkron S, Strouse JJ, Wilson R, et al. Systematic review: hydroxyurea for the treatment of adults with sickle cell disease. Ann Intern Med. 2008;148:939–55.
24. Ashby RL, Gabe R, Ali S, et al. Clinical and cost-effectiveness of compression hosiery versus compression bandages in treatment of venous leg ulcers (venous leg ulcer study IV, VenUS IV): a randomized controlled trial. Lancet. 2014;383:871–9.
25. Barwell JR, Davies CE, Deacon J, et al. Comparison of surgery and compression with compression alone in chronic venous ulceration (ESCHAR study): randomised controlled trial. Lancet. 2004;363:1854–9.
26. Weinzweig N, Schuler J, Marschall M, Koshy M. Lower limb salvage by microvascular free-tissue transfer in patients with homozygous sickle cell disease. Plast Reconstr Surg. 1995;96:1154–61.
27. Mauck KF, Asi N, Undavalli C, et al. Systematic review and meta-analysis of surgical interventions versus conservative therapy for venous ulcers. J Vasc Surg. 2014;60:60S–70S.
28. Gohel MS, Heatley F, Liu X, et al. A randomized trial of early endovenous ablation in venous ulceration. N Engl J Med. 2018;378:2105–14.
29. Holm JS, Toyserkani NM, Sorensen JA. Adipose-derived stem cells for treatment of chronic ulcers: current status. Stem Cell Res Ther. 2018;9:142.
30. Burgos-Alonso N, Lobato I, Hernández I, et al. Adjuvant biological therapies in chronic leg ulcers. Int J Mol Sci. 2017;18:E2561.

31. Meneses JV, Fortuna V, de Souza ES, et al. Autologous stem cell-based therapy for sickle cell leg ulcer: a pilot study. Br J Haematol. 2016;175:949–55.
32. Connor JL Jr, Minniti CP, Tisdale JF, Hsieh MM. Sickle cell anemia and comorbid leg ulcer treated with curative peripheral blood stem cell transplantation. Int J Low Extrem Wounds. 2017;16:56–9.
33. White J, Ivins N, Wilkes A, Carolan-Rees G, Harding KG. Non-contact low-frequency ultrasound therapy compared with UK standard of care for venous leg ulcers: a single-centre, assessor-blinded, randomised controlled trial. Int Wound J. 2016;13:833–42.
34. Dumville JC, Land L, Evans D, Peinemann F. Negative pressure wound therapy for treating leg ulcers. Cochrane Database Syst Rev. 2015;7:CD011354.

Pyoderma Gangrenosum

19

Harikrishna K. R. Nair

19.1 Introduction

Pyoderma gangrenosum (PG) was introduced by Brunsting et al. in 1930 [1]. These patients had intractable ulcers with underlying ulcerative colitis and empyema. The assessment is important in pyoderma gangrenosum as the diagnosis is difficult but crucial in the comprehensive management especially when there are multiple clinical variants [2].

Pyoderma gangrenosum which is a rare inflammatory condition is not caused by infection or ischaemia. There is neutrophilic dermatosis with painful skin ulceration which later form scars. The Health Related Quality of Life (HrQOL) of the patient is often affected due to the nature of the presentation.

The incidence of PG is 3–10 cases per million people per year [3]. PG can affect all ages especially female patients.

19.2 Pathophysiology

The pathogenesis of PG is complex and involves genetic mutations, neutrophil dysfunction, immune dysregulation, and abnormal inflammatory responses. Some lesions of pyoderma gangrenosum have been found to have a proliferation of clonal T-cells supporting the possibility of an aberrant T-cell response [4]. In PG there is inflammation and is noted to have many inflammatory cells and mediators such as Interleukin 23 which contribute to the clinical manifestation of this disease.

H. K. R. Nair (✉)
Wound Care Unit, Kuala Lumpur Hospital, Kuala Lumpur, Malaysia

A. K. Khanna, S. K. Tiwary (eds.), *Uncommon Ulcers of the Extremities*, https://doi.org/10.1007/978-981-99-1782-2_19

19.3 Common Features

- Inflammatory papule, pustule, nodule or vesicle which erodes to form an ulcer.
- Inflammatory reaction.
- Pain.
- Arthralgia.
- Lethargy.
- Healing by scarring (secondary intention).
- Pathergy (surgical procedures can exacerbate this condition).

19.4 Heidi

History: It should be taken comprehensively. Associated comorbid conditions such as inflammatory bowel disease and leukaemia should be asked in the history. Past or current history of similar conditions, polyarthritis or immune diseases such as rheumatoid artritis, mixed connective tissue disease, etc. are also important.

19.4.1 Examination

There are four variants:

- Classical or ulcerative.
- Pustular.
- Bullous.
- Vegetative or granulomatous [5].

Differential diagnosis includes vasculitis, calciphylaxis, malignancy, infection, drug eruptions, etc.

19.4.2 Investigations

- Full blood test.
- Erythrocyte Sedimentation Rate and C-Reactive Protein.
- Anti-Nuclear Antibody or factor, Rheumatoid factor, and immunological screen.
- Chest X-Ray to note any lung pathology.
- Liver function test to exclude hepatitis or liver pathology.
- Skin biopsy to support the pathophysiology of an inflammatory condition with succinct history and examination is important with a proper exclusion of the other differential diagnosis.
- There are no definitive blood, serology or histopathological investigations.

19.4.3 Diagnosis

- The diagnosis is made after careful history, physical examination with a skin biopsy which are not confirmatory but gives you a high index of suspicion. PG is a diagnosis of exclusion [6].
- The Delphi consensus of international experts by [7] includes a single major criterion and eight minor criteria. At least the major criterion and four minor criteria are necessary for diagnosis of PG.

  1 major criterion: —biopsy of ulcer edge demonstrating neutrophilic infiltrate.
  8 minor criteria:

1. exclusion of infection,
2. pathergy,
3. history of inflammatory bowel disease or inflammatory arthritis,
4. history of papule, pustule, or vesicle ulcerating within 4 days of appearing,
5. peripheral erythema, undermining border, and tenderness at ulceration site,
6. multiple ulcerations, at least 1 on an anterior lower leg,
7. cribriform or "wrinkled paper" scar(s) at healed ulcer sites,
8. decreased ulcer size within 1 month of initiating immunosuppressive medication(s).

19.4.4 Intervention

19.4.4.1 Topical

Proper wound care with advanced dressings, topical corticosteroids, cromolyn sodium 2%, nitrogen mustard, 5-aminosalicylic acid and tacrolimus or pimecrolimus.

19.4.4.2 Systemic

Corticosteroids, cyclosporine, mycophenolate mofetil, azathioprine, dapsone, tacrolimus, cyclophosphamide, chlorambucil, thalidomide, tumor necrosis factor-alpha (TNF-alpha) inhibitors, and nicotine. Intravenous (IV) therapies include pulsed methylprednisolone, pulsed cyclophosphamide, infliximab, IV immunoglobulin, and ustekinumab. Interleukin 23, phosphodiesterase 4 inhibitors, along with the newer Janus kinase inhibitors and intravenous immune globulin are other biologic agents under trials [8].

19.4.5 Pain

Pain is the fifth vital sign and has to managed with appropriate analgesia according to the pain ladder. The pain will reduce when the wound improves with the immunopathic dressings.

19.4.6 Wound Care Management

19.4.6.1 Wound Assessment

Local Assessment involves the assessment of the wound which looks at the

1. Wound bed.
   (a) assess for necrotic, granulation, slough, and epithelial tissue,
   (b) assess for infection or bacterial bioburden and inflammation,
   (c) assess the exudate and odour,
   (d) wound bed preparation paradigm involves the management of the bacterial burden, debridement, and exudate or moisture management. This paradigm has been used quite extensively for the past 23 years. [9].
2. Wound edges: assess for undermining and condition of the margin.
3. Surrounding skin: assess for the colour, moisture, suppleness, and the Harikrishna Periwound Skin Classification can be utilized. The periwound skin is from the edge up to about 4 cm. The periwound skin has to be managed well to allow the keratinocytes to move in from the periphery to allow wound healing.
4. The wound size has to be measured and this involves the length, width, and depth which gives you a volumetric measurement. The wound also should be photographed digitally for proper documentation [10].

Under the Wound Bed Preparation concept is TIME. TIME has been used since 2003 till now to assess the wound bed and plan a proper management of the wound.

T	Tissue
I	Infection or inflammation
M	Moisture imbalance
E	Epidermal margin
S	Surrounding skin or Periwound

The 2015 Harikrishna Periwound Skin Classification system [10] in Table 19.1 illustrates the proper way of classifying the periwound area when assessing the surrounding skin. The periwound is from the edge up to 4 cm.

Table 19.1 HPSC Periwound condition

Class 0 Normal
Class 1 Fibrous tissue/tissue at risk
Class 2A Exudate centred with desiccation
Class 2B Exudate centred with maceration
Class 2C Exudate centred with allergy
Class 3 Inflammation without infection
Class 4 Inflammation with infection
Class 5 Atypical (senescent cells/cancer/subcutaneous emphysema)

19.4.7 Cleansing Solutions

- Water for irrigation.
- Normal saline.

Non-toxic wound cleansers:

- PHMB (PolyHexaMethyl Biguanide) with Betaine.
- Superoxide Solution.
- Octenidine Dihydrochloride.
- Nanocopper.
- Hypochlorous Acid spray.

19.4.8 Dressings

Immunopathic dressings are the main dressings considered.

These dressings are those that reduce the inflammation in the wound such as

- Collagen such as sheets, gel, ointments, etc.
- Polymeric membrane dressings.
- Sucralfate or urgostart.

Antimicrobial dressings such as silver, copper, iodine-based products are only used if we suspect there is an infection in the wound bed. However, in PG the predominant cause is a proinflammatory condition and there is an elevated protease activity with increased interleukin and MMPs. This has to be managed as shown in Fig. 19.1.

Patient was also started on oral prednisolone for her Mixed Connective Tissue Disease associated with the pyoderma gangrenosum

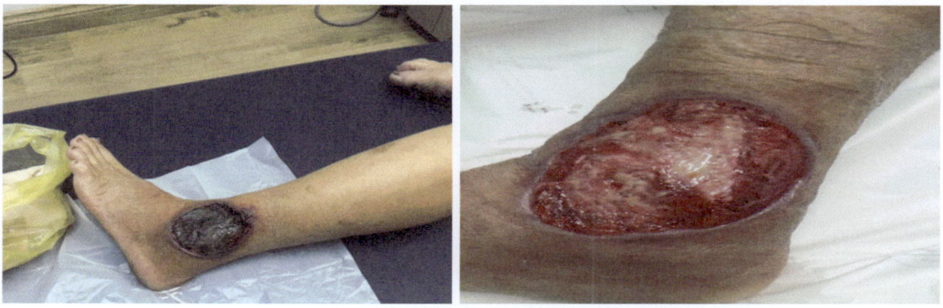

Fig. 19.1 The wound was treated with polymeric membrane dressing and noted improvement with 1 week (courtesy of the Wound Care Unit, Kuala Lumpur Hospital).

19.4.9 Surgery

Acute PG should not be debrided as there will be tissue death and necrosis and the wound will become bigger. Pathergy is the cause of this. Refrain from surgical or sharp debridement in cases of acute pyoderma gangrenosum.

References

1. Brunsting L, et al. Pyoderma (echthyma) gangrenosum: clinical and experimental observations in five cases occurring in adults. Arch Dermatol Syphilol. 1930;22(4):655–80. https://doi.org/10.1001/archderm.1930.01440160053009.
2. Alavi A, Sajic D, Cerci FB, Ghazarian D, Rosenbach M, Jorizzo J. Neutrophilic dermatoses: an update. Am J Clin Dermatol. 2014;15(5):413–23.
3. Ruocco E, et al. Pyoderma gangrenosum: an updated review. J Eur Acad Dermatol Venereol. 2009;23(9):1008–17.
4. Marzano AV, Trevisan V, Gattorno M, Ceccherini I, de Simone C, Crosti C. Pyogenic arthritis, pyoderma gangrenosum, acne, and hidradenitis suppurativa (PAPASH): a new autoinflammatory syndrome associated with a novel mutation of the PSTPIP1 gene. JAMA Dermatol. 2013;149(6):762–4.
5. Powell FC, Hackett BC, Wallach D. Pyoderma gangrenosum. In: Goldsmith LA, Katz SI, Gilchrest BA, et al., editors. Fitzpatrick's dermatology in general medicine, vol. 1. 8th ed. New York: McGraw-Hill Companies; 2012. p. 371.
6. Patel F, Fitzmaurice S, Duong C, et al. Effective strategies for the management of pyoderma gangrenosum: a comprehensive review. Acta Derm Venereol. 2015;95(5):525–31.
7. Maverakis E, Ma C, Shinkai K, et al. Diagnostic criteria of ulcerative pyoderma Gangrenosum: a Delphi consensus of international experts. JAMA Dermatol. 2018;154(4):461–6. https://doi.org/10.1001/jamadermatol.2017.5980.
8. Harikrishna, et al. Atypical wounds. Selangor Darul Ehsan: Uniquelink Dot Print Sdn Bhd; 2021.
9. Sibbald G. Preparing the wound bed for healing- debridement, bacterial burden and exudate management. Ostomy Wound Manage. 2000;46(1):14–22.
10. Nair HKR. Compendium of wound care dressings and other modalities. 4th ed. Kuala Lumpur: Malaysian Society of Wounds Care Professionals; 2017.

Necrotizing Fasciitis of the Extremities 20

Sandeep Raj Pandey, Jai Prakash Jaiswal,
Angampally Rajeev, and Ayman Khalil

20.1 Background

Necrotizing fasciitis (NF) is a rapidly progressive inflammatory infection of the fascia, with secondary necrosis of the subcutaneous tissues [1]. NF has also been referred to as hemolytic streptococcal gangrene, Meleney ulcer, acute dermal gangrene, hospital gangrene, suppurative fasciitis, and synergistic necrotizing cellulitis.

NF of the extremities may occur as a complication of a variety of surgical procedures or medical conditions, including cardiac catheterization [2], injury, and vein sclerotherapy [3]. It may also be idiopathic. The causative bacteria may be aerobic, anaerobic, or mixed flora [4] (Figs. 20.1 and 20.2).

S. R. Pandey (✉) · J. P. Jaiswal
Norvic Int'l Hospital, Kathmandu, Nepal

A. Rajeev
Heart and vascular care of Georgia, Newnan, USA

A. Khalil
AMC hospital, Hurghada, Egypt

A. K. Khanna, S. K. Tiwary (eds.), *Uncommon Ulcers of the Extremities*,
https://doi.org/10.1007/978-981-99-1782-2_20

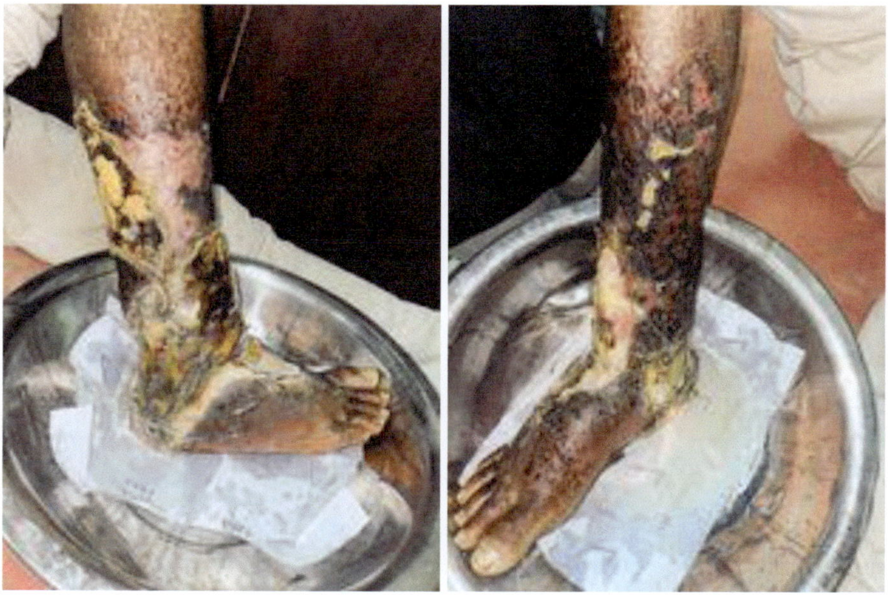

Figs. 20.1 and 20.2 Right lower extremity NF in a diabetic who got COVID-19 and his leg wound was not much cared during COVID-19 management

20.2 Pathophysiology

NF is characterized by widespread necrosis of the subcutaneous tissue and the fascia. Although the pathogenesis of necrotizing fasciitis is still open to speculation, the rapid and destructive clinical course of necrotizing fasciitis is thought to be due to multi-bacterial symbiosis and synergy. In 1990s, media popularized that NF was caused by "flesh-eating bacteria" [5] (Figs. 20.3 and 20.4).

In recent two decades, researchers have found that NF is usually polymicrobial rather than monomicrobial which was mainly by group A beta-hemolytics Streptococcus [6]. NF is usually associated with an underlying cause, such as diabetes, [7] atherosclerotic vascular disease, or venous insufficiency with edema.

Anaerobic bacteria are present in most necrotizing soft tissue infections, usually in combination with aerobic gram-negative organisms. Anaerobic organisms proliferate in an environment of local tissue hypoxia in those patients with trauma, recent surgery, or medical compromise.

Along group A hemolytic streptococci and *Staphylococcus aureus,* other aerobic and anaerobic pathogens may be present in NF, including the following:

- *Bacteroides.*
- *Clostridium.*
- *Peptostreptococcus.*
- Enterobacteriaceae.
- Coliforms (e.g., *Escherichia coli*).
- *Proteus.*

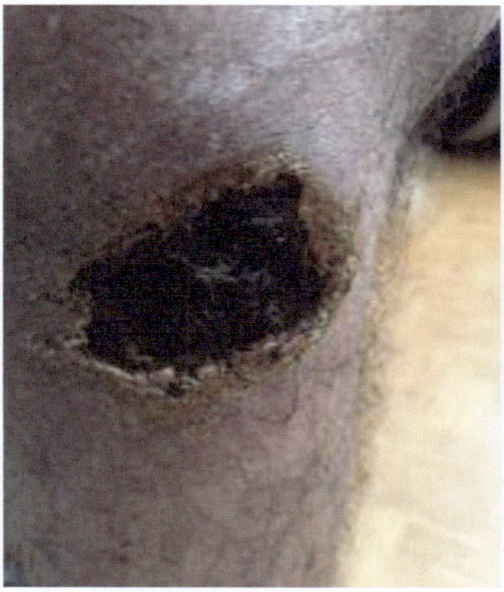
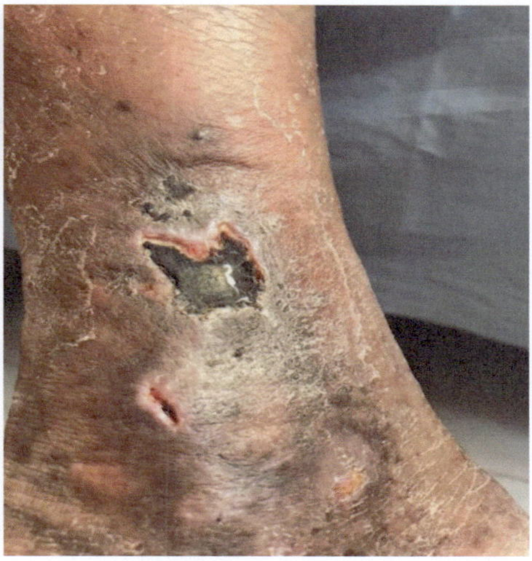

Figs. 20.3 and 20.4 NF post-foam sclerotherapy

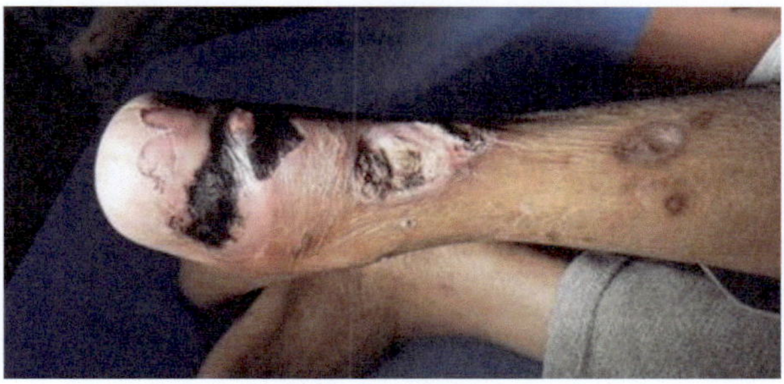

Fig. 20.5 NF of posterior ankle and lower leg in a diabetic

- *Pseudomonas.*
- *Klebsiella.*

Severe myositis accompanying septic NF may be caused by a Panton-Valentine leukocidin–positive *S aureus* strain [8].

Although NF most frequently develops after trauma that compromises skin integrity, it may rarely develop in a healthy person after minor trauma such as an isolated shoulder sprain that occurred without a break in skin barrier [9] (Fig. 20.5).

20.3 Etiology

NF may occur due to surgical procedures causing local tissue injury and bacterial invasion. These procedures include surgery for intraperitoneal infections and drainage of ischiorectal and perianal abscesses. Intramuscular injections and intravenous infusions may lead to NF of extremities.

Minor insect bites may set the stage for NF. Streptococci introduced into the wounds may be prominent initially, but the bacteriologic pattern changes with hypoxia-induced proliferation of anaerobes.

Local ischemia and hypoxia can occur in patients with systemic illnesses (e.g., diabetes). Host defenses can be compromised by underlying systemic diseases favoring the development of these infections. Diabetes or cancer have been described in >90% of cases of progressive bacterial gangrene.

A study by Hung et al. suggested that liver cirrhosis is an independent risk factor for NF. In a retrospective analysis of hospital data, the investigators determined the incidence of NF development in 40,802 patients with cirrhosis and 40,865 control patients, over a 3-year follow-up period after each patient's initial hospitalization. NF occurred during follow-up in 299 patients with cirrhosis (0.7%) and in 160 control patients (0.4%), giving patients with cirrhosis a hazard ratio of 1.98 for NF. It was also found that the risk of NF greater in patients with complicated cirrhosis than in those with the non-complicated type (hazard ratio 1.32) [10].

Studies have shown a possible relationship between the use of NSAIDs, such as ibuprofen, and the development of NF during varicella infections. Additional studies are needed to establish whether ibuprofen use has a causal role in the development of necrotizing fasciitis and its complications during varicella infections. This has not previously been described.

Group A beta-hemolytic streptococci have historically been noted as a cause of NF, but *Haemophilus aphrophilus* and *S. aureus* are also associated with the condition, and some patients have mixed infections involving multiple species of bacteria, including mycobacteria, as well as fungi [11, 12].

20.4 Clinical Presentation

20.4.1 History

Diagnosis of NF can be difficult and requires a high degree of suspicion. In many cases of NF, antecedent trauma or surgery can be identified. Surprisingly, the initial lesion is often trivial, such as an insect bite, minor abrasion, boil, or injection site. Idiopathic cases are not uncommon, however.

Hallmark symptom of NF can be intense pain and tenderness over the involved skin and underlying muscle [13]. The intensity of the pain often causes suspicion of a torn or ruptured muscle. The local pain may progress to anesthesia over several hours to days.

Other indicative findings include edema extending beyond the area of erythema, skin vesicles, and crepitus. The fascial planes and muscle groups cannot be detected by palpation.

A history of comorbid factors, including diabetes, should be sought in all cases of suspected NF. A retrospective, multicenter study by van Stigt et al. of 58 patients with NF found CVD to be the most common comorbidity (39.7% of patients) [14].

20.4.2 Physical Examination

Early in the disease course, the patient may look deceptively well; unfortunately, this may interfere with early detection, which is key to a favorable outcome. Soon, however, the patient will usually begin to appear moderately to severely toxic.

Typically, the infection begins with an area of erythema that quickly spreads over a course of hours to days. The redness quickly spreads, and its margins move out into normal skin without being raised or sharply demarcated. As the infection progresses, the skin near the site of insult develops a dusky or purplish discoloration. Multiple identical patches expand to produce a large area of gangrenous skin, as the erythema continues to spread.

Iwata et al. reported that 2 of 3 patients who lacked inflammatory signs such as redness and heat experienced fulminant progression of NF and death [15]. The initial necrosis appears as a massive undermining of the skin and subcutaneous layer. If the skin is open, gloved fingers can pass easily between the two layers and may reveal yellowish green necrotic fascia. If the skin is unbroken, a scalpel incision will reveal it.

The normal skin and subcutaneous tissue become loosened from the rapidly spreading deeper necrotic fascia that is a great distance from the initiating wound. Fascial necrosis is typically more advanced than the appearance suggests.

Anesthesia in the involved region may be detected, and it usually is caused by thrombosis of the subcutaneous blood vessels, leading to necrosis of nerve fibers.

Without treatment, secondary involvement of deeper muscle layers may occur, resulting in myositis or myonecrosis. Normally, however, the muscular layer remains healthy red with normal bleeding muscle under the yellowish green fascia.

Usually, the most important signs are tissue necrosis, putrid discharge, bullae, severe pain, gas production, rapid burrowing through fascial planes, and lack of classic tissue inflammatory signs.

Usually, some degree of intravascular volume loss is detectable on clinical examination. Other general signs, such as fever and severe systemic reactions, may be present.

Local crepitation can occur in more than one half of patients. This is an infrequent finding, specific but not sensitive, particularly in cases of nonclostridial NF.

20.5 Complications

- *Septic shock with CV collapse.*
- *Renal failure.*
- *Scarring with cosmetic deformity.*
- *Limb loss.*
- *Sepsis.*
- *Toxic shock syndrome*(TSS).

Metastatic cutaneous plaques may occur in necrotizing fasciitis. Septicemia is typical and leads to severe systemic toxicity and rapid death unless appropriately treated.

20.6 Differential Diagnoses

- Cellulitis
- Gas Gangrene
- Streptococcal Toxic Shock Syndrome.

20.7 Approach Considerations

20.7.1 Laboratory Evaluation

- CBC with differential.
- Serum chemistry studies.
- ABG analysis.
- Urinalysis.
- Blood and tissue cultures.

New techniques: rapid streptococcal diagnostic kits and a PCR assay for tissue specimens that tests for the genes for streptococcal pyrogenic exotoxin produced by group A streptococci.

20.7.2 Imaging

B-mode and color Doppler USG, contrast-enhanced CT, or MRI can promote early diagnosis of NF [16]. In addition, these studies permit visualization of the location of the rapidly spreading infection. More importantly, MRI or CT scan delineation of the extent of NF may be useful in directing rapid surgical debridement.

Plain radiographs, often obtained to detect soft tissue gas that is sometimes present in polymicrobial or clostridial necrotizing fasciitis, are of no value in the diagnosis of necrotizing infections.[17] Indeed, nondiagnostic plain radiographs may even hinder the diagnosis of necrotizing infection (Fig. 20.6).

20.7.2.1 CT and MRI

CT scanning can pinpoint the anatomic site of involvement by demonstrating necrosis with asymmetrical fascial thickening and the presence of gas in the tissues. However, note that early on, CT scan findings may be minimal (Fig. 20.7).

While no published, well-controlled, clinical trial has compared the efficacy of various diagnostic imaging modalities in the diagnosis of necrotizing infections, MRI is the preferred technique to detect soft tissue infection because of its

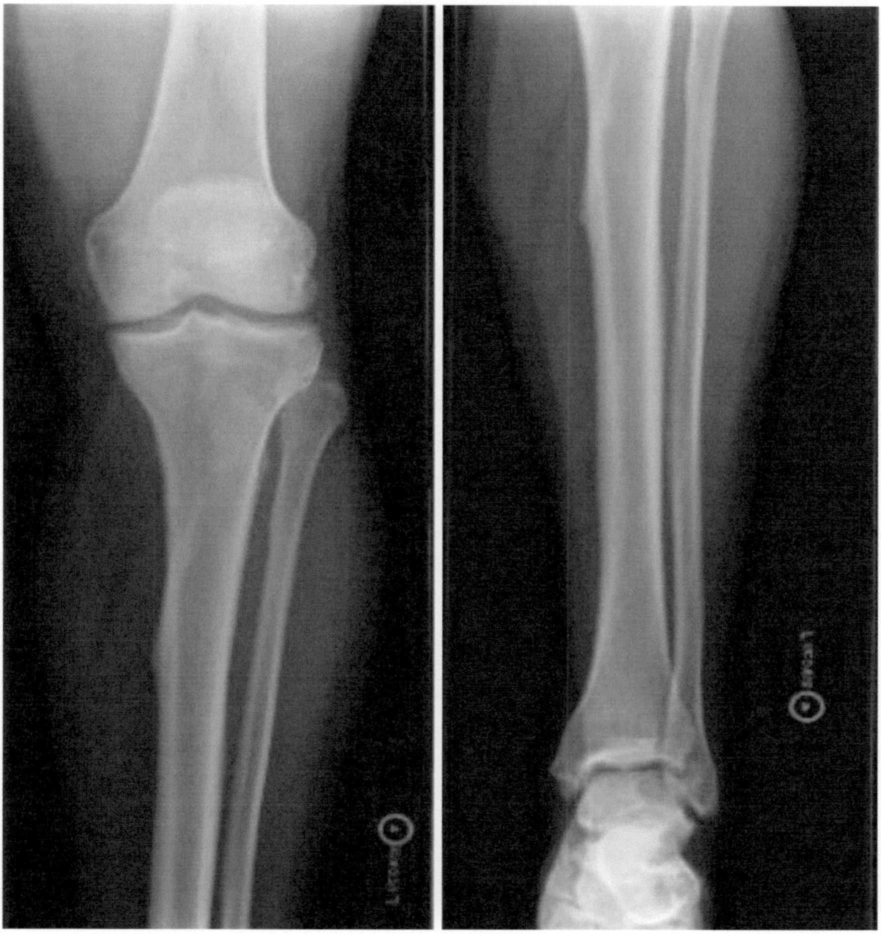

Fig. 20.6 Drug-indued NF showing mild tibial plafond spurring

Fig. 20.7 CT of drug induced NF showing small amount of gas and subcutaneous fat edema in anterior and lateral leg

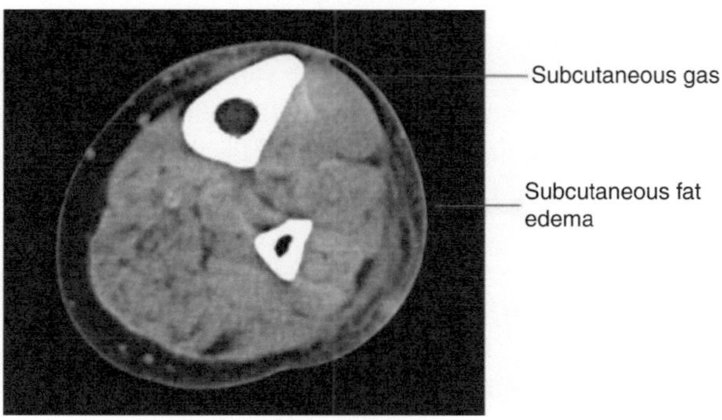

unsurpassed soft tissue contrast and sensitivity in detecting soft tissue fluid, its spatial resolution, and its multiplanar capabilities [18].

20.7.3 Finger Test and Biopsy

The finger test should be used in the diagnosis of patients who present with NF [19]. The area of suspected involvement is first infiltrated with local anesthesia. A 2-cm incision is made in the skin down to the deep fascia. Lack of bleeding is a sign of NF. On some occasions, a dishwater-colored fluid is noticed seeping from the wound.

A gentle, probing maneuver with the index finger covered by a sterile powder-free surgical double-glove puncture indication system is then performed at the level of the deep fascia. If the tissues dissect with minimal resistance, the finger test is positive.

Tissue biopsies are then sent for frozen section analysis. The characteristic histologic findings are obliterative vasculitis of the subcutaneous vessels, acute inflammation, and subcutaneous tissue necrosis. If either the finger test or rapid frozen section analysis is positive or if the patient has progressive clinical findings consistent with NF, immediate operative treatment must be initiated.

20.7.3.1 Excisional Deep Skin Biopsy

Excisional deep skin biopsy may be helpful in diagnosing and identifying the causative organisms [20]. Specimens can be taken from the spreading periphery of the necrotizing infection or the deeper tissues, reached only in surgical debridement, to obtain proper cultures for microorganisms.

Avoid doing this procedure from the actual necrosis or granulating center, as many bacteria that neither cause nor add to the infection would be detected.

20.7.4 Aspiration and Gram Stain

20.7.5 Histologic Findings

Sections from NF tissue show superficial fascial necrosis with blood vessels occluded by thrombi. A dense infiltration of neutrophils may be observed in deeper parts of the subcutaneous tissue and fascia. Subcutaneous fat necrosis and vasculitis are also evident. Eccrine glands and ducts may be necrotic.

20.8 Management

20.8.1 Surgical Debridement

Surgery is the primary treatment for NF. Surgeons must be consulted early in the care of these patients, as early and aggressive surgical debridement of necrotic tissue can be life-saving [21]. In addition, early surgical treatment may minimize tissue loss, eliminating the need for amputation of the infected extremity.

There should be wide, extensive debridement of all tissues that can be easily elevated off the fascia with gentle pressure. Wide debridement of all necrotic and poorly perfused tissues is associated with more rapid clinical improvement.

After the initial debridement, the wound must be carefully examined. Hemodynamic instability is usually present after surgery, and it may cause progressive skin necrosis. After debridement, the patient may return as often as necessary for further surgical debridement. The anesthesiologist is an important member of the operative team because continued resuscitative efforts are undertaken during the operative procedure.

The surgical regimen can be summarized as follows:

- Surgical incisions should be deep and extend beyond the areas of necrosis until viable tissue is reached.
- The entire necrotic area should be excised.
- The wound should be well irrigated.
- Hemostasis should be maintained, and the wound should be kept open.
- Surgical debridement and evaluations should be repeated almost on a daily basis.
- The wound should be inspected in the operating room.

20.8.1.1 Double Gloving

During surgery, all operating room personnel should wear a powder-free double-glove hole indication system (i.e., including an underglove with distinct color that becomes apparent when the outer glove is punctured in the presence of fluid). This protects the staff as well as the patient from exposure to potentially deadly bloodborne viral infections [22].

The US Food and Drug Administration (FDA) only requires that the leakage rate of sterile surgical gloves does not exceed 1.5%. This high frequency of glove holes is an invitation to the spread of deadly bloodborne infections between operating room personnel and the patient.

20.8.2 Dressings

Following each debridement of the necrotic tissue, daily antibiotic dressings are recommended [23]. Silver sulfadiazine (Silvadene) remains the most popular antimicrobial cream. This agent has broad-spectrum antibacterial activity and is associated with relatively few complications in these wounds.

The current formulation of silver sulfadiazine contains a lipid-soluble carrier, polypropylene glycol, which has certain disadvantages, including pseudoeschar formation. When this antibacterial agent is formulated with poloxamer 188, the silver sulfadiazine can be washed easily from the wound because of its water solubility, making dressing changes considerably more comfortable.

If the patient is allergic to sulfa, alternative agents include Polysporin, Bacitracin, and Bactroban. While these agents are relatively inexpensive, they may induce allergies.

Mafenide is an alternate agent that penetrates eschar more effectively than silver sulfadiazine. Consequently, it is frequently used on infected wounds that do not respond to silver sulfadiazine. Use mafenide with caution because it can induce metabolic acidosis.

The Acticoat brand of barrier dressings provides the beneficial antimicrobial properties of the silver ion by coating the dressing material with a thin, soluble silver film. This dressing appears to maintain antibacterial levels of silver ions in the wound for up to 5 days. Because Acticoat can remain on the wound for up to 5 days, the patient is spared the pain and expense associated with the dressing changes. Additional studies are now under way to determine the ultimate benefit of this product.

20.8.3 Soft Tissue Reconstruction

Once all of the affected tissues have been debrided, soft tissue reconstruction can be considered. In the authors' experience, this may take at least two debridements. When the debridement involves relatively small (< 25%) body surface areas, skin grafts, and flaps can provide coverage. When donor-site availability is limited, alternatives to standard skin graft construction must be considered, including Integra artificial skin (Integra Life Sciences, Plainsboro, NJ) and AlloDerm (LifeCell Corporation, Blanchburg, NJ) [24] (Figs. 20.8–20.10)

20.8.4 Antimicrobial Therapy

Empiric antibiotics should be started immediately. Initial antimicrobial therapy should be broad-based to cover aerobic gram-positive and gram-negative organisms and anaerobes. A foul smell in the lesion strongly suggests the presence of anaerobic organisms. The maximum doses of the antibiotics should be used, with consideration of the patient's weight and liver and renal status (Figs. 20.11–20.18).

Antibiotic therapy is a key consideration. Possible regimens include a combination of penicillin G and an aminoglycoside (if renal function permits), as well as clindamycin (to cover streptococci, staphylococci, gram-negative bacilli, and anaerobes).

A more specifically targeted antibiotic regimen may be begun after the results of initial gram-stained smear, culture, and sensitivities are available.

Although some necrotizing infections may still be susceptible to penicillin, clindamycin is the treatment of choice for necrotizing infections, for the following reasons [17].

- Unlike penicillin, the efficacy of clindamycin is not affected by the inoculum size or stage of bacterial growth [25, 26].
- Clindamycin is a potent suppressor of bacterial toxin synthesis [27, 28].
- Subinhibitory concentrations of clindamycin facilitate the phagocytosis of GABS [16].

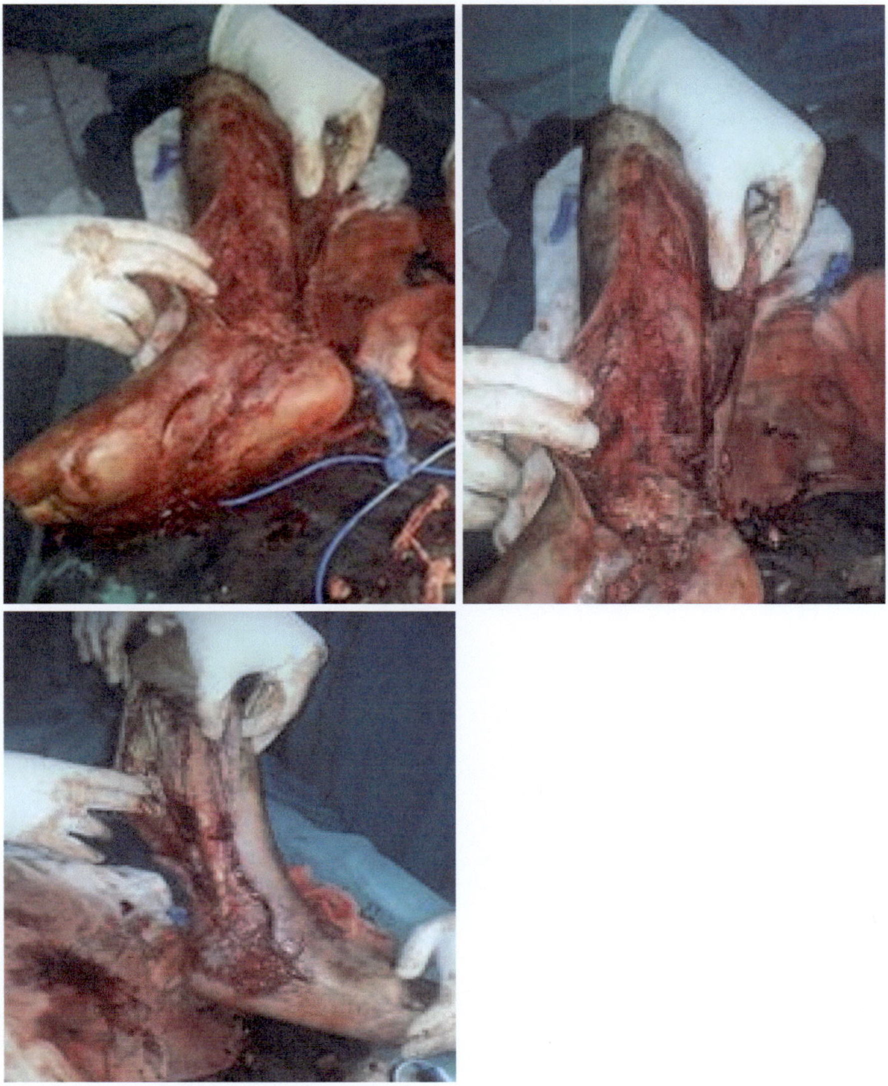

Figs. 20.8–20.10 Aggressive surgical debridement of NF in a diabetic patient

- Clindamycin reduces the synthesis of penicillin-binding protein, which, in addition to being a target for penicillin, is also an enzyme involved in cell wall synthesis and degradation [26].
- Clindamycin has a longer postantibiotic effect than β-lactins such as penicillin [28].
- Clindamycin suppresses lipopolysaccharide-induced mononuclear synthesis of tumor necrosis factor-α (TNF-α) [29].

Consequently, the success of clindamycin also may be related to its ability to modulate the immune response [30].

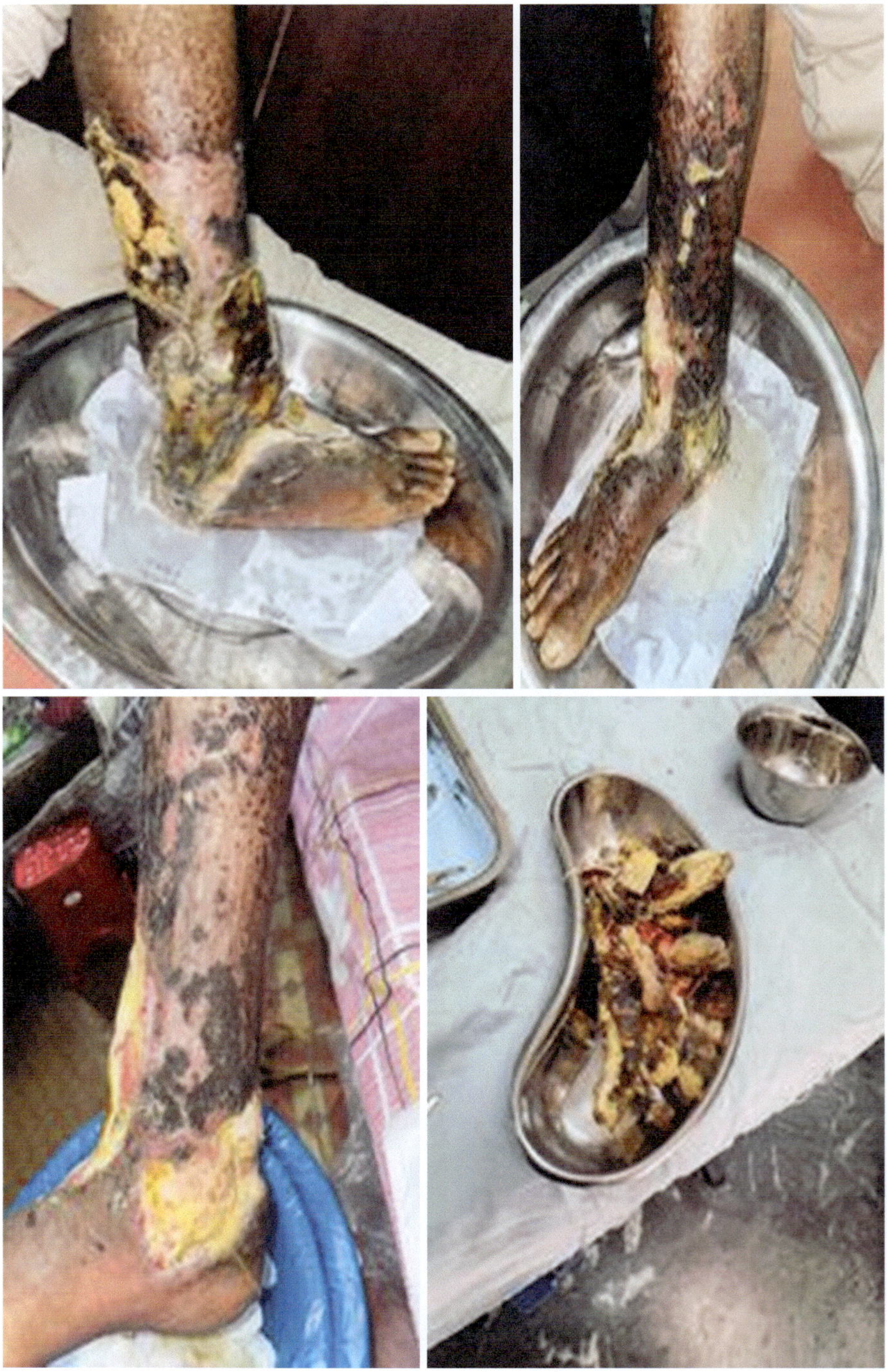

Figs. 20.11–20.18 Excised Necrotic Eschars in NF Leg Followed by Daily Dressings Showing Good Vascularity & Healing Well

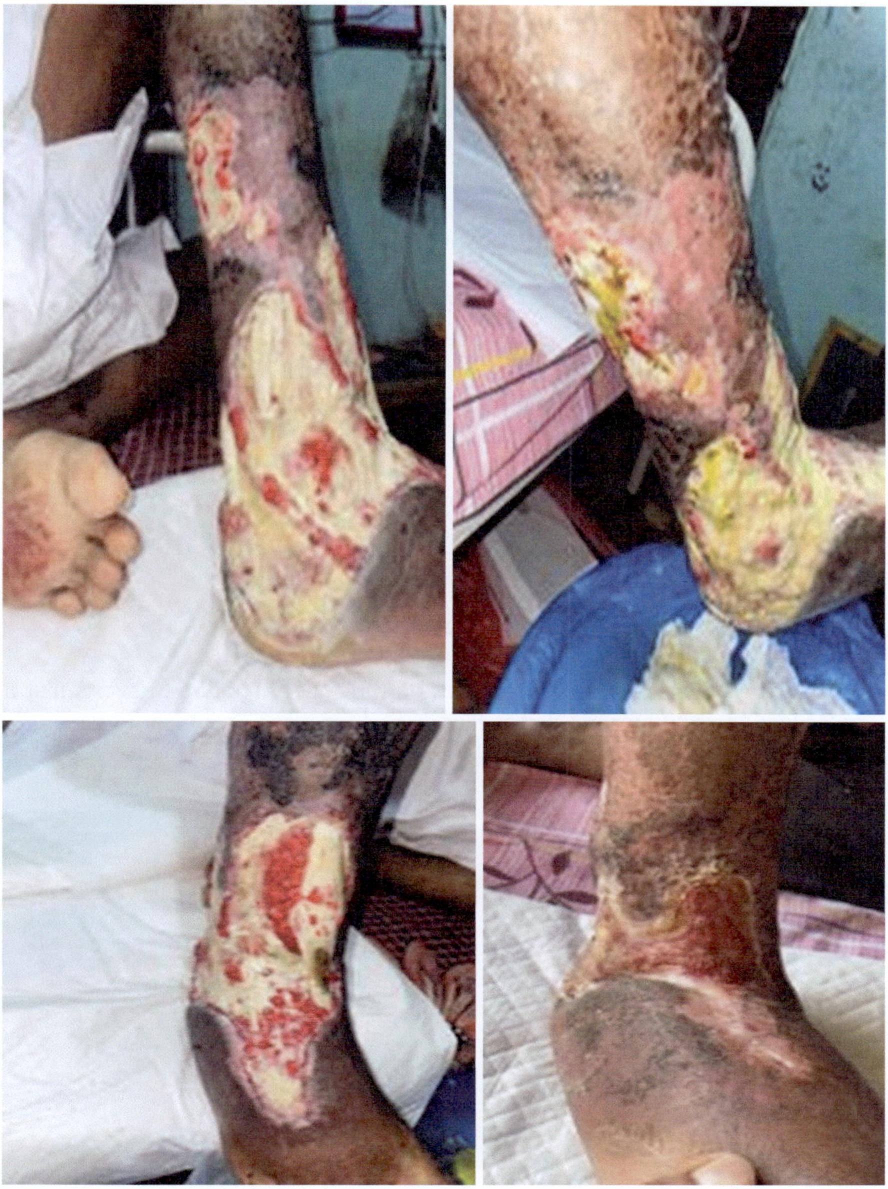

Figs. 20.11–20.18 (continued)

Broad-spectrum beta-lactam drugs such as imipenem cover aerobes, including *Pseudomonas* species. Ampicillin sulbactam also has broad-spectrum coverage, but it does not cover *Pseudomonas* species; however, NF caused by *Pseudomonas aeruginosa* is unusual [31].

If staphylococci or gram-negative rods are involved, vancomycin and other antibiotics to treat gram-negative organisms other than aminoglycosides may be required. The use of vancomycin to treat methicillin-resistant *Staphylococcus aureus* (MRSA) may depend on the clinical situation. It's use may depend on whether a naso-cranial infection is present, or it may need to be avoided in patients who are likely to be carriers of MRSA (e.g., those with diabetes, those who use illicit drugs, those undergoing hemodialysis).

20.8.5 Fluid, Nutritional Support, IVIG (Intravenous Immunoglobulin)

Because of persistent hypotension and diffuse capillary leak, massive amounts of intravenous fluids may be necessary after the patient is admitted to the hospital. Nutritional support is also an integral part of treatment for patients with NF. This supplementation should be initiated as soon as hemodynamic stability is achieved. Enteral feeding should be established as soon as possible to offset the catabolism associated with large open wounds.

Successful use of IVIG has been reported in the treatment of streptococcal TSS [32, 33].

20.8.6 Hyperbaric Oxygen Therapy (HBOT)

HBOT May Be Considered, if Available [34, 35]. The Literature Suggests that it Can Reduce Mortality when Used as Part of an Aggressive Treatment Regimen for NF [36] (Figs. 20.19, 20.20 and 20.21).

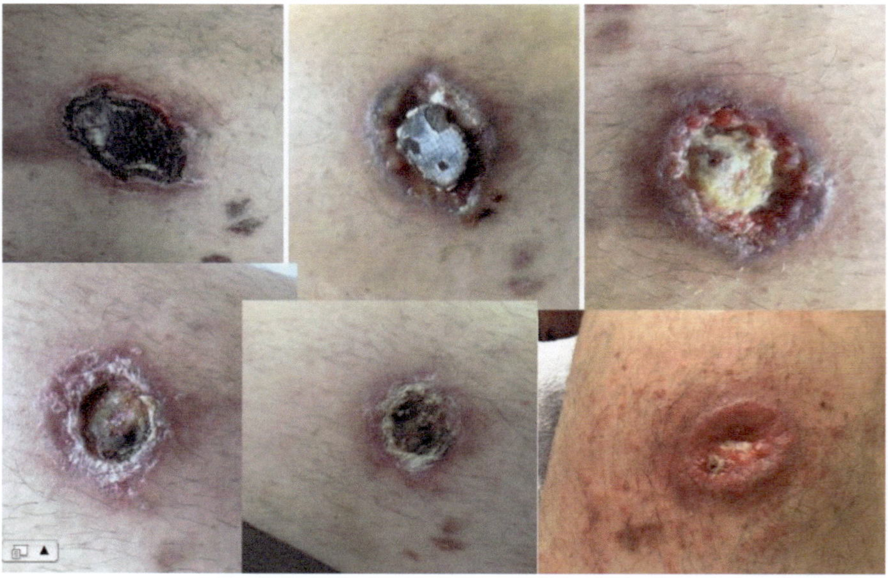

Fig. 20.19 Healing NF of leg caused by sclerotherapy

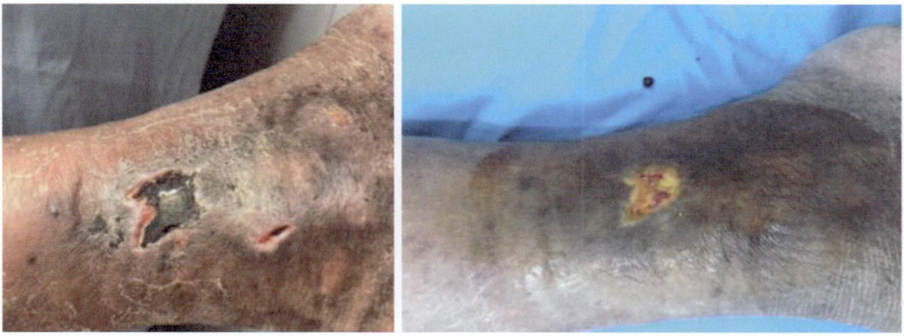

Fig. 20.20 Healing NF of ankle caused by sclerotherapy

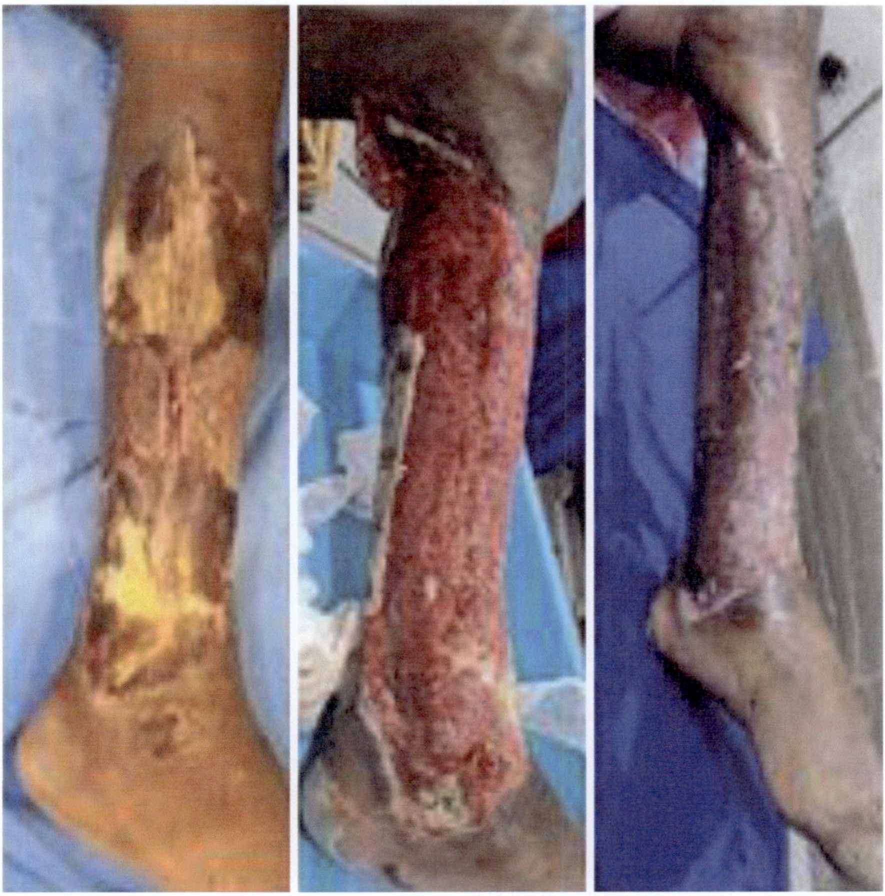

Fig. 20.21 Healed NF of lateral leg

References

1. Misiakos EP, Bagias G, Patapis P, Sotiropoulos D, Kanavidis P, Machairas A. Current concepts in the management of necrotizing fasciitis. Front Surg. 2014;1:36.
2. Federman DG, Kravetz JD, Kirsner RS. Necrotizing fasciitis and cardiac catheterization. Cutis. 2004;73(1):49–52.
3. Chan HT, Low J, Wilson L, Harris OC, Cheng AC, Athan E. Case cluster of necrotizing fasciitis and cellulitis associated with vein sclerotherapy. Emerg Infect Dis. 2008;14(1):180–1.
4. Kihiczak GG, Schwartz RA, Kapila R. Necrotizing fasciitis: a deadly infection. J Eur Acad Dermatol Venereol. 2006;20(4):365–9.
5. Quirk WF Jr, Sternbach G. Joseph Jones: infection with flesh eating bacteria. J Emerg Med. 1996;14(6):747–53.
6. Rouse TM, Malangoni MA, Schulte WJ. Necrotizing fasciitis: a preventable disaster. Surgery. 1982;92(4):765–70.
7. Bahebeck J, Sobgui E, Loic F, Nonga BN, Mbanya JC, Sosso M. Limb-threatening and life-threatening diabetic extremities: clinical patterns and outcomes in 56 patients. J Foot Ankle Surg. 2010;49(1):43–6.
8. Lehman D, Tseng CW, Eells S, et al. Staphylococcus aureus Panton-valentine leukocidin targets muscle tissues in a child with myositis and necrotizing fasciitis. Clin Infect Dis. 2010;50(1):69–72.
9. Kim HJ, Kim DH, Ko DH. Coagulase-positive staphylococcal necrotizing fasciitis subsequent to shoulder sprain in a healthy woman. Clin Orthop Surg. 2010;2(4):256–9.
10. Hung TH, Tsai CC, Tsai CC, et al. Liver cirrhosis as a real risk factor for necrotising fasciitis: a three-year population-based follow-up study. Singap Med J. 2014;55(7):378–82.
11. Sendi P, Johansson L, Dahesh S, et al. Bacterial phenotype variants in group B streptococcal toxic shock syndrome. Emerg Infect Dis. 2009;15(2):223–32.
12. Tang WM, Ho PL, Yau WP, Wong JW, Yip DK. Report of 2 fatal cases of adult necrotizing fasciitis and toxic shock syndrome caused by Streptococcus agalactiae. Clin Infect Dis. 2000;31(4):E15–7.
13. Olafsson EJ, Zeni T, Wilkes DS. A 46-year-old man with excruciating shoulder pain. Chest. 2005;127(3):1039–44.
14. van Stigt SF, de Vries J, Bijker JB, et al. Review of 58 patients with necrotizing fasciitis in The Netherlands. World J Emerg Surg. 2016;11:21.
15. Iwata Y, Sato S, Murase Y, et al. Five cases of necrotizing fasciitis: lack of skin inflammatory signs as a clinical clue for the fulminant type. J Dermatol. 2008;35(11):719–25.
16. Drake DB, Woods JA, Bill TJ, et al. Magnetic resonance imaging in the early diagnosis of group a beta streptococcal necrotizing fasciitis: a case report. J Emerg Med. 1998;16(3):403–7.
17. Namias N, Martin L, Matos L, Sleeman D, Snowdon B. Symposium: necrotizing fasciitis. Contemp Surg. 1996;49:167–78.
18. Beltran J, McGhee RB, Shaffer PB, et al. Experimental infections of the musculoskeletal system: evaluation with MR imaging and Tc-99m MDP and Ga-67 scintigraphy. Radiology. 1988;167(1):167–72.
19. Childers BJ, Potyondy LD, Nachreiner R, et al. Necrotizing fasciitis: a fourteen-year retrospective study of 163 consecutive patients. Am Surg. 2002;68(2):109–16.
20. Bakleh M, Wold LE, Mandrekar JN, Harmsen WS, Dimashkieh HH, Baddour LM. Correlation of histopathologic findings with clinical outcome in necrotizing fasciitis. Clin Infect Dis. 2005;40(3):410–4.
21. Hakkarainen TW, Kopari NM, Pham TN, Evans HL. Necrotizing soft tissue infections: review and current concepts in treatment, systems of care, and outcomes. Curr Probl Surg. 2014;51(8):344–62.
22. Edlich RF, Wind TC, Heather CL, Thacker JG. Reliability and performance of innovative surgical double-glove hole puncture indication systems. J Long-Term Eff Med Implants. 2003;13(2):69–83.

23. Gear AJ, Hellewell TB, Wright HR, et al. A new silver sulfadiazine water soluble gel. Burns. 1997;23(5):387–91.
24. Frame JD, Still J, Lakhel-LeCoadou A, et al. Use of dermal regeneration template in contracture release procedures: a multicenter evaluation. Plast Reconstr Surg. 2004;113(5):1330–8.
25. Stevens DL, Yan S, Bryant AE. Penicillin-binding protein expression at different growth stages determines penicillin efficacy in vitro and in vivo: an explanation for the inoculum effect. J Infect Dis. 1993;167(6):1401–5.
26. Yan S, Bohach GA, Stevens DL. Persistent acylation of high-molecular-weight penicillin-binding proteins by penicillin induces the postantibiotic effect in streptococcus pyogenes. J Infect Dis. 1994;170(3):609–14.
27. Gemmell CG, Peterson PK, Schmeling D, et al. Potentiation of opsonization and phagocytosis of streptococcus pyogenes following growth in the presence of clindamycin. J Clin Invest. 1981;67(5):1249–56.
28. Stevens DL, Bryant AE, Yan S. Invasive group a streptococcal infection: new concepts in antibiotic treatment. Int J Antimicrob Agent. 1994;4:297–301.
29. Stevens DL, Bryant AE, Hackett SP. Antibiotic effects on bacterial viability, toxin production, and host response. Clin Infect Dis. 1995;20(Suppl 2):S154–7.
30. Edlich RF, Winters KL, Woodard CR, Britt LD, Long WB 3rd. Massive soft tissue infections: necrotizing fasciitis and purpura fulminans. J Long-Term Eff Med Implants. 2005;15(1):57–65.
31. Lota AS, Altaf F, Shetty R, Courtney S, McKenna P, Iyer S. A case of necrotising fasciitis caused by Pseudomonas aeruginosa. J Bone Joint Surg Br. 2010;92(2):284–5.
32. Barry W, Hudgins L, Donta ST, Pesanti EL. Intravenous immunoglobulin therapy for toxic shock syndrome. JAMA. 1992;267(24):3315–6.
33. Yong JM. Necrotising fasciitis. Lancet. 1994;343(8910):1427.
34. Korhonen K. Hyperbaric oxygen therapy in acute necrotizing infections with a special reference to the effects on tissue gas tensions. Ann Chir Gynaecol Suppl. 2000;897:36.
35. Korhonen K, Kuttila K, Niinikoski J. Tissue gas tensions in patients with necrotising fasciitis and healthy controls during treatment with hyperbaric oxygen: a clinical study. Eur J Surg. 2000;166(7):530–4.
36. Green RJ, Dafoe DC, Raffin TA. Necrotizing fasciitis. Chest. 1996;110(1):219–29.

Vasculitis

21

Shantonu Kumar Ghosh

Vasculitis is a term used to describe a group of uncommon diseases which produce inflammatory changes and necrosis in the blood vessel walls. Loss of integrity leads to bleeding and compromise of the lumen leads to tissue ischemia and necrosis [1]. In 1994, the definition of vasculitis was proposed at an international consensus conference as "Vasculitis is the inflammation of vessel wall, resulting in vascular damage and a wide variety of clinical signs and symptoms" [2].

Vasculitis may occur as a primary process or may be secondary to another underlying disease, e.g., Rheumatoid Arthritis (RA), Systemic Lupus Erythematosus (SLE) or Sjögren's syndrome. The outcome of this inflammation depends on the size, type, and location of the vessels involved. Inflammation can affect the aorta and its branches or may affect medium sized arteries through to small arteries, venules, and arterioles [3]. Though ulcers are also evident in large vessel vasculitis, the small vessel vasculitis is most associated with cutaneous changes, including nail fold infarct and leg ulceration. General features such as fever, weight loss, and anorexia may accompany widespread inflammation, which cause significant morbidity and mortality. Patients with Rheumatoid Arthritis (RA) are predisposed to developing chronic leg ulcers. Thurtle and Cawley [4] found that 9% of patients with RA had a leg ulcer at some time, and 0.6–8% of inpatients with RA have an active leg ulcer, compared to 1% prevalence in the general adult population.

S. K. Ghosh (✉)
Department of Vascular Surgery, National Institute of Cardiovascular Diseases and Hospital, Dhaka, Bangladesh

A. K. Khanna, S. K. Tiwary (eds.), *Uncommon Ulcers of the Extremities*,
https://doi.org/10.1007/978-981-99-1782-2_21

Table 21.1 Types of systemic vasculitis

Type of vessel involved	Primary	Secondary
Large-vessel vasculitis	Giant-cell arteritis	Aortitis associated with RA
	Takayasu's arteritis	Infection (tuberculosis, syphilis)
Medium-sized-vessel vasculitis	Polyarteritis nodosa	HBV associated PAN
	Kawasaki's disease	
Small-vessel vasculitis, ANCA associated	Granulomatosis with polyangiitis (Wegener's), c-ANCA associated	Drugs: Propylthiouracil Hydralazine
	Microscopic polyangiitis, p-ANCA associated	
	Eosinophilic granulomatosis with polyangiitis (Churg-Strauss syndrome), p-ANCA associated	
Small-vessel vasculitis, immune complex associated	IgA vasculitis (Henoch-Schonlein purpura) (IgAV)	RA, SLE, Sjogren's syndrome
	Cryoglobulinaemic vasculitis (non-HCV)	Serum sickness
	Anti-GBM disease	Cryoglobulinaemic vasculitis (HCV)
	Hypocomplementemic vasculitis	Drug induced: Sulfonamides, Penicillins, thiazide diuretics
Variable	Behçet's disease	Drugs: Cocaine
	Cogan's syndrome	

Adapted from [19, 20]

21.1 Classification

The development of a standard classification of different types of vasculitis was challenging for clinicians involved in diagnosis and management [5, 6]. First diagnostic classification was proposed by Zeek et al. [7] in 1950 based on the size of vessel. In 1990, American college of Rheumatology published a classification based on clinical and histopathologic criteria. However, all these classifications could not overcome the difficulties posed by overlapping clinical features. Later Carlson et al. [8] proposed a framework for classifying cutaneous vasculitides that included clinical features, histopathologic criteria, laboratory findings, and relationship of different etiologies (Table 21.1).

21.2 Etiology and Pathogenesis

The development of the different types of vasculitis is affected by many factors. One of these is the deposition of circulating immune complexes within vessel walls, a mechanism implicated in hypersensitivity vasculitis. Potential antigens include drugs and chemicals as well as infectious agents such as viruses or bacteria. Interacting with the complement system, the immune complex deposition stimulates the production of chemotactic factors, vasoactive amines (histamine), and proinflammatory cytokines (interleukin 1, tumor necrosis factor), which in turn induce the expression of adhesion molecules on endothelial cells (intracellular adhesion molecule-1, vascular cell adhesion molecule-1, P-selectin, and E-selectin). The hypothesis is that this phenomenon promotes the recruitment of neutrophils, which subsequently degranulate by binding with the Fc portion of the deposited antibodies and release reactive oxygen species, collagenase, and elastase, which trigger fibrinoid necrosis of the vessel walls [9].

21.3 Role of ANCA

Antineutrophil cytoplasmic antibodies (ANCA) also play a role in the development of vasculitis. ANCA are autoantibodies directed primarily against the cytoplasmic protein anti- gens proteinase 3 (PR3) and myeloperoxidase. On indirect immunofluorescence, these antigens adopt a fluoroscopic pattern that is either perinuclear (p-ANCA), cytoplasmic (c-ANCA), or atypical. The atypical pattern (x-ANCA or a-ANCA) includes features common to both. Although most c-ANCA recognize PR3 and most p-ANCA recognize myeloperoxidase, a percentage of p-ANCA are directed against other components of primary cytoplasmic granules, such as elastase and cathepsin, or components of the secondary granules, such as lactoferrin [10]. These antibodies activate and trigger the degranulation of polymorphonuclear cells, promoting their adhesion to the endothelial cells and the generation of reactive oxygen species. However, a positive ANCA test result should be interpreted with caution because the presence of ANCA is also associated with infectious diseases (malaria and human immunodeficiency virus [HIV]), gastrointestinal diseases (inflammatory bowel disease, autoimmune hepatitis, primary biliary cirrhosis), and connective tissue diseases (lupus erythematosus, rheumatoid arthritis), and they are occasionally found in healthy individuals [11].

Other factors that may be related to the pathophysiology of systemic vasculitis are antiendothelial cell antibodies, which are also involved in the development of other autoimmune connective tissue diseases through direct and indirect action on the vascular endothelium [12]. Furthermore, a number of authors have described genetic polymorphisms that are associated, to a greater or lesser degree, with an increased risk of developing autoimmune diseases. Two examples are the case of the CD18 gene, associated with microscopic polyangiitis and the Churg-Strauss syndrome [13], and human leukocyte antigens A2, A11, and B35 alleles, associated with Henoch-Schönlein purpura [14].

21.4 Clinical Features

The different types of vasculitis give rise to a variety of primary lesions. The morphology of these lesions depends on vessel size, the anatomical site affected, and the stage of development of the lesion.

The most common primary lesions are purpuric macules or papules (palpable purpura) secondary to the involvement of the small caliber blood vessels of the skin. Other lesions that may occur include hemorrhagic blisters, pustules, urticarial or annular plaques, and nodules of varying depths that can become ulcerated. The nodules may be associated with livedo reticularis and represent damage to the vessels of the deep dermis and hypodermis. All of these lesions are found more frequently on the lower limbs, probably owing to hemodynamic factors. Cutaneous involvement in sites other than the lower limbs and the presence of nodular lesions, livedo reticularis, and ulcers are indications of vasculitis with systemic involvement. Irrespective of the underlying process or trigger, any vasculitis of the skin may be accompanied by fever, fatigue, or joint pain [15] (Table 21.2).

Circulating immune complexes (antibody/antigen) deposit in the blood vessel walls, causing inflammation that may be segmental or may involve the entire vessel.

Table 21.2 Common symptoms

Name	Typical vessels involved	Symptoms
Churg-Strauss syndrome	Small and medium vessel	Three stages: • Airway inflammation, asthma, allergic rhinitis • Hypereosinophilia • Vasculitis with tissue necrosis
Giant cell arteritis	Temporal and cranial arteries	Headaches, temporal pain, visual disturbances, scalp sensitivity, dry cough with respiratory symptoms, fever, upper extremity weakness, and sensory changes
Henoch-Schönlein purpura	Small vessels	Purpura, arthritis, abdominal pain (usually in children)
Immune complex–associated vasculitis	Small vessels to neurons	Peripheral neuropathy
Microscopic polyangiitis	Small vessels to organs	Ischemia, hemorrhage, loss of organ function
Polyarteritis nodosa	Small and medium arteries	Subcutaneous nodules or projections of lesions; fever, chills, tachycardia, arthralgia, myositis, motor, and sensory neuropathies
Primary angiitis of the CNS	Small and medium vessels in the brain and spinal cord	Brain: Headache, altered mental status, focal CNS deficits; spinal cord: Lower extremity weakness, bladder dysfunction
Takayasu's arteritis	Aorta, aorta branches, pulmonary arteries	Inflammatory phase with flu-like symptoms, pulseless upper extremity, claudication, renal artery disease
Wegener's granulomatosis (granulomatosis with polyangiitis)	Small and medium vessels	Organ failure (lung and kidneys), variable including skin, depending on the vessels involved

Adapted from [21]

At the site of inflammation, varying degrees of cellular inflammation and resulting necrosis or scarring occur in one or more layers of the vessel wall, and inflammation in the media of the muscular artery tends to destroy the internal elastic lamina [16]. Leukocytoclastic vasculitis describe findings in small-vessel vasculitis, refers to the breakdown of inflammatory cells that leaves small nuclear fragments in and around the vessels. Vasculitic inflammation tends to be transmural, rarely necrotizing, and non-granulomatous. Resolution of the inflammation tends to result in fibrosis and intimal hypertrophy, which in combination with secondary clot formation can narrow the arterial lumen and account for the ischemia or necrosis of the tissue supplied by the affected vessels [17].

21.4.1 Vasculitis Ulcer

Clinical presentation of cutaneous vasculitis, which varies depending on the arterial involvement, includes palpable purpura, livedo reticularis, pain, skin lesions with or without nodules, and tissue necrosis. It may present as one large necrotic lesion or several small lesions, but all are full thickness after debridement. Systemic symptoms may also be present and usually relate to kidney, lung, or gastrointestinal tract involvement. On some occasions, signs of vasculitis in other organs (e.g., symptoms of a CVA or lung disease) may appear at the same time that skin lesions appear. Characteristically, vasculitic ulcers are deep, with a punched out appearance, often with a reddish or bluish tinge around the edge. They are often extremely painful, and may deteriorate rapidly (Fig. 21.1). There may also be an accompanying

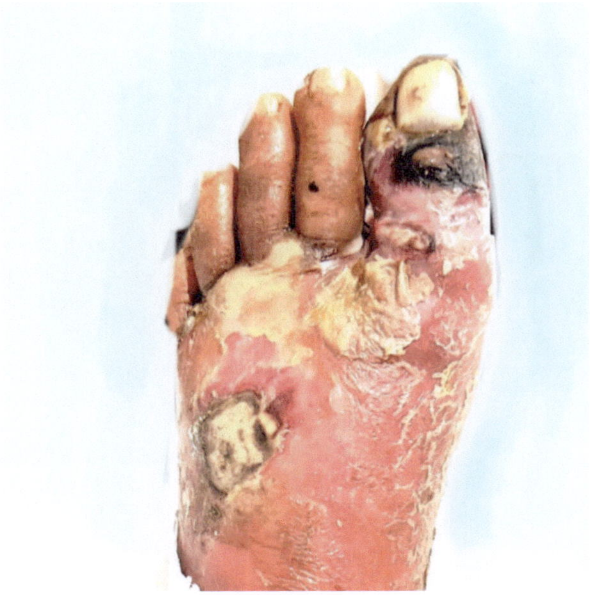

Fig. 21.1 Vasculitic ulcer and gangrene

palpable purpuric rash. One very distinctive characteristic for differential diagnosis from chronic venous wounds is the exquisite pain that occurs with vasculitis, making the initial local treatment very tedious.

21.4.2 Giant Cell Arteritis (GCA)

It is the commonest vasculitis affecting the elderly. Headache is the most common symptom occurring in >60% of patients, typically felt over the temporal areas. Temporal arteries may be tender non-pulsatile and thickened (Fig. 21.2). In 30% cases jaw claudication, pain in tongue or jaw may be present. Acute visual loss occurs in as many as 20% of patients due to anterior ischemic optic neuropathy and central retinal artery occlusion. Constitutional features, including fever, fatigue, anorexia, weight loss, and depression are present in majority of cases. In severe cases, segmental scalp necrosis or tongue infarction may be present. Extracranial arteries involved in GCA are axillary artery, subclavian artery, and aorta.

Fig. 21.2 Giant cell arteries (temporal artery)

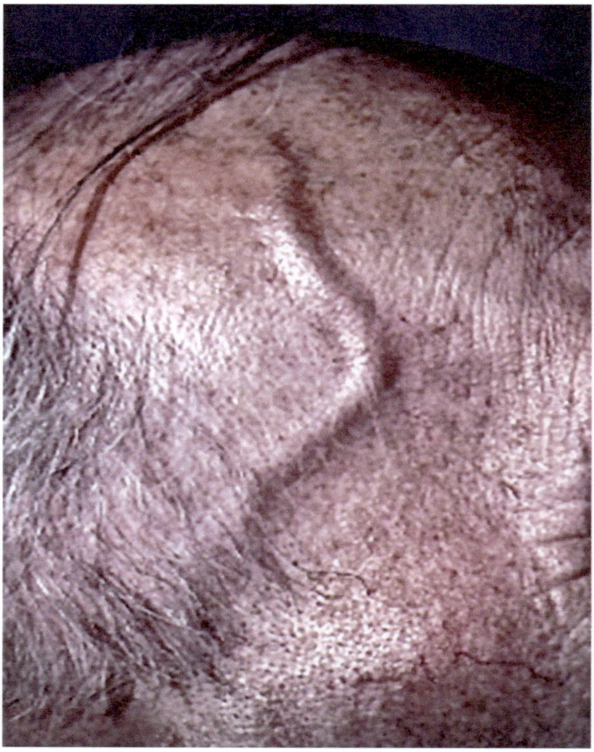

21.4.3 Takayasu Arteritis (TA)

It is a granulomatous necrotizing vasculitis affecting large vessels. In acute inflammatory phase there is adventitial thickening, cellular infiltration of the tunica media, with local destruction of the vascular smooth muscle. The intima becomes fibrosed, which leads to vessel stenosis [18]. TA is characterized by stenosis, occlusion and sometimes aneurysm formation of large arteries. Most common findings at presentation are absence or asymmetry of peripheral pulses, non-recordable blood pressure, claudication of arm or legs, transient visual disturbance scotoma, blurring or diplopia. In limbs, it frequently develops ischemia of limbs, occasionally of all four (Figs. 21.3 and 21.4).

21.4.4 Polyarteritis Nodosa (PAN)

It is a rare medium vessel vasculitis that is often associated with Hepatitis B Virus (HBV-PAN) infection. It is not associated with ANCA. Typically, the patient experiences constitutional features of fever, malaise, weight loss, and diffuse aching, along with manifestations of multisystem involvement such as peripheral neuropathy and an asymmetric polyarthritis. Cutaneous lesions include infarctions, ulcerations, livedo reticularis, subcutaneous nodules, and ischemic changes of the distal digits (Fig. 21.5).

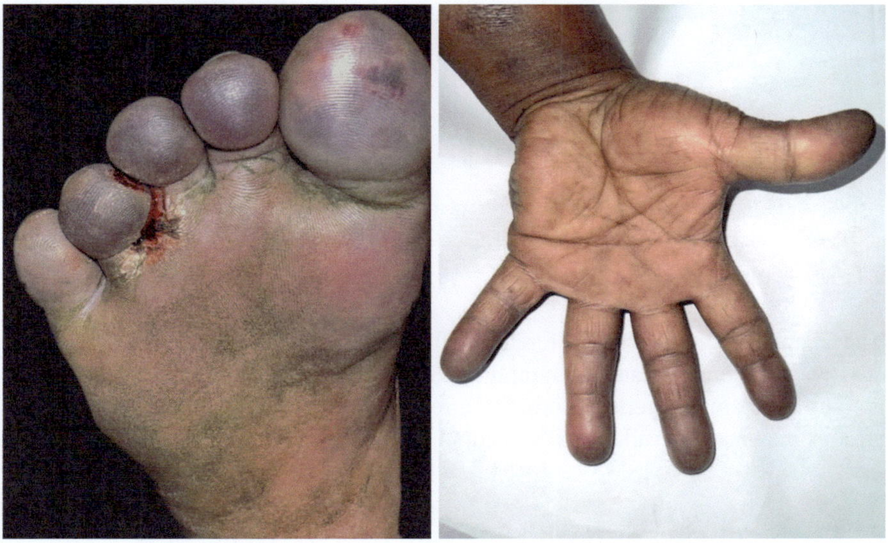

Fig. 21.3 Takayasu arteritis

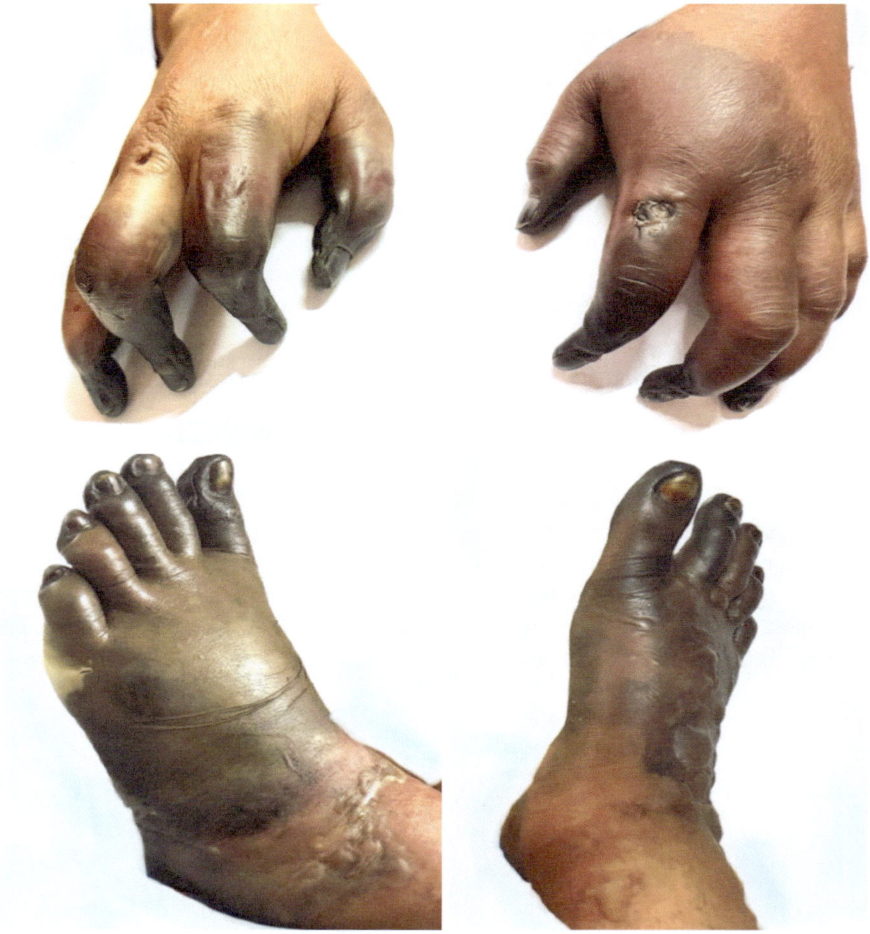

Fig. 21.4 Ischemia of all limbs of Takayasu arteritis

21.4.5 Kawasaki Disease (KD)

The Chapel Hill consensus conference defined Kawasaki disease as Arteritis associated with the mucocutaneous lymph node syndrome and predominantly affecting medium and small arteries. Coronary arteries are often involved. Aorta and large arteries may be involved. Usually occurs in infants and young children [18].

21.4.6 Granulomatosis with Polyangiitis-GPA (Wegener's)

Necrotizing granulomatous inflammation usually involving the upper and lower respiratory tract, and necrotizing vasculitis affecting predominantly small and medium vessels, e.g., capillaries, venules, arterioles, arteries, and veins (Fig. 21.6).

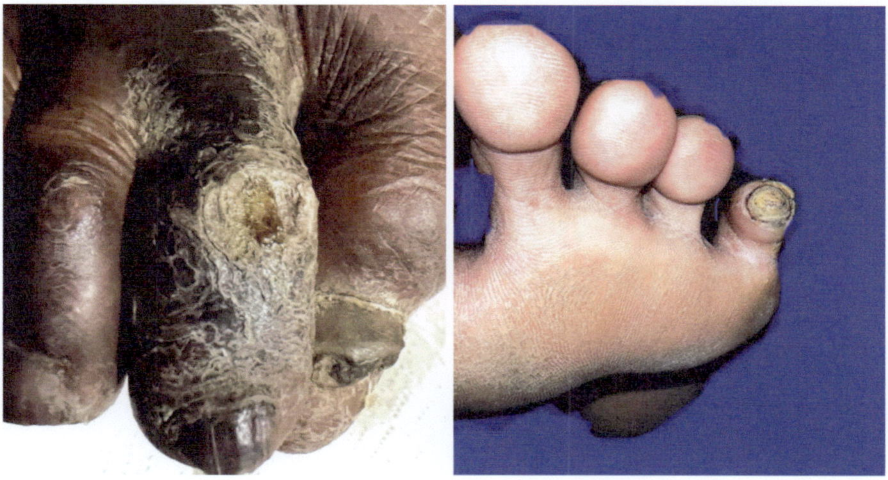

Fig. 21.5 Digital gangrene of polyarteritis nodosa

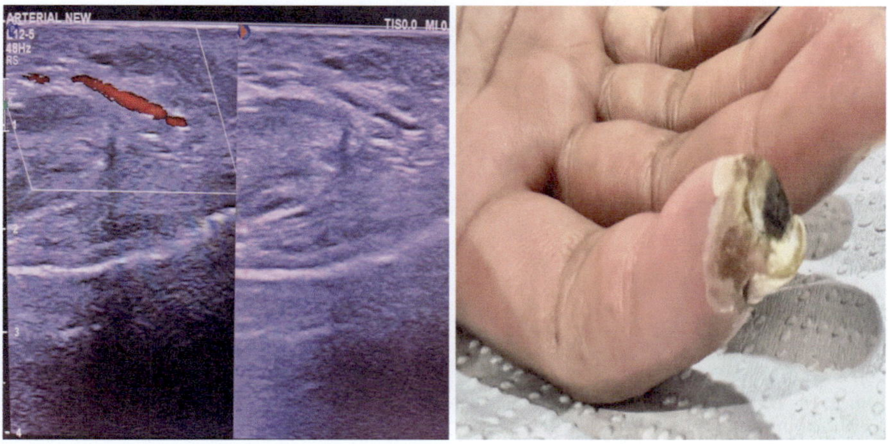

Fig. 21.6 Digital gangrene of Granulomatosis with polyangiitis

It is associated with ANCA, specifically PR3 [18]. Common pulmonary symptoms include cough, hemoptysis, and dyspnea. 40% patients may have skin involvement such as palpable purpura, digital gangrene (Fig. 21.7). Typical ENT symptoms include epistaxis, nasal crusting, sinusitis, and nasal collapse. Small bowel ischemia is a rare gastrointestinal manifestation.

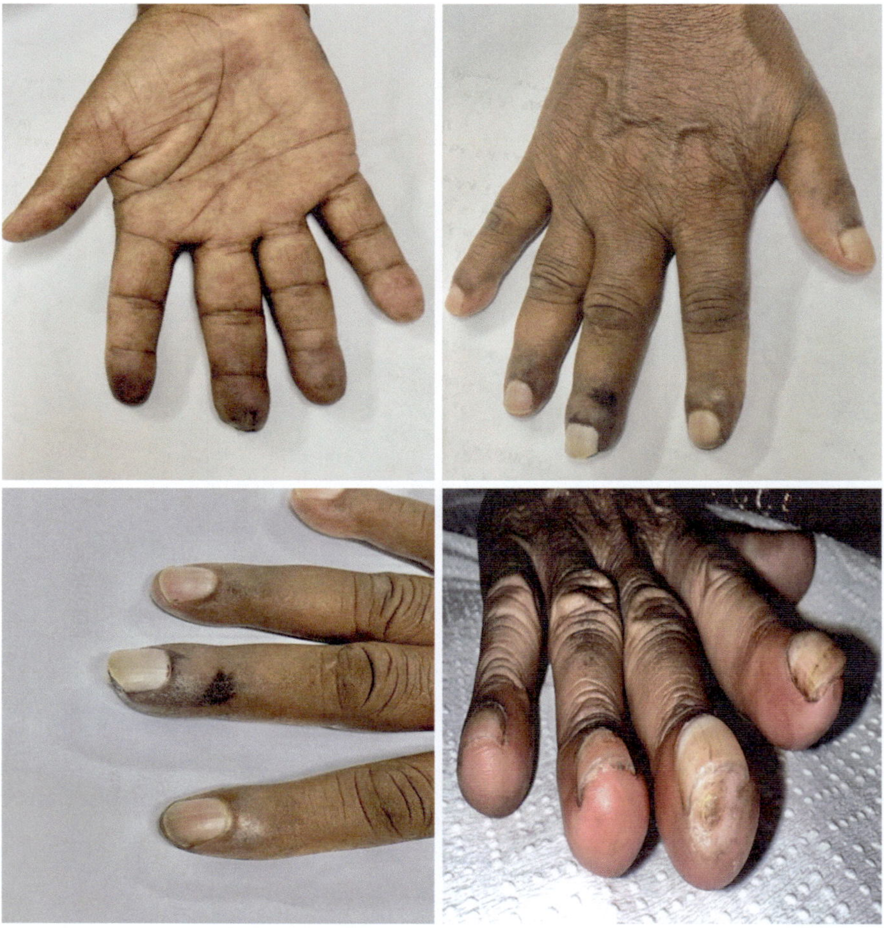

Fig. 21.7 Digital gangrene of Granulomatosis with polyangiitis

21.4.7 Microscopic Polyangiitis (MPA)

It is an ANCA associated necrotizing vasculitis, with few or no immune deposits, predominantly affecting small vessels (i.e., capillaries, venules, or arterioles). Necrotizing arteritis involving small- and medium-sized arteries may be present [18]. Necrotizing glomerulonephritis is very common. Pulmonary capillaritis often occurs leading to life threatening massive pulmonary hemorrhage. Granulomatous inflammation is absent. Skin involvement is frequent, typically a purpuric rash. Nailbed infarcts, splinter hemorrhages, livedo, infarction, or ulceration can occur.

21.4.8 Eosinophilic Granulomatosis with Polyangiitis-EGPA (Churg-Strauss Syndrome)

Eosinophil-rich and necrotizing granulomatous inflammation often involving the respiratory tract, and necrotizing vasculitis predominantly affecting small to medium vessels and associated with asthma and eosinophilia. ANCA is more frequent when glomerulonephritis is present [18]. Asthma, usually late-onset (mean age 50 years), is a cardinal feature of the disease and seen in the majority of cases (>95%). Skin involvement is seen in 40–70% of patients and is one of the most common features of the vasculitic phase of EGPA. Palpable purpura (50%) commonly occurs on the lower extremities. Cutaneous or subcutaneous nodules (30%) are the most distinctive skin lesions of EGPA (Fig. 21.8). These red or violaceous lesions occur primarily on the scalp and the limbs or hands and feet and are often bilateral and symmetrical.

21.4.9 IgA Vasculitis (Henoch-Schönlein Purpura) (IgAV)

Vasculitis, with IgA1-dominant immune deposits, affecting small vessels (predominantly capillaries, venules, or arterioles) [18]. IgA vasculitis is a predominantly childhood vasculitic syndrome. It can occur from 6 months of age onward. The classical features of IgA vasculitis are a triad of rash, gastrointestinal upset, and joint pain. The classical rash of IgA vasculitis is usually the first sign of the disease. It is an erythematous papular rash which develops into a palpable purpura (Fig. 21.9). The usual distribution is on the dependent and pressure-bearing areas of the lower limbs and buttocks. The rash is usually symmetrical and does not blanch with pressure. Skin necrosis may be seen in areas of severe cutaneous hemorrhage, and is more common in adults.

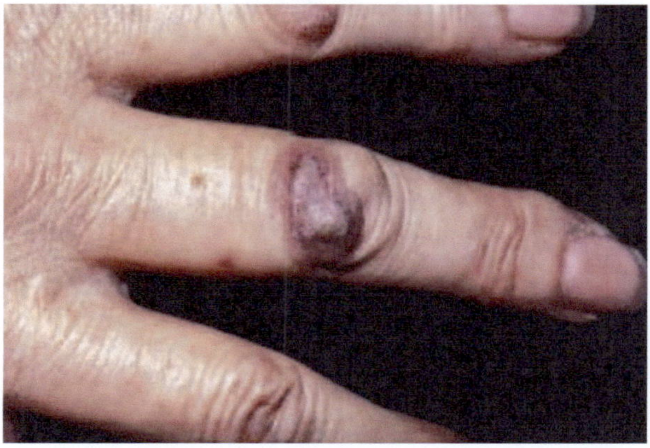

Fig. 21.8 Eosinophilic granulomatosis with polyangiitis-EGPA (Churg-Strauss syndrome)

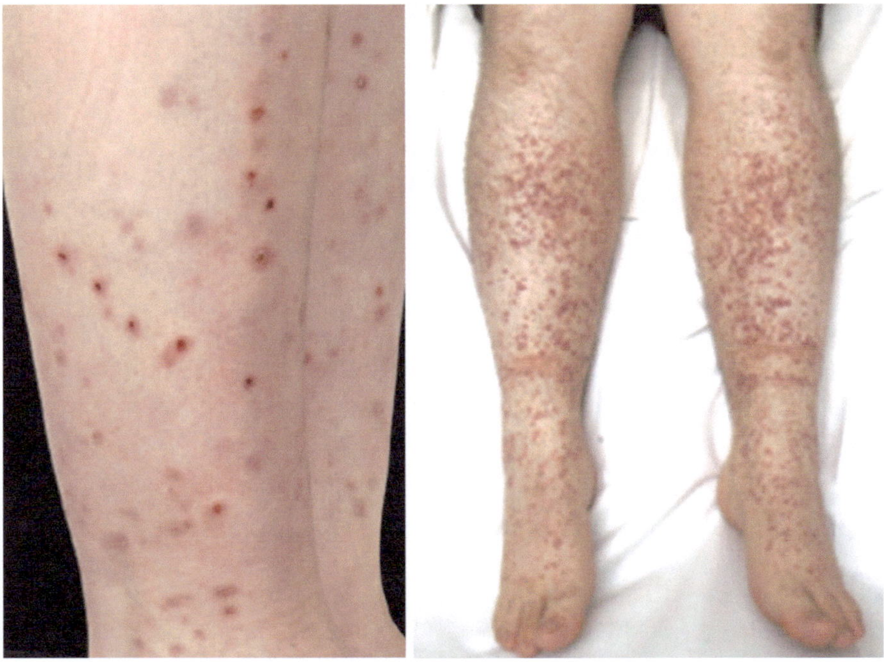

Fig. 21.9 Erythematous papular rash of IgA vasculitis (Henoch-Schönlein purpura)

Fig. 21.10 Oral aphthous ulceration in Behçet's disease

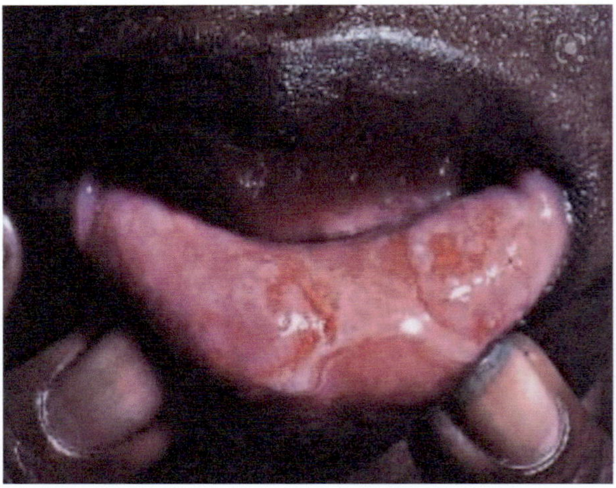

21.4.10 Behçet's Disease (BD)

It is a multisystem disease; generally recognized to be a triad of anterior uveitis usually resulting in a hypopyon, oral aphthous ulceration (Fig. 21.10), and genital ulceration. Recurrent oral ulceration is usually the first symptom. Genital ulceration in males is usually scrotal, on the shaft of penis or on the glans penis. In females, the labia majora and minora can be ulcerated. The ulcers have a punched-out appearance. They can be larger, more painful, and deeper than the oral ulcers. Genital ulcers are resistant to treatment, more likely to get infected, and usually heal with scarring. Behçet's disease can involve any part of the vascular tree—aortitis, pulmonary arterial involvement, medium-sized vessel involvement, leukocytoclastic vasculitis, portal vein thrombosis, deep venous thrombosis, dural sinus thrombosis are all a feature of Behçet's disease.

21.5 Laboratory Investigations (Table 21.3)

1. Complete blood count: Leukocytosis, neutrophilia, high platelet count.
2. Renal function: Abnormal serum creatinine in small vessel vasculitis. Compromised renal function in medium and large vessel disease due to renal arterial or suprarenal aorta involvement. Urinary protein estimation and urine protein/ creatinine ratio may be used to assess prognosis.
3. Liver function: Liver transaminases and alkaline phosphatase may be abnormal. Hepatitis due to HBV and HCV are associated with polyarteritis nodosa and cryoglobulinemic vasculitis.
4. Inflammatory markers: ESR and CRP elevated.
5. Immunology tests: (a) Antineutrophil cytoplasmic antibody test, (b) Rheumatoid factor, (c) Complement (C3 and C4) consumption, (d) Immunoglobulin subclass IgG4 level.
6. Histopathology (Table 21.4).
7. Imaging: X-ray, Duplex scanning, CT Angiogram, MR Angiogram, conventional Angiogram, Digital Substraction Angiogram, PET-CT scan.

Table 21.3 Laboratory tests for vasculitis

May increase	May decrease
Blood tests	
Erythrocyte sedimentation rate C-reactive protein Platelets White cell count	Hemoglobin Serum proteins
Specific immunological test	
Rheumatoid factor (RF) is positive in 60–80% of patients with rheumatoid arthritis. May be positive in other autoimmune conditions, e.g., Sjögren's syndrome	
Antinuclear antibody (ANA) suggests the presence of an underlying connective tissue disorder	
Complement. Low serum complement may be present in certain vasculitic conditions	
A positive test for antineutrophil cytoplasmic antibodies (ANCA) may indicate systemic vasculitis, e.g., polyarteritis, Wegener's granulomatosis, etc.	

Adapted from [22]

Table 21.4 Histologic criteria for diagnosis

Histologic definition	
Inflammatory process affecting the vessel wall. Two criteria must be met: 1. Inflammatory infiltrate in the vessel wall 2. Damage in the form of fibrin deposition and/or endothelial necrosis	
Histopathologic criteria for vasculitis	
Major Neutrophils and karyorrhexis (nuclear dust) Necrosis and fibrin deposition	
Minor	
Endothelial cell swelling Hemorrhage Thrombosis Necrosis Calcinosis	Epidermal vesicles Histiocytes Eosinophils Aneurysms

Adapted from [23]

21.6 Principles of Treatment

Treatment of any vasculitis depends on the etiology, extent, and severity of the disease. Treatment may be divided into remission induction, maintenance, and long-term follow-up [19].

21.6.1 Remission Induction

Large Vessel Disease Large vessel vasculitis (TAK and GCA) can be treated with oral Prednisolone. In critical cases intravenous Methyl Prednisolone can be used. Low dose Aspirin can be used in GCA.

Medium Vessel Disease PAN with HBV is treated with antivirals and plasma exchange. Non-HBV-associated PAN requires immunosuppression with Glucocorticoids and Cyclophosphamide. KD is treated with Immunoglobulin along with Glucocorticoids.

Small Vessel Vasculitis ANCA associated vasculitides is treated with Cyclophosphamide or Rituximab.

21.6.2 Maintenance Therapy

Mostly required for AAV. Maintenance therapy is usually started at 3 month of treatment and continued for 6–12 months with Cyclophosphamide. Then it is substituted with Methotrexate or Azathioprine [19].

21.6.3 Long-Term Follow-Up

As there is a high risk of relapse even after many years of successful remission induction, regular long-term follow-up should be carried out.

21.7 Treatment of Secondary Vasculitis

For secondary vasculitic disorders, treating the underlying comorbidity (e.g., infection, drug use, cancer, or autoimmune disorder) is crucial. Remission of life- or organ-threatening disorders is induced by using cytotoxic immunosuppressants (e.g., cyclophosphamide) and high-dose corticosteroids, usually for 3–6 months, until remission occurs or until the disease activity is acceptably reduced. Adjusted treatment to maintain remission takes longer, usually 1–2 years. During this period, the goal is to eliminate corticosteroids, reduce the dosage, or use less potent immune suppressants if needed. After tapering or eliminating corticosteroids, methotrexate or azathioprine can be substituted to maintain remission.

21.8 Management of Ulcer

Initial treatment of wounds caused by vasculitis is extremely difficult because of the pain. The principles of standard wound care (debride necrotic tissue, treat inflammation and infection, apply moist wound dressings, nurture the edges) are recommended. Topical lidocaine helps reduce pain during treatments, non-contact low-frequency ultrasound helps mobilize cellular activity and interstitial fluids, and compression therapy helps manage the edema that occurs in the lower extremities because of the inflammation and decreased mobility. Non-adherent dressings that promote autolysis of the necrotic tissue (e.g., X-Cell, Medline, Mundelein, IL) are excellent initially, especially in reducing pain levels with dressing changes. Silicone-backed foam dressings are helpful in absorbing exudate as well as in reducing pain. If the patient is on steroids, local vitamin A can be used to negate the effects of steroids. As the acute inflammation recedes, pain levels decrease, and wound healing progresses to proliferation, treatment can be more aggressive with the goals of full re-epithelialization and return to prior level of function.

References

1. Langford CA. Chronic immunosuppressive therapy for systemic vasculitis. Curr Opin Rheumatol. 1997;9(1):41–7.
2. Jennette JC, et al. Nomenclature of systemic vasculitides. Proposal of an international consensus conference. Arthritis Rheum. 1994;37:187–92.
3. Scott G. Vasculitis. In: Butler R, Jayson M, editors. Collected reports on the rheumatic diseases. Chesterfield: Arthritis and Rheumatisim Council for Research; 1995. p. 105–8.

4. Thurtle OA, Cawley MI. The frequency of leg ulceration in rheumatoid arthritis: a survey. J Rheumatol. 1983;10(3):507–9.
5. Ghersetich I, Comacchi C, Jorizzo JL, Katsambas A, Lotti TM. Proposal for a working classification of cutaneous vasculitis. Clin Dermatol. 1999;17:499–503.
6. Jennette JC, Falk RJ. Do vasculitis categorization systems really matter? Curr Rheumatol Rep. 2000;2:430–8.
7. Zeek PM. Periarteritis nodosa and other forms of necrotizing angiitis. N Engl J Med. 1953;248:764–72.
8. Carlson JA, Cavaliere LF, Grant-Kels JM. Cutaneous vasculitis: diagnosis and management. Clin Dermatol. 2006;24:414–29.
9. Sunderkötter C. Vasculitis of small blood vessels some riddles about IgA and about the complexity of transmigration. Exp Dermatol. 2009;18:91–6.
10. Radice A, Sinico RA. Antineutrophil cytoplasmic antibodies (ANCA). Autoimmunity. 2005;38:93–103.
11. Cui Z, Zhao MH, Segelmark M, Hellmark T. Natural autoantibodies to myeloperoxidase, proteinase 3, and the glomerular basement membrane are present in normal individuals. Kidney Int. 2010;78:590–7.
12. Guilpain P, Mouthon L. Antiendothelial cell antibodies in vasculitis-associated systemic diseases. Clin Rev Allergy Immunol. 2008;35:59–65.
13. Meller S, Jagiello P, Borgmann S, Fricke H, Epplen JT, Gencik M. Novel SNPs in the CD18 gene validate the association with MPO-ANCA+ vasculitis. Genes Immun. 2001;2:269–72.
14. Peru H, Soylemezoglu O, Gonen S, Cetinyurek A, Bakkaloglu SA, Buyan N, et al. HLA class 1 associations in Henoch Schonlein purpura: increased and decreased frequencies. Clin Rheumatol. 2008;27:5–10.
15. Sais G, Vidaller A, Jucgla A, Servitje O, Condom E, Peyr J. Prognostic factors in leukocytoclastic vasculitis. Arch Dermatol. 1998;134:309–15.
16. Lawley TJ, Kubota Y. Vasculitis. Dermotol Clin. 1990;8(4):681–7.
17. Fauci A, Braunwalk E, Isselbacher KT, et al. Harrison's principles of internal medicine. New York: McGraw-Hill; 1998. p. 989–91, 1004–19
18. Jennette JC, Falk RJ, Bacon PA, Basu N, Cid MC, Ferrario F, et al. 2012 revised International Chapel Hill consensus conference nomenclature of vasculitides. Arthritis Rheum. 2013;65(1):1–11.
19. Watts RA, Scott DGI, Mukhtyar C. Vasculitis in clinical practice. 2nd ed. Cham: Springer; 2015. p. 7–13.
20. Warrington KJ, Cooper JRLT. Vasculitis and other uncommon arteriopathies. In: Cronenwett JL, Johnston KW, editors. Rutherford's vascular surgery. 8th ed. Philadelphia, USA: Elsevier Saunders; 2014. p. 1154–66.
21. Hamm R. Why isn't this wound healing? In: Schiffman M, editor. Recent clinical techniques, results, and research in wounds. Springer; 2018.
22. Armitage M, Roberts J. Caring for patients with leg ulcers and a vasculitic leg condition. Br J Community Nurs. 2004;Suppl:S16–22.
23. Pulido-Perez A, Aviles-Izquierdo JA, Suarez-Fernandez R. Cutaneous vasculitis. Actas Dermosifiliogr. 2012;103(3):179–91.

22 Marjolin's Ulcer

Madhuri Gore

22.1 Introduction

Malignant ulcer developing most often in burn scar is a rare lesion. The term Marjolin's ulcer was coined by Da Costa [1] but such lesions were also observed and described by Dypuytren and much before that by Celsus in the first century AD [2, 3]. The debate about which histological type of malignancy occurring in scar be called Marjolin's ulcer is still ongoing. The description of classical Marjolin's ulcer appears appropriate for squamous cell carcinoma. As proposed by some, other variants of malignancies occurring in scar should be included in the group called scar tissue carcinomas and not Marjolin's ulcer [2]. Still other group of workers is of the opinion that the term Marjolin's ulcer should be an all-encompassing term applied to all histological types of malignancies that occur in scar tissue and chronic wounds. Therefore, no consensus has been reached yet and the debate is still on. The changes responsible for the development of malignancy are not clear, awareness about its occurrence and hence timely diagnosis is rare and studies including large number of cases are not available. All these factors make Marjolin's ulcer (MU) an enigma though it has been described almost 200 years ago.

22.2 Predisposing Factors

Marjolin's ulcer is a rare condition that occurs due to malignant degeneration in a long-standing scar tissue or chronic wound. The most common scar in which this change develops is burn scar (Fig. 22.1). Longer the time taken for healing of the burn wound, more is the possibility of development of malignancy in the scar.

M. Gore (✉)
LTMMC and LTMGH, Consultant Surgeon, Dr. Gores' Clinic, Mumbai, India

A. K. Khanna, S. K. Tiwary (eds.), *Uncommon Ulcers of the Extremities*,
https://doi.org/10.1007/978-981-99-1782-2_22

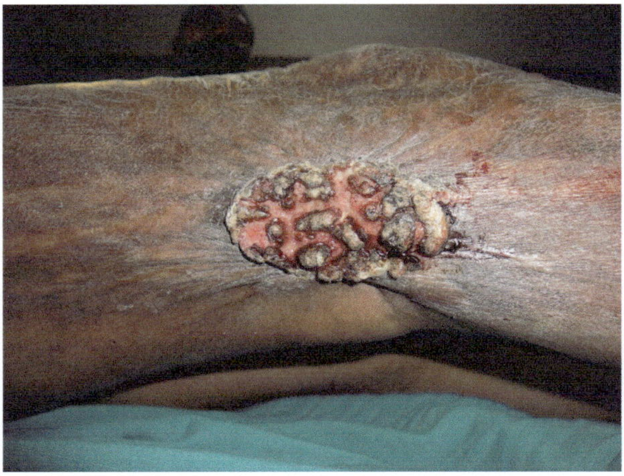

Fig. 22.1 Showing ulcerative lesion involving burn scar on lateral aspect of right knee. (Photograph curtesy Dr. Ajay Khanna)

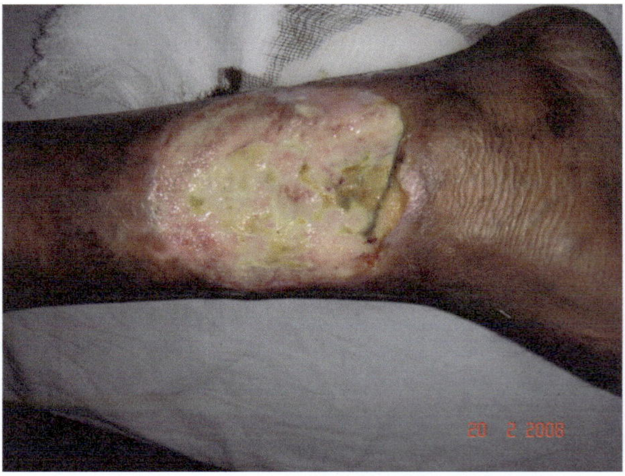

Fig. 22.2 Showing ulcerative MU developing in chronic non-healing ulcer due to chronic osteomyelitis of right lower extremity. (Photograph curtesy Dr. Ajay Khanna)

Hence it is appropriate that while treating wounds that don't heal in 3 weeks (which usually happens with deep partial thickness and full thickness burn wounds) wound closure should be achieved by resorting to either split thickness skin graft or flap as indicated [4]. The incidence of development of Marjolin's ulcer in burn scar can be 0.77–2% [5].

Any type of trauma resulting in unstable scar with recurrent breakdown is also likely to develop malignant transformation especially if it is on the flexor aspect of joints and under tension. Chronic non-healing ulcers such as venous ulcer [6] and other chronic ulcers such as decubitus ulcer, ulcer due to chronic osteomyelitis (Fig. 22.2) have been reported to have 1.7% incidence [7] of undergoing malignant change. Scars including donor site scars, vaccination scar, scars following Lupus lesions, amputation stump scar, scar due to radiotherapy (Table 22.1) are other probable locations where Marjolin's ulcer may originate [8]. In general scars of wounds left to heal by secondary intention and are unstable are likely to undergo malignant transformation.

Table 22.1 Predisposing factors

1. Burn scar
2. Chronic wounds
3. Unstable scars with recurrent ulceration
4. Chronic osteomyelitis
5. Flexor aspect scars
6. Pressure sore
7. Venous ulcer
8. Vaccination scar
9. Lupus lesion scars
10. Donor site scar
11. Postradiation scar

The most common locations of Marjolin's ulcer are lower extremities, heel, plantar aspect of foot. But it has also been reported to occur over upper extremities, scalp, face, buttocks, trunk and rarely on breasts [9].

This pathological condition can affect individuals of any gender, age or race. Men have been reported to be three times more prone than women though some believe that this observation is because a greater number of males receive burn injury [3]. It has been detected in young children (11 years), but the average age of majority of the patients is 59 years. Younger the age at the time of initial injury, longer is the latency period. The average latency period is 30–35 years in chronic variety [8]. Occurrence of initial trauma at advanced age leads to development of malignancy in the scar after shorter latency period. A study from Tanzania reported shorter latency period of about 10 years between initial burn injury and development of malignant change in scar [9]. An acute variety of M.U. in which the change occurs within 1 year of initial injury has been observed but is rare [5, 8].

22.3 Classification

The lesion can be classified based on the time lapse between initial trauma and detection of malignant change, morphological appearance and histopathology of the lesion and the extent of the spread as given in Table 22.2.

Commonly the duration between initial trauma and development of malignancy is 32 years with the range of latency period reported as 11–75 years and this type is categorized as "Chronic". Rarely the change occurs as early as within 1 year of initial trauma and is then termed as "Acute" [8].

Though the lesion carries the name Marjolin's ULCER, it may not always appear as an ulcer. Morphologically the lesion may be a papillary, exophytic growth which is usually well differentiated. This type is rare and has lesser malignant potential. The commonest variety has an indurated, ulcerative or flat appearance, is poorly differentiated and it infiltrates deeper tissue. This type spreads to lymph nodes rapidly and being aggressive recurrence is common. This variety carries poor prognosis [10].

Table 22.2 Classification

1. Duration of latency period
A. Acute
B. Chronic
2. Morphological appearance
A. Exophytic, proliferative
B. Flat, ulcerative, infiltrating
3. Histological types
A. Squamous cell carcinoma
B. Basal cell carcinoma
C. Malignant melanoma
D. Sarcoma—Liposarcoma, osteogenic sarcoma
4. Extent
Tumour (T): Size, local spread affecting adjacent tissues, structures
Lymph nodal involvement (N)—Mobile, fixed, perinodal tissue involvement
Distant metastasis (M)

Though conventionally the term Marjolin's ulcer refers to Squamous Cell Carcinoma (SCC) occurring in a scar or chronic wound, other histological types of carcinomas and rarely sarcoma may also occur in scar tissue. These could be Basal Cell Carcinoma (BCC), Malignant Melanoma (MM) and sarcoma such as—Liposarcoma [10], Fibrosarcoma [9]. Some workers in this field suggest that only SCC occurring in a scar be called Marjolin's ulcer and all other histological types should be included under the term Scar Carcinoma [2]. The debate is still on.

Based on the tumour size, extent of local spread, involvement of lymph nodes and presence or absence of distant metastasis, Marjolin's ulcer can also be classified using standard Tumour Nodes metastasis (TNM) classification [8]. No specific classification has been recommended as yet.

22.4 Etiopathology

The chronicity of wound healing process as seen in wounds allowed to heal by secondary intention, recurrent ulceration in unstable scar and chronic non-healing wounds—has been associated with increased possibility of the development of malignant change in the scar or persistent wound. Though the process that leads to malignancy is not yet clear, following processes in these scars or wounds are the most likely responsible factors.

1. Chronic inflammation and repeated attempt at healing: Unstable scars and chronic non-healing wounds have persistence of inflammatory process with abnormality of its mediators including matrix metalloproteinases and components of scar such as collagen. Recurrent breakdown of scar generates stimulus

for cellular multiplication to achieve wound healing along with release of multiple cytokines and growth factors. Ongoing attempt at healing may give rise to multiple cell mutation and malignant change [10].

2. Toxins and co-carcinogens: Presence of toxins in necrotic tissue in non-healing chronic wounds, infection and effect of co-carcinogens such as repeated physical and chemical injury in unstable scars may lead to malignant change and proliferation of latent malignant cells [5, 11].
3. Immune isolation: In the presence of normal immune response, when cell mutation occurs it is recognized by immune system as non-self and immune response is mounted accordingly leading to destruction of mutated cell. But scar tissue has significant fibrosis with destruction of lymphatics and blood vessels. Hence normal immune response is affected in the scar tissue leading to immune isolation of the area. This allows the malignant change to escape recognition by immune system and the multiplication of abnormal cell continues unopposed leading to the development of malignancy [11].

   Aberration of immune response which is present in autoimmune conditions such as Lupus probably explains the development of malignancy in scars of Lupus ulcers.
4. Immune escape in Scar tissue: The scar resulting after a full thickness skin loss has decreased population of Langerhans cells that are responsible for detecting immune aberration [12]. Exposure of scar to Ultraviolet radiation causes further decrease in the number of Langerhans cells. This hampers the ability of scar tissue to detect immunological aberration. It is also proposed that Ultraviolet radiation also leads to changes in the p53 gene leading to loss of its inhibitory role on tumour growth [11].
5. Genetic changes: In patients with Marjolin's ulcer, researchers have reported the presence of HLA DR4 which is known to be associated with malignancy. Aberration in the p53 gene due to a homozygous deletion has been detected in patients who develop this malignancy [13]. This along with mutation in FAS in the region of apoptosis appears to predispose malignant degeneration in the scar [11–13]. Further support to this theory of genetic predisposition is provided by identification of changes in transcription that lead to differential expression of genes in squamous cells in both SCC and Marjolin's ulcer [13].
6. It has been proposed that at the time of initial trauma, epithelial element get implanted in the dermis. These epithelial cells undergo disorganized regeneration and multiplication in the unusual environment of dermis giving rise to malignant change [14].

   Several researchers such as Virchow, Friedwald and Rouse, Saffioti and Shubik, Ribet, Treves and Pack, Castillo and Goldsmith and others have all contributed to above explanations for the malignant change leading to Marjolin's ulcer [14]. It appears that a combination of changes in genetic configuration, microenvironment of the wound, immunological aberration and external factors leads to development of Marjolin's ulcer.

In sub-Saharan Africa this malignancy has been reported to occur at younger age and with short latency period [15]. The reason for this observation could be a combination of increased susceptibility due to genetic differences, environmental factors and suboptimal initial medical care.

22.5 Histopathology

Squamous cell carcinoma (SCC) is the most common histological type (97.6%) [15]. Morphologically ulcerative variety with infiltration of deeper tissues is more common [9, 14, 16] compared to proliferative, exophytic (Fig. 22.3) and it carries poorer prognosis. Besides SCC, basal cell carcinoma, malignant melanoma, sarcoma and tumours arising from other rare cell types (adenocarcinoma) in variable order have been reported in different studies [3, 9, 15, 17, 18]. Dermatofibrosarcoma protuberans appearing as a nodule has been reported by Fei Xiang [18]. Basosquamous—a combination of basal and squamous cell carcinoma as well as a mix of melanoma and squamous cell carcinoma (which may be named melanosquamous) have been described [14]. The confirmation of diagnosis should be obtained by performing multiple punch biopsies from periphery and centre of the lesion [8].

The commonest variety of squamous cell carcinoma seen in Marjolin's ulcer is spinocellular type histologically [8]. Minimal keratinization and evidence of chronic inflammation is the peculiarity of Marjolin's as it occurs in scar or chronic non-healing wound. Other features such as keratin pearl formation and pleomorphic appearance of pseudoglandular pattern are seen on histology. Perineural infiltration (23.08%) and lymphatic and vascular permeation (30.77%) are common [19] explaining the high incidence of nodal involvement and local recurrence. A feature that may cause confusion is the presence of pseudoepitheliomatous hyperplasia which often seen in chronic ulcers too [14]. But malignant changes such as de-differentiation, invasion of basement membrane may occur in such areas of

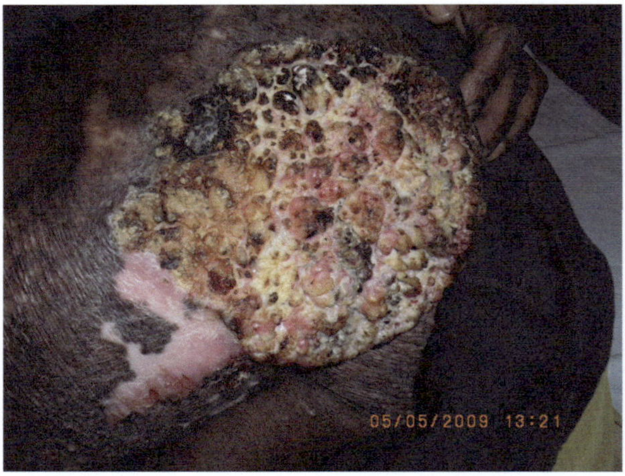

Fig. 22.3 Showing exophytic, proliferative growth involving burn scar on left gluteal region. (Photograph curtesy Dr. Ajay Khanna)

hyperplasia as well. Hence to avoid mis-diagnosis, multiple biopsies from various areas need to be taken from the lesion [14]. Squamous cell carcinoma of verrucous variety is also noted in some lesions [8]. Poorly differentiated growths show decreased inflammatory response.

The lesions show variable degree of cellular differentiation and can be graded depending on extent of differentiation [8]. With large number of poorly differentiated cells, tumours with pathological grade III are more aggressive, spread faster, and have poor prognosis. The gradation may direct the treatment plan as discussed later.

Grade I: More than 75% of the cells are differentiated.
Grade II: 25–75% of the cells are differentiated.
Grade III: Less than 25% of the cells are differentiated.

In the event of full thickness skin loss at the initial injury, the scar tissue is not likely to have basal cells and melanocytes. Hence basal cell carcinoma (BCC) and malignant melanoma (MM) are less likely to develop in the scar tissue [3]. Presence of these varieties may be explained on the basis of the theory of implantation of epithelial elements into deeper tissues at the time of initial injury [14]. BCC and MM may develop if the initial injury is superficial and the skin appendages are spared [20] or if MU develops in an area which had been skin grafted previously [18]. BCC has also been observed to be more common in acute variety of Marjolin's ulcer [11]. In one study the histological variety of the lesion was found to be different at different locations on the body, e.g., over head, neck, and lower limbs SCC was more common, face lesion was often BCC and dermatofibrosarcoma protuberans was predominant on trunk [18].

22.6 Presentation

Marjolin's ulcer is very likely to go unsuspected and undiagnosed for prolonged period as it is viewed as a chronic non-healing ulcer. The history and clinical findings that would suggest the malignant change in the scar or chronic wound need to be sought vigilantly. These are as follows.

Location of ulcer: Maximum number of Marjolin's ulcers are located in scars or non-healing wounds on lower extremities (42.1%), followed by head, face (34.5%); upper extremities; trunk in the order of frequency [14, 18].

Initial injury: The possibility of development of Marjolin's ulcer in a scar following full thickness ungrafted flame burn is maximum (76.5%). This risk has been reported to be about 8.1% in chronic non-healing wounds due to non-burn injury, 6.3% in ulcers due to chronic venous insufficiency and 2.6% in chronic osteomyelitis [11]. The decubitus ulcer carries the least risk which is less than 0.5%. Hence the history of causative factor of the initial trauma needs to be sought along with the information about time taken and method used for the wound to heal.

Change in scar: Development of burning sensation and itching in an old, previously asymptomatic scar, appearance of vesicle or blister over the scar with intact surface [2] should raise a doubt. These symptoms may be neglected by the patient and hence not reported. But these may appear in pre-ulceration period and should be asked about specifically.

Repeated breakdown of a scar particularly on flexor aspect, any change in thick, firm hypopigmented scar [14] including itching, post-burn scar and scar over junctional area of mobile and immobile part of body [14], development of nodule or induration in the scar [8]—all these changes should be checked for in the scar. It should also be noted that ulceration occurring in a chronic scar for the first time has high possibility of being malignant [2].

Change in ulcer: The following changes occurring in the ulcer are highly suggestive of development of malignancy—failure of ulcer to heal within 3 months [8], increase in the size of the ulcer after initial response to treatment, flat ulcer with indurated, elevated margin [9], appearance of excessive hyper granulating tissue [8], involvement of adjacent normal skin due to expansion of the ulcer [12], partial healing of ulcer with persistence of remaining part of ulcerated lesion, necrotic tissue on floor of ulcer with blood clot [14], change in the appearance of wound to an exophytic, proliferative ulcer, unsatisfactory response of the ulcer despite appropriate, optimal care [14].

Pain: Increasing pain or appearance of recent onset pain at the ulcer site has been a symptom consistently reported and observed in multiple studies [8, 9, 12].

Exudate from ulcer: Increase in exudate from the ulcer, purulent, foul smelling discharge, bleeding from ulcer on contact, formation of excessive crust over the ulcer [8, 12]—these findings should raise strong suspicion of malignant change.

Regional lymphadenopathy: This may be due to chronic inflammation associated with non-healing ulcer. But it should not be neglected and multiple biopsies from ulcer edge and centre should be obtained and studied.

In order to avoid delay in detection and appropriate treatment of malignant transformation of scar or chronic wound, it is essential to have high level of suspicion. Besides detailed history, clinical examination must be performed to check for ulceration, induration and nodule formation [12]. The clinical diagnosis may often be misleading as the ulcer commonly appears benign [14]. Hence multiple biopsies from the lesion are necessary for early diagnosis [9]. The features on histopathological examination also may be confounding because of difficulty in differentiating between changes due to chronic ulceration and inflammation and malignancy. The outcome of delay in diagnosis could be need for limb amputation, occurrence of metastasis and poor prognosis.

22.7 Investigations

22.7.1 For Confirmation of Diagnosis

Biopsy: It is mandatory to obtain histological confirmation when diagnosis of Marjolin's ulcer is suspected. The change usually begins at the margin and hence biopsies should be taken from the most suspicious peripheral areas and from the centre of the ulcer too.

It is important to include deeper tissue from subcutaneous region in the biopsy to get information about invasion and to avoid missing the diagnosis [13].

The pathology could be multifocal and so may be missed even by multiple biopsies. Hence it has been suggested that whenever feasible complete ulcer should be excised and subjected to histological examination. This would decrease the possibility of false negative report [14].

22.7.2 For Assessment of Extent of Spread

At the time of diagnosis 20–36% of patients have metastasis [21]. The metastases are commonly seen in distant lymph nodes, brain, kidneys, lung and liver [8]. To plan appropriate treatment, it is important to investigate for extent of primary and presence and location of metastasis initially. Various imaging techniques are useful for this purpose.

Radiographs: Invasion of underlying bone has been reported in 32.9% of the lesions [18]. This incidence was observed to be maximum in lesions on head and neck. On X-ray, the bony involvement may be evident as periosteal reaction (Fig. 22.4) which is often seen as bone lamellation and bone destruction [8]. Smith et al. observed significantly large sized soft tissue masses on X-ray along with multiple types of non-specific periosteal reactions, the commonest being lamellation

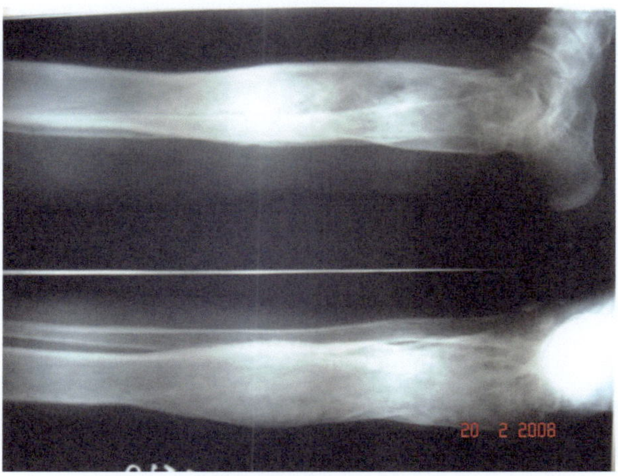

Fig. 22.4 Showing radiograph of lower limb with MU associated with chronic osteomyelitis with periosteal reaction and bone dysplasia. (Photograph curtesy Dr. Ajay Khanna)

[22]. Solid periosteal reaction seen with venous insufficiency and changes associated with chronic osteomyelitis were rarely seen in this study. But all these changes were observed to be non-specific and did not help in reaching the diagnosis.

Radiograph of chest is routinely performed.

Bone scan: This is useful in demonstrating bone erosion in cases with chronic osteomyelitis [8]. But in today's era of MRI and PET scan it is rarely performed or needed.

Ultrasonography: It is useful for the evaluation of regional lymph nodes (palpable or non-palpable) and for initial evaluation of intraabdominal structures.

Computed tomography: Computed tomography (CT) helps to assess bony involvement more thoroughly and with greater sensitivity than plain radiograph [8, 14]. It also provides information about involvement of deeper tissues. CT scan of brain is an integral part of metastatic work up.

Magnetic resonance imaging (MRI): MRI provides information about extent of bone as well as soft tissue involvement better than CT [14]. The details about depth, margins, extent of tumour, involvement of bone marrow along with condition of nearby neurovascular structures can be obtained from MRI [13]. This is useful in deciding the most appropriate surgical option. Performing optimal biopsies may be difficult in suspected Marjolin's in a large sacral sore. In such a situation MRI provides information about extent and level of soft tissue involvement. It also enables to judge the severity of inflammation [11].

Surprisingly, Smith et al. commented that they found CT and MRI studies informative but these were not essential for treatment of the patient [21].

Positron emission tomography CT (PET CT): This imaging technique allows differentiation between benign chronic inflammatory changes and changes associated with malignancy, i.e., Marjolin's ulcer. It provides information about the depth of invasion of deeper tissues which compares and correlates well with that judged surgically and histologically [13]. This quality is of great advantage in deciding the extent and depth of excision while performing surgery.

PET CT can be replaced by PET-MRI as has been done in other malignant lesions, the advantage being lesser dose of radiation. But PET-MRI is not yet routinely used for diagnosis of Marjolin's ulcer [13].

Sentinel lymph node biopsy (SLNB): With high incidence of lymph nodal metastasis at diagnosis, the role of SLNB appears important for detection of latent spread in regional lymph nodes [11]. SLNB has been reported to be successful in detecting occult metastasis in 83% of the patients [23] leading to lymphadenectomy and so more complete surgical resection.

22.8 Treatment

MU is a rare pathology and so there is no single centre that has accrued experience of treating large number of patients. The largest series the author has come across includes 187 patients [16]. This is probably the reason for the absence of a recommended uniform treatment protocol as yet [13]. Surgery remains the main treatment modality with some common and some differing approaches. The role of radiotherapy and chemotherapy is still under evaluation and is rather unclear.

1. Surgery
   (a) **Wide local excision**—Complete excision of the Marjolin's ulcer along with surrounding wide zone of tumour free tissue is the most essential component of surgical procedure and there are no diverse opinions about it [3, 8, 10, 11, 14, 21]. The excision should address all three dimensions of the ulcer and periphery as well as depth need to be considered while planning the extent of resection. With the presence of invasion of deeper tissue, excision including only deep fascia [11] may not be adequate and then it needs to be extended to include muscle as well as bone too if invasion is either suspected [18] or confirmed on investigation. The discrepancy in different studies is mainly regarding the extent of margin around the tumour and views about excision of complete scar which contains the MU.
      - **Margin**—Different studies have recommended different extents of surgical margin from 2 cm [11], 2–4 cm [14], 2–5 cm [12], 3–5 cm [10]. No controlled clinical trial has been reported yet so as to reach a consensus. MU in decubitus ulcer is more aggressive and a tumour free margin of up to 5 cm has been advocated [11] while 2.5 cm margin of healthy tissue has been suggested for recurrent MU [14]. All the margins of excised specimen including those in depth must be examined histologically and further excision or if necessary amputation proximal to the lesion should be performed if any margin is found positive for malignant cells. The use of electrocautery has been advocated during skin incision as well as three-dimensional excision so as to control entry of malignant cells in the lymphatics and blood vessels that open up if knife is used [8].
      - **Resection of scar**—This is another topic of controversy. Detection of multiple foci of malignant degeneration in the same scar suggests that it would be logical to excise the complete scar along with MU with the hope of controlling development of recurrence or second primary lesion [14]. But in the opinion of Aydogdu et al. the uninvolved scar tissue with fewer or absent lymphatics and blood vessels provides protection from spread of malignant cells. This should not be disturbed by complete excision of the scar tissue as it may promote lymph nodal and distant metastasis [24]. It is suggested that this approach may be considered while treating MU detected early in its course.
      - **Mohs's micrographic surgery**—To overcome the uncertainty about having clear margin [3] and for avoiding unnecessary loss of healthy tissue due to excision, Moh's micrographic surgical principles can be applied particularly when the lesion is on cosmetically and functionally important areas such as face. This procedure demands significant time, training of surgeon and expensive equipment. The excised tissue is sub-

jected to histological examination immediately and the result of examination guides the need for further excision. With reported 90% cure rate at 5 years following this surgery, it is now considered the gold standard [8] and is recommended over wide excision which has 76% survival at 5 years. With the drawbacks such as expenses, time required and lack of trained surgeons, this procedure is being performed in select cases at specialized centres at present.

(b) **Wound closure**—After wide excision of the lesion the defect created needs to be closed by an appropriately chosen method. On a very rare occasion primary wound closure with approximation of wound edges may be possible if the lesion is very small in size. But most of the times the defect created demands one of the following options available for closure. The views about the choice of the method vary.

- **Split thickness skin graft/Full thickness skin graft**—The method most commonly used for wound closure after wide excision of MU is split thickness skin grafting (STSG). It is an easy procedure and allows satisfactory observation of the site for the detection of local recurrence during follow-up [12]. But split thickness skin graft itself is prone for contraction and for development of contracture if applied over a joint. To avoid this situation, the use of full thickness skin graft has been advocated over joints [3]. Split thickness or full thickness skin graft may be applied as a temporary, initial method of wound closure to aid observation of the area of resection. A disadvantage of split thickness skin graft is that it may undergo necrosis if the area needs to be subjected to radiotherapy in future for control of local recurrence.
- **Replacement of STSG with flap closure**—Most of the local recurrences have been observed to develop within 1 year of surgical excision [18]. As mentioned above STSG allows for easy surveillance for local recurrence. Hence it appears logical to perform initial closure of defect with STSG and observe for at least 1 year [12, 14]. In the absence of recurrence, the STSG should then be replaced by a fasciocutaneous or myocutaneous flap for definitive closure. This approach would probably be most appropriate for large size lesions with high histological grade of tumour.
- **Immediate flap closure**—Several reports now suggest that primary use of appropriate flap to close the defect at the time of wide excision has certain advantages. Flap closure becomes essential when the wound bed created by excision is not suitable for application of a skin graft [14]. Flap closure overcomes the possibility of contracture effectively. It provides significant volume of soft tissue and aids reduction of stretch and searing force which is the main reason for recurrent ulceration after reconstruction. Local transposition flaps may be suitable at appropriate location. But use of free flap for tissue transfer has been observed to be more effective for this purpose. Shobhit Sharma et al. have described the advantage of free anterolateral thigh flap in avoiding limb shortening and improving limb function in patients with MU around the knee [25]. This

method of reconstruction allows radical excision of MU without compromise and prevents amputation. Aydogdu et al. [24] have also reported advantages of use of free flap in reconstruction following excision of MU. MU with larger than 10 cm diameter is more likely to have positive margins due to compromised extent of excision and the incidence of local recurrence following excision is high in MU. These patients often need to receive radiotherapy. If the defect has been closed using free flap, it is able to tolerate the radiation better than STSG which may undergo necrosis [25]. Using leg arteries distal to popliteal trifurcation, perforator based free flaps can also be used to close defects over the leg.

Use of free flaps for tissue transfer or local transposition flap is now recommended for closure of defect with significant soft tissue loss and over joints after excision of MU and it provides the advantage of allowing more radical excision which should help control recurrence and metastasis particularly in early stage [13]. It has also been observed to avoid amputation.

(c) **Regional lymph nodes**—The main path for MU to metastasize is via lymphatic channels to lymph nodes and then to distant nodes and organs. This makes the scheduling of regional lymphadenectomy a key issue while performing surgery for MU. There is no doubt that lymph nodal dissection has to be performed when nodal involvement is confirmed [11].

- **Concomitant regional lymphadenectomy**:

  In a patient with lesion suspicious of MU, the regional lymph nodes must be diligently examined clinically. If those are palpable, enlarged, perceived to be metastatic on examination, confirmation of the suspicion must be sought by one or more of following methods—

  - Ultrasound examination to evaluate the changes in the nodes suggestive of malignant spread, performance of ultrasound guided needle cytology/biopsy of node for examination.
  - PET CT scan to detect the uptake and performance of CT guided needle biopsy if the location of the node demands this approach.
  - Lymph node biopsy for histological examination.

    With confirmation obtained from any of the above investigations, lymphadenectomy is definitely indicated. Some studies have recommended lymphadenectomy along with wide excision of the primary lesion when regional lymph nodes are palpably enlarged [8]. The lymphadenectomy of clinically palpable regional lymph nodes without performing SLNB for confirmation has not been recommended if the MU histology is malignant melanoma [9].

- **Delayed regional lymphadenectomy**:

  If the primary lesion is more than 10 cm in diameter and the histology reveals high grade of malignancy, regional lymphadenectomy has been advised after a 2–4 weeks period of observation [3]. Some authors have suggested performing regional lymph node biopsy in all patients with MU particularly when the primary tumour is poorly differentiated and then proceeding with lymphadenectomy if the histology reveals lymph nodal involvement [8]. With the advent of PET CT and SLNB, probably this approach will now be needed in areas where the socioeconomic conditions and available health care facilities do not permit use of sophisticated methodology.

- **Prophylactic regional lymphadenectomy**:

  The performance of prophylactic regional lymphadenectomy in clinically node negative patients is the issue with controversial opinions. If only wide local excision is performed, the incidence of development of regional lymph node metastasis or distant spread is 15–75% and 50% of these affect the lymph nodes. Almost 90% of these appears within 3 years of detection [21] leading to increased morbidity and mortality. Considering this data, some have advocated performance of prophylactic lymphadenectomy along with wide local excision of MU in all the patients [14] or atleast in patients having MU with high grade of malignancy [8]. As regional nodal involvement is more common at presentation with primary lesion on the lower extremity, some have suggested this approach for patients with MU on lower extremity and in those requiring amputation due to involvement of bone, joint or neurovascular structures [3]. But as available data does not show significant difference in the incidence of recurrence with or without prophylactic lymphadenectomy, many do not favour performance of prophylactic lymphadenectomy for non-palpable lymph nodes [8].

  The concept of sentinel lymph node biopsy to judge the status of regional lymph nodes though initially applied to patients with malignant melanoma, is now used with SCC too [21]. This method has been shown to have good sensitivity [23] leading to its recommendation for detection of occult metastasis in the regional lymph nodes and subsequent lymphadenectomy [12, 13]. But despite its success in detecting occult metastasis in lymph nodes, consensus about the routine use of SLNB in clinically node negative patients of MU has not yet been reached [13]. Kanth et al. state that the available evidence does not clearly define the efficacy of SLNB and lymphadenectomy with non-palpable lymph nodes [26]. Therefore, the confusion continues.

  Other investigation that can help detect the presence of occult metastasis in non-palpable regional lymph nodes is PET CT. Fei Xiang [18] reported that in 11 patients PET CT performed to detect lymph nodal metastasis showed positive result leading to lymphadenectomy of these clinically non-palpable nodes. But on histopathological examination only in two patients the nodes showed the evidence of malignant metastasis. This experience indicates possibility of false positive findings on PET CT. Thus, again creating debate about the performance of preventive lymphadenectomy of non-palpable regional lymph nodes.

  At present the opinion seems to be that the incidence of recurrence is not affected by performance of prophylactic lymphadenectomy and hence, it is not indicated for this purpose [18]. It is suggested that if the MU is on lower extremity (which has higher incidence of nodal involvement) and/or the tumour pathology reveals high grade of malignancy; then prophylactic lymphadenectomy should be considered [18].

Therefore, it can be concluded that multiple factors should be taken into consideration while taking the decision about lymphadenectomy of non-palpable regional lymph nodes. Besides the systemic condition of the patient other factors include location of the lesion, size of the lesion, extent of invasion of deeper tissues, histological grade of the malignancy and the findings on imaging study of the lymph node.

(d) **Amputation**—The most common location for occurrence of MU is lower extremity. If after wide excision and wound closure the limb causes difficulty in the mobility of patient, the limb becomes a liability. In this situation amputation at appropriate level and provision of prosthesis with rehabilitation is recommended. Amputation is also indicated with recurrence of MU after wide excision, involvement of bone, joint space and /or deeper tissues including neurovascular structures [3]. More than 10 cm diameter MU with poorly differentiated malignancy and extensive scarring or deformity of the involved extremity and possibility of unsatisfactory function after limited surgical procedure would also lead to the decision of performing amputation [11, 12, 17].

(e) **Hemicorporectomy**—MU developing in pressure ulcer has been reported to be aggressive. The patients prone for development of pressure sores generally suffer from poor nutritional and immunological status. The situation worsens with development of malignant change in the pressure sore. Excision with adequate margin and reconstruction with appropriate flap is often impractical. In such a challenging situation hemicorporectomy which involves amputation of both lower extremities and sex organs may be the only choice available [11].

(f) **Hemipelvectomy**—Hemipelvectomy may have to be considered if completion of adequate radical excision is difficult due to involvement of bone or joint and/or the resection if completed is likely to lead to severe impairment of limb function [13] and amputation is not a suitable choice.

2. Radiotherapy

The role of radiotherapy in treatment of MU is as yet rather ill defined. The response to radiotherapy on this pathology in area with significant fibrosis has not been observed to be encouraging [14]. The decision to administer adjuvant radiotherapy may be taken based on degree of malignancy, location of MU and large extent of the lesion [11] and involvement of lymph nodes [8] or patient refusal to undergo surgery. Tumours with high grade of malignancy and large extent of growth may achieve better control with adjuvant radiotherapy. In patients with unfavourable prognostic factors or presence of distant metastasis either neoadjuvant or adjuvant radiotherapy may be used with the aim of achieving better disease control. Radiation may be the only treatment possible if the lesion cannot be excised completely either due to its large size or location and if the patient refuses surgical resection.

Radiotherapy has also been observed to be useful in providing palliation while treating inoperable tumours. In situations such as development of local recurrence, detection of positive margins after wide excision, lesion larger than 10 cm diameter; radiotherapy has been shown to be of benefit [24].

MU involving head and neck with lymph nodal metastasis on node dissection, presence of lymph nodal metastasis that is inoperable, association of positive lymph nodes on dissection with high grade malignancy and lesion larger than 10 cm diameter—radiotherapy has been recommended in these situations [8].

After wide excision if the wound closure has been achieved by application of split thickness skin graft, there is a possibility of development of skin necrosis following radiotherapy. Hence if radiotherapy is likely to be needed as adjuvant therapy, the wound closure should be achieved using a myocutaneous of fasciocutaneous flap [11].

Therefore, radiotherapy is a modality which may be of benefit in the following situations.

(a) Primary lesion—Size larger than 10 cm diameter, incomplete excision, extensive local recurrence, associated with distant metastasis, palliation in non-resectable disease.
(b) Inoperable lymph node metastasis, positive nodes on dissection with high grade malignancy
(c) Refusal of surgical excision.

3. Chemotherapy

The efficacy of chemotherapy in MU is still being evaluated. The area of origin of MU has poor vascularity as it is a scar tissue. Hence chemotherapeutic agents administered systemically have poor assess to the lesion and hence poor response too [14]. To overcome this barrier adjuvant intra-arterial limb perfusion of chemotherapeutic agent (Methotrexate) has been reported to be useful in patients with MU with SCC [8, 14].Multidrug chemotherapy with administration of four cycles of Methotrexate, Bleomycin and Cisplatinum combination has been used in patients with distant metastasis and expected poor prognosis [9]. For small size MU topical application of 5-fluorouracil has been found to be useful. But no conclusive recommendation has been made yet.

Adjuvant chemotherapy has been proposed for patients diagnosed to have metastasis in the regional lymph nodes at detection [3].This appears logical as this factor is an important determinant of the prognosis. Use of sentinel lymph node biopsy has been suggested in patients who do not have clinical evidence of regional node involvement. The outcome of SLNB could be of use in deciding the need for adjuvant chemotherapy [10]. Chemotherapy has also been tried in patients with widespread disease and while treating MU occurring in pressure sore. The outcome has not been consistent or predictable [10].

In the absence of adequate evidence to have uniform guidelines, the general opinion is to take the decision about adjuvant chemotherapy after consideration of multiple factors in each patient [11]. At present this treatment modality is generally considered in patients with guarded prognosis due to recurrence or metastasis or in patients who are either unsuitable or unwilling for any type of surgical procedure [8].

Therefore, in the absence of any established evidence and guidelines, radiotherapy or chemotherapy is not routinely resorted to while treating MU. The response of MU to these modalities is unpredictable and poor. These therapies particularly radiation is resorted to in almost desperate situations when surgery is an unsuitable or inadequate option [13].

4. Use of newer technology—The following newer technologies are presently under evaluation so as to add refinement to surgical procedure [8].
   (a) Cryosurgery
   (b) Carbon dioxide laser
   (c) Intralesional interferon
   (d) Photodynamic therapy

22.9 Suggested Treatment Protocol

Available data suggests that the prognosis is encouraging following surgical management when the lymph nodes are not involved. At the other end of the spectrum, in advance stage of the disease the outcome remains poor despite the use of combination of therapeutic modalities [3]. Hence it is very desirable that appropriate planning and execution of radical excision, prophylactic lymphadenectomy and adjuvant therapy be done before the disease reaches advanced stage. The experience with SLNB in MU is limited at present [23] and same observation applies to the false positive results with PET CT [18]. In the opinion of the author more data needs to be accrued before drawing any conclusion. Taking into consideration experiences and recommendations expressed in various studies, the following treatment protocol is being suggested.

1. After complete history and clinical examination, confirmation of malignancy, its histological type and pathological grading should be obtained using multiple biopsies from the suspicious lesion.
2. Necessary investigations (MRI, PET CT, Ultrasound or CT guided needle biopsy) should be performed to evaluate the extent of invasion and metastatic spread.
3. Based on above information the patients can be categorized into following groups and customized treatment protocol should be implemented.

   Group I: Tumour size less than 10 cm diameter, no palpable lymphadenopathy, well differentiated lesion on histology, negative result for nodal or distant uptake on PET CT—Mohs micrographic surgical technique should be used to ensure wide local excision with negative margins and closure of defect should be achieved with STSG or with use of appropriate flap particularly if lesion is on flexor aspect of joint.

Group II: Tumour size less than 10 cm diameter, palpable lymphadenopathy, well differentiated lesion on histology, positive result for nodal uptake on PET CT—Confirmation of nodal involvement with needle biopsy, wide local excision with at least 2.5 cm tumour free margin (confirmed histologically), lymphadenectomy and closure of defect with STSG or appropriate flap. Adjuvant therapy to be considered.

Group III: Tumour size more than 10 cm diameter, no palpable lymphadenopathy, poorly differentiated lesion on histology, negative result for nodal or distant uptake on PET CT—Wide local excision with at least 2.5 cm three-dimensional margin, SLNB and if positive then performance of lymphadenectomy and closure of defect with STSG or preferably by use of flap. Histological confirmation of negative margins is mandatory.

If the lesion is on the lower extremity, prophylactic lymphadenectomy even without SLNB would be advisable. Adjuvant radiotherapy is suggested for prevention of local recurrence.

Group IV: Tumour size more than 10 cm diameter, palpable lymphadenopathy, poorly differentiated lesion on histology, Positive result for nodal or distant uptake on PET CT—Neo-adjuvant radiotherapy or chemotherapy followed by wide local excision with at least 2.5 cm three-dimensional tumour free margin, lymphadenectomy and closure of defect preferably with free tissue transfer in view of need for adjuvant radiotherapy. Histological confirmation of negative margins is mandatory.

If the lesion is on the lower extremity, the use of free tissue transfer for closure of defect is certainly indicated so as to avoid compromised resection, limb shortening and probability of amputation. Adjuvant radiotherapy is suggested for the prevention of local recurrence.

Group V: Tumour location on lower extremity, tumour size more than 10 cm diameter, any status of lymph nodes clinically and/or on PET CT, poorly differentiated lesion on histology, involvement of deeper structures such as joint cavity, neurovascular bundle, presence of extensive scarring, possibility of compromised local resection or creation of instability—Amputation of limb proximal to the lesion with regional lymphadenectomy or hemipelvectomy is suggested.

Hemicorporectomy is another major ablative procedure that may be conducted to obtain radical excision in patients with MU in sacral pressure ulcer.

Regular close follow-up of all patients is mandatory for detection of local recurrence, nodal or distant spread.

Adjuvant therapy: The indications for use of radiotherapy have been defined with some clarity and have been elaborated upon earlier. The use of chemotherapeutic agents is not clear yet and it is mainly used in patients with poor prognosis, advanced disease and unfit/reluctant to undergo surgery.

22.10 Prognosis

The observations reported in multiple studies indicate that Marjolin's ulcer is a particularly aggressive malignancy. This is apparent from its tendency to develop local recurrence, presence of metastasis at diagnosis, appearance of metastasis after treatment of primary lesion and higher mortality with shorter survival period in comparison to SCC occurring due to other causes. Various factors that influence the outcome have been identified.

1. Local recurrence:

   Following excision local recurrence (Fig. 22.5) has been reported in 20–50% of patients [8, 9]. Chun-Yuan Huang has quoted lower incidence (10.8–37%) of local recurrence [3]. The difference in incidence could be because no standardized protocol has yet been recommended addressing the margin to be excised around the lesion.98% of the recurrences have been observed to occur within first 3 years after diagnosis [8]. Despite the aggressive nature of the malignancy, the growth of tumour is slow. Distant metastases may occur in the absence of local recurrence after wide excision [3].
2. Metastasis at diagnosis and follow-up:

   The presence of regional lymph nodal metastasis at the time of diagnosis of MU is an important indicator of poor prognosis. This status has been detected in 20–36% of MU. The lymph node involvement rate is higher [20] and overall incidence of metastases is also higher (53.8%) [3] when the MU is in lower extremity. The possibility of development of metastasis in lymph nodes and other organs is 15–75% if wide excision of the primary lesion is the only surgery performed. About 50% of these metastases occur in regional lymph nodes as lymphadenectomy has not been performed at the time of first surgery. The most (92%) of these nodal metastases present within a time period of 3 years from detection of MU [20]. This data suggests that wide excision alone is not ade-

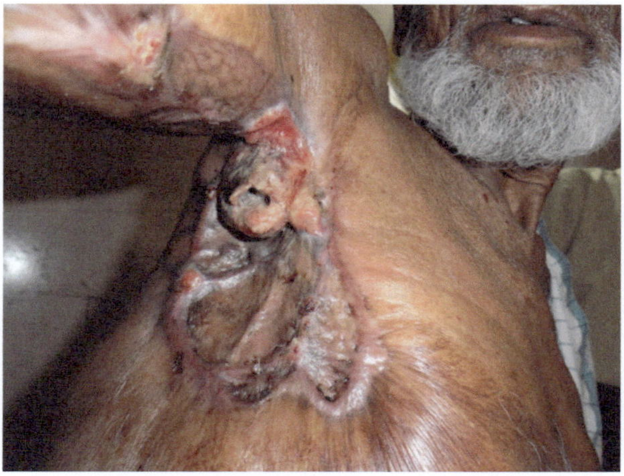

Fig. 22.5 Showing local recurrence of Marjolin's ulcer following local wide excision and STSG of lesion involving post burn scar in right axilla. (Photograph curtesy Dr. Ajay Khanna)

quate in achieving disease control. The role of sentinel lymph node biopsy (SLNB) appears important in guiding the need to perform lymph nodal clearance along with wide excision of primary. The presence of lymph node metastasis has been identified as the most important determinant of prognosis and outcome [14]. Distant metastases observed in the absence of local recurrence may be due to the presence of micro metastasis in regional lymph nodes or breaking of the barrier of scar tissue during excision of primary. As the scar tissue is excised it allows the malignant cells to gain access to blood vessels so as to reach distant organs [3].

Extremely close observation at follow-up has been recommended in young patients with MU of high pathological grade. The risk of development of local recurrence and nodal metastasis has been reported to be high in this group [27].

3. Mortality:

   After detection of MU the possibility of survival at 3 years has been reported as 65–75% [10]. About 34% are likely to survive at 10 years [8]. The reported 5 year survival varies widely between 52% and 80% [3]. But the presence of regional lymph node involvement brings down the 3-year survival rate to 35–50% [8]. Other study has identified regional lymph node involvement at diagnosis as predictor of death within 2 years while yet another study predicts mortality of 66% at 2 years attributable to metastatic or local disease [10]. One study reports that the patients without regional lymphadenopathy had median survival period of 66 months, while those with regional lymphadenopathy the median survival duration dropped to 16 months [3]. Overall the conclusion is that presence of regional lymph node metastasis is the main determinant of duration of survival. As more than 95% of patients with metastasis report within first year after diagnosis one can presume that if patient survives for 3 years without nodal metastasis, then the possibility of long-term survival is likely to be good [8].

   Location of MU is also an important factor influencing mortality. In patients who develop MU in decubitus ulcer the mortality at 2 years is 80% if only local excision is performed [10].

   Better prognosis has been observed in lesions that are well differentiated and so are less aggressive. In this group the 5-year survival is 40–69% and is somewhat better in those subjected to amputation of involved extremity [8].

   A rather dismal observation made by Chun-Yuan Huang [3] is that the mortality reported in the recent studies barely differs from the one (28.5%) reported by Treves and Pack in 1930. This probably indicates that no significant improvement has occurred in the treatment of this pathology over all these years. This certainly deserves attention.

4. Comparison with conventional SCC:

   The behaviour and outcome of SCC that occurs in scar tissue or chronic non-healing wounds differs from the conventional SCC (generally attributed to exposure to actinic rays) mainly in terms of incidence, local recurrence, regional lymph nodal involvement and mortality (Table 22.3). SCC is the commonest type of carcinoma identified in MU while BCC is the most commonly identified carcinoma among conventional skin tumours [3]. Development of metastasis is

Table 22.3 Differences between SCC MU and conventional SCC [3]

Observation	SCC MU	Conventional SCC
Age	50 years	65–70 years
Latency period	30 years	10 years
Incidence	75% of MU	16% of skin cancers
Location	Scar tissue, chronic wound Lower extremity	Exposed body parts Head, face
Aetiology	Multifactorial	Exposure to actinic rays—mainly
Behaviour	More aggressive	Less aggressive
Metastatic spread	More likely	Less likely
Local recurrence	10.8–37%	1.3–18.7%
Regional lymph nodal involvement	5.6–60%	0.5–16%
Incidence of metastasis from primary in lower extremity	53.8%	2–5%
Mortality	21–38%	1%

Table 22.4 Factors affecting prognosis [3, 11–14]

Prognostic factor	Poor prognosis	Better prognosis
Latency period	Long latency period More than 5 years	Short latency period Less than 5 years
Location	Lower extremity involvement	Upper extremity, head, neck, trunk involvement
Initial cause of trauma	Pressure sore	Burns and other trauma
Type of growth	Ulcerative, infiltrating	Proliferative, Exophytic
Involvement of deeper tissue	More than 4 mm	Less than 4 mm
Diameter of tumour	More than 2 cm/10 cm	Less than 2 cm/10 cm
Degree of differentiation	Poorly differentiated	Well differentiated
Peritumoral T lymphocyte infiltration	Scanty	Dense
Local recurrence	Present	Absent
Regional lymph nodal involvement	Present at diagnosis	Absent at diagnosis
Metastasis	Present	Absent

ten times more likely with SCC in MU as compared to conventional SCC [3]. Overall the prognosis is worse with SCC in MU compared to SCC due to other aetiology.

Such an obvious difference is not found in BCC or MM occurring in scar tissue and conventional BCC and MM.

5. Factors influencing prognosis:

The prognosis of MU is dependent on multiple factors including grade of tumour, type of growth, location, size, presence of metastasis, histology, etc. Observations collated from different studies [3, 11–14] have been detailed in Table 22.4.

Some discrepancy has been observed within different studies regarding the critical diameter of the tumour that affects the prognosis. One report states that tumour size larger than 2 cm has poor prognosis [14], while other study observes that tumour larger than 10 cm diameter is associated with poorer prognosis [3]. But it is certain that larger the tumour, worse is the prognosis. The presence of good peritumoral T cell lymphocyte infiltration indicates good immune response and so is associated with better prognosis. The factors that certainly affect the prognosis adversely are histological grade of tumour indicating severity of de-differentiation, involvement of lower extremity and most importantly presence of regional lymph nodal metastasis at presentation.

22.11 Prevention

Marjolin's ulcer is a rare but aggressive malignant lesion with high incidence of metastasis at diagnosis and overall poor prognosis. The detection of malignant change is often delayed and the histopathology of biopsy may mislead causing further delay in confirmation. The pathogenesis is not completely clear. The treatment protocol is not yet standardized. In this situation adoption of methods of primary prevention and high level of suspicion with focussed attempts to achieve early diagnosis are the appropriate steps towards prevention. The preventive measures have been enlisted in Table 22.5.

1. Burns—Burn scar is the commonest site of origin of Marjolin's ulcer. Closure of the burn wound should be obtained at the earliest either by epithelisation or for deep burns by excision and early skin grafting. Use of skin allografts, skin substitutes, cultured epithelia—all have their role in aiding wound closure. Development of malignancy has rarely been reported in burn wound that had been closed by successful skin grafting [3].
2. Chronic wounds—The possibility of chronic wound developing malignancy is 0.1–2.5% [12]. Infection in chronic wounds should be appropriately treated. Wounds that do not heal within 3 weeks [8] should be excised and skin grafting

Table 22.5 Preventive measures

1. Early wound closure of burn and chronic wounds
2. Scar follow up and management
3. Regional lymphadenopathy
4. Regular scar biopsy
5. Multidisciplinary team
6. Oncology awareness
7. Patient education
8. Molecular and genetic studies

should be done. Wounds causing pain, having unusual morphology, with foul smelling discharge and resistant to appropriate treatment should be subjected to multiple biopsies from margins and centre [11].

3. Venous ulcers—In patients with chronic venous insufficiency if the venous ulcers do not heal within 3 months despite treatment, multiple biopsies should be taken from margins and centre of non-healing ulcers as 2.4% of venous ulcers may develop malignant degeneration [11].
4. Scars—Scars particularly burn scars developing recurrent breakdown, scars on flexor aspect of joints prone to repeated tension/stretching injury, thick and hypopigmented scars, inelastic scars over mobile areas should be completely excised and skin graft or flap should be used to obtain closure with supple tissue. Post burn contractures should be released so as to avoid repeated trauma and breakdown [3]. Use of pressure garment or compression bandage over scars should be recommended.
5. Monitoring scar and regional nodes: All scars should be regularly monitored and if detected to have recent onset itching, breakdown; multiple biopsies should be done to obtain histology. Assessment of regional lymph nodes should be performed regularly for the detection of lymphadenopathy [11].
6. Protection from exposure to sun rays—Scars on scalp can be excised and grafted as well as protected by using wig, cloth and exposure to chemicals should be avoided [12, 14]. All scars should be protected from sun rays using sunscreen protection creams, covers and avoidance of exposure.
7. Regular multiple punch biopsies—For early detection of this aggressive malignancy, some workers have recommended performance of multiple punch biopsies from margin and centre of the scar or chronic wound at yearly follow-up.
8. Multidisciplinary approach—Obtaining early wound closure, conducting regular follow up of patients with wounds and scars with keen vigilance for any change, taking rapid, appropriate action for suspected pathology and ensuring complete rehabilitation of the patient—such comprehensive approach needs care by a multidisciplinary team [11]. Establishment of special clinics for chronic leg ulcers would be of help in prevention, early detection and development of standardized protocol for treatment of MU with the hope of improving the prognosis.
9. High level of oncology awareness—To develop acute alertness about malignant transformation in a scar or non-healing wound and to take the necessary action for detection and management of MU, development of high level of oncology awareness needs to be inculcated in health care personnel including paramedics and wound care specialists.
10. Health education—The patient with particularly burn scar, chronic non-healing wound and family members of such a patient should be informed about the possibility of malignant transformation in the lesion. Counselling should be conducted about the need for regular follow-up and reporting of any symptom or change occurring in the lesion. This health education is likely to help in early detection of malignant degeneration.

11. Studies at genetic and molecular level—Association of MU with HLA DR4, aberration in p53 gene and mutation of FAS gene has been detected [3]. Changes in mediators of chronic inflammation have been found to be responsible for modification of microenvironment. It needs to be seen whether this knowledge helps in identifying scars that are more likely to develop malignancy. Such an identification may be of help in early detection and successful treatment of this pathology in years to come.

22.12 Conclusion

Marjolin's ulcer is a rare malignancy that develops most often in a postburn scar. Unstable scars and other types of non-healing wounds are also likely to be the sites of origin. Some studies have reported male predominance. The latent period between initial trauma and detection of malignancy varies significantly and has been reported to be shorter in studies from Africa, Nigeria and Southwest China [14, 15, 18] probably due to ethnic variations. The lower extremity is the most commonly affected body part and SCC is the most common histological type. But this SCC behaves more aggressively in comparison to original SCC. After histological confirmation by biopsy, local wide excision of lesion with confirmation of tumour free margins and closure of defect using STSG or appropriate flap is the main stay of treatment. Lymphadenectomy is performed for clinically palpable nodes or with large tumour of high grade of malignancy. Amputation of limb, hemipelvectomy, hemicorporectomy are procedures resorted to when radical excision without creation of instability is not possible. Adjuvant treatment such as radiotherapy and chemotherapy has limited role in desperate situations. Despite treatment, the incidence of local recurrence and lymph nodal as well as distant metastasis remains high. The patients need to be under meticulous follow up throughout their life. Diligent implementation of preventive measures and high level of alertness for early detection and treatment of the malignant lesion are the main recourses for improving the outcome at present.

References

1. Tian J, Zou J-P, Xiang X-F, Tang J-B, Cheng B. Marjolin's ulcer: a case report and literature review. World Acad Sci J. 2021;3(5):1–6. https://doi.org/10.3892/wasj.2020.76.
2. Nanze Y, Long X, Lujan-Hernandez JR, Hassan KZ, Bai M, Wang Y, Wang X, Zha R. Marjolin's ulcer: a preventable malignancy arising from scars. World J Surg Oncol. 2013;11:313–9. http://www.wjso.com/content/11/1/313
3. Huang C-Y, Feng C-H, Hsiao Y-C, Chuang SS, Yang J-Y. Burn scar carcinoma. J Dermatol Treat. 2010;21(6):350–6. https://doi.org/10.3109/09546630903386580.
4. Das KK, Chakaraborty A, Rahman A, Khandkar S. Incidences of malignancy in chronic burn scar ulcers: experience from Bangladesh. Burns. 2015;41(6):1315–21. https://doi.org/10.1016/j.burns.2015.02.008. Epub 2015 Feb 21. PMID: 25716761
5. Copcu E. Marjolin's ulcer: a preventable complication of burns? Plast Reconstr Surg. 2009;124(1):156e–64e. https://doi.org/10.1097/PRS.0b013e3181a8082e. PMID: 19568055.

6. Baldursson BT, Hedblad MA, Beitner H, Lindelöf B. Squamous cell carcinoma complicating chronic venous leg ulceration: a study of the histopathology, course and survival in 25 patients. Br J Dermatol. 1999;140(6):1148–52. https://doi.org/10.1046/j.1365-2133.1999.02879.x. PMID: 10354087.
7. Trent JT, Kirsner RS. Wounds and malignancy. Adv Skin Wound Care. 2003;16(1):31–4.
8. Pekarek B, Buck S, Osher L. A comprehensive review on Marjolin's ulcers: diagnosis and treatment. J Am Col Certif Wound Spec. 2011;3:60–4.
9. Chalya PL, Mabula JB, Rambau P, et al. Marjolin's ulcers at a university teaching hospital in Northwestern Tanzania: a retrospective review of 56 cases. World J Surg Oncol. 2012;10:38. http://www.wjso.com/content/10/1/38. https://doi.org/10.1186/1477-7819-10-38.
10. Khan K, Giannone AL, Mehrabi E, Khan A, Giannone RE. Marjolin's ulcer complicating a pressure sore: the clock is ticking. Am J Case Rep. 2016;17:111–4. https://doi.org/10.12659/AJCR.896352. PMCID: PMC4763807. PMID: 26898816.
11. Bazaliński D, Przybek-Mita J, Barańska B, Więch P. Marjolin's ulcer in chronic wounds—review of available literature. Contemp Oncol (Pozn). 2017;21(3):197–202. https://doi.org/10.5114/wo.2017.70109.
12. Challa VR, Deshmane V, Reddy MBA. A retrospective study of Marjolin's ulcer over an eleven year period. J Cutan Aesthet Surg. 2014;7(3):155–9. https://doi.org/10.4103/0974-2077.146667. PMCID: PMC4271295. PMID: 25538436.
13. Tian J, Zou J-P, Xiang X-F, Tang J-B, Cheng B. Marjolin's ulcer: a case report and literature review. World Acad Sci J. 2021;3:5. https://doi.org/10.3892/wasj.2020.76.
14. Opara KO, Otene IC. Marjolin's ulcers: a review. Niger Health J. 2011;11(4):107–11.
15. Nthumba PM. Marjolin's ulcers in sub Saharan Africa. World J Surg. 2010;34:2272–7. https://doi.org/10.1007/s00268-010-0727-6.
16. Liu Z, Zhou Y, Zhang P, Zhang M, Ren L, Zeng J, Zhou J, Liang P, Huang X. Analysis of clinical characteristics of 187 patients with Marjolin's ulcers. Zhonghua Shao Shang Za Zhi. 2016;32(5):293–8. https://doi.org/10.3760/cma.j.issn.1009-2587.2016.05.009. PMID: 27188488.
17. Tian J, Liang P, Zhang P, Liu Z, Zhou J, Ren L. Experience of diagnosis and treatment for 89 patients with Marjolin's ulcers in lower limbs. Zhong Nan Da Xue Xue Bao Yi Xue Ban. 2019;44(2):180–5. https://doi.org/10.11817/j.issn.1672-7347.2019.02.010. PMID: 30837387.
18. Xiang F, Song H-P, Huang Y-S. Clinical features and treatment of 140 cases of Marjolin's ulcer at a major burn center in southwest China. Exp Ther Med. 2019;17(5):3403–10. https://doi.org/10.3892/etm.2019.7364.
19. Burusapat C, Wanichjaroen N, Wongprakob N, Satayasoontorn K. Characteristics of Marjolin's ulcers in 21st century: a retrospective study, systematic review, and surgical guideline recommendation. J Burn Care Res. 2021;42(2):152–66. https://doi.org/10.1093/jbcr/iraa196. PMID: 33128365.
20. Ochenduszkiewicz U, Matkowski R, Szynglarewicz B, Kornafel J. Marjolin's ulcer: malignant neoplasm arising in scars. Rep Pract Oncol Radiother. 2006;11(3):135–8.
21. Cobey FC, Engrav LH, Klein MB, Isom CN, David R. Byrd brief report: sentinel lymph node dissection and burn scar carcinoma sentinel node and burn scar carcinoma. Burns. 2008;34:271–4.
22. Smith J, Mello LF, Nogueira Neto NC, Meohas W, Pinto LW, Campos VA, Barcellos MG, Fiod NJ, Rezende JF, Cabral CE. Malignancy in chronic ulcers and scars of the leg (Marjolin's ulcer): a study of 21 patients. Skelet Radiol. 2001;30(6):331–7. https://doi.org/10.1007/s002560100355. PMID: 11465774.
23. Eastman AL, Erdman WA, Lindberg GM, Hunt JL, Purdue GF, Fleming JB. Sentinel lymph node biopsy identifies occult nodal metastases in patients with Marjolin's ulcer. J Burn Care Rehabil. 2004;25(3):241–5. https://doi.org/10.1097/01.bcr.0000124791.17426.58. PMID: 15273464.
24. Aydoğdu E, Yildirim S, Aköz T. Is surgery an effective and adequate treatment in advanced Marjolin's ulcer? Burns. 2005;31(4):421–31. https://doi.org/10.1016/j.burns.2005.02.008. Epub 2005 Apr 1. PMID: 15896503.

25. Sharma S, Das N, Gupta V, Bera S, Bisht N. Lower extremity Marjolin's ulcer reconstruction with free anterolateral thigh flap: a case series of 11 patients. Cureus. 2020;12(11):e11392. https://doi.org/10.7759/cureus.11392.
26. Kanth AM, Heiman AJ, Nair L, Giammarino A, Carpenter C, Ricci JA, Patel A. Current trends in management of Marjolin's ulcer: a systematic review. J Burn Care Res. 2021;42(2):144–51. https://doi.org/10.1093/jbcr/iraa128. PMID: 32805009.
27. Metwally IH, Roshdy A, Saleh SS, Ezzat M. Epidemiology and predictors of recurrence of Marjolin's ulcer: experience from Mansoura Universityxs. Ann R Coll Surg Engl. 2017;99(3):245–9. (ISSN: 1478-7083).

23 Malignant Melanoma

Satyendra Kumar Tiwary

23.1 Introduction

A lower extremity ulcer is full thickness skin loss with progression into chronic wound, which shows no tendency to heal after 3 months of appropriate treatment or is still not fully healed at 12 months [1]. Chronic wounds may be of malignant etiology and as high as 10.4% incidence has been reported [2]. Malignant melanoma is a malignancy of aggressive behavior that develops when melanin-producing melanocytes originating from the neural crest undergo malignant transformation. Melanoma can develop in other places where neural crest cells migrate, such as the gastrointestinal system and the brain, and is most commonly found on the skin [3].

23.2 Epidemiology

Indian subcontinent has relatively low incidence of malignant melanoma as well as poor statistical data, whereas American Cancer Society data estimates that in the USA, a total of 106,110 cutaneous melanomas were expected to be diagnosed in 2021, according to estimations (62,260 in male and 43,850 in female) [4]. Although melanoma accounts for only about 1% of skin cancers, considering the aggressive behavior, it is the cause of the great majority of skin cancer deaths. According to the American Cancer Society, 7180 people in the USA (4600 males and 2580 women) will lose their life to melanoma in 2021 [4]. Unlike other solid tumors that target elderly folks, malignant melanoma is known for striking youthful and middle-aged people. It is most frequent in individuals under the age of 55, and it is more common

S. K. Tiwary (✉)
Department of General Surgery, Institute of Medical Sciences, Banaras Hindu University, Varanasi, India

A. K. Khanna, S. K. Tiwary (eds.), *Uncommon Ulcers of the Extremities*,
https://doi.org/10.1007/978-981-99-1782-2_23

in women, and it is responsible for the third-highest number of deaths among all malignancies [5].

23.3 Etiology

- **Precursor lesions:** Certain precursor lesions are more likely to transform into melanoma as compared to normal healthy skin. Important among them are:
  - Common acquired nevus
  - Dysplastic nevus
  - Congenital nevus
  - Cellular blue nevus
- **Family history:** A positive family history is found in 5–10% of patients; at least one affected relative is linked to a 2.2-fold increased risk.
- **Genetics:** CDKN2A (p16), CDK4, RB1, CDKN2A (p19), PTEN/MMAC1, and rasCDKN2A (p16) appear to be notably relevant in both sporadic and hereditary melanomas.
- **Personal characteristics:** Skin response to sunlight (easily burnt); freckling; benign and/or dysplastic melanocytic nevi (number indicates a stronger link than size); immunosuppressive conditions (transplantation patients, hematologic malignancies) all enhance the risk of melanoma [3].
- **Ultraviolet radiations and sun exposure:** UVA and UVB radiation has a carcinogenic effect that can lead to melanoma. There are numerous mechanisms at work, including inhibition of the immune system. There are numerous methods, including suppression of the skin's immune system, promotion of melanocyte cell proliferation, creation of free radicals, and DNA damage in melanocytes. Sunscreen prevents UVB; however, sunscreen users are more exposed to UVA than the general public. Low latitude, blistering sunburns, and tanning bed use all contribute to increased exposure and subsequent melanoma formation.
- **Atypical mole syndrome (B-K mole syndrome/dysplastic nevus syndrome/familial atypical multiple mole melanoma)**: Melanoma risk rises by 10.7% every 10 years (vs. 0.62% of controls). Depending on the number of family members affected, a higher risk of melanoma exists (nearly 100% risk if two or more relatives have dysplastic nevi and melanoma).
- **Parkinson's disease:** Parkinson's disease (PD) is a neurological disorder that affects millions of people worldwide. When compared to healthy people, those with Parkinson's disease have a nearly four-fold greater risk of malignant melanoma [6].
- **Socioeconomic status**: Lower socioeconomic level, like other diseases, has been associated with more advanced disease at the time of identification.

23.4 Pathophysiology

Melanomas can arise from a pre-existing precursor lesion or from healthy skin. De novo melanoma refers to a malignant melanoma that develops in healthy skin. Many of these melanomas are caused by UV radiation from the sun, and they can appear on both exposed and unexposed parts of the skin, such as the palms, soles (Fig. 23.1), and perineum. Melanoma has two growth phases in its history: radial and vertical. Malignant cells proliferate radially in the epidermis during the early radial growth phase. Most melanomas eventually move to the vertical growth phase, in which malignant cells infiltrate the dermis and develop the potential to spread [7].

Lesions are categorized clinically based on their depth as follows:

- 1 mm or less (thin)
- 1–4 mm (moderate)
- >4 mm (thick)

The four major forms of melanomas are as follows, based on their growth patterns:

- In the early stages, the **superficial spreading melanoma** (70%) is normally flat, but it can become uneven and raised. Variegated colors, peripheral notches, and indentations characterize the average size of 2 cm in diameter.
- **Nodular melanoma (15–30%)** is often blue-black in color; however, it may be pigmentless in some cases.
- **Melanoma lentigo maligna (4–10%)**: The lesions are typically more than 3 cm in diameter, flat, and tan, with pronounced border notching; they start off as little, freckle-like lesions.
- **Acral lentiginous melanoma** is a type of lentiginous melanoma (2–8%). Flat, tan, or brown stains with uneven borders may form on the palms and soles; subungual lesions can be dark or black, with ulcerations in advanced stages.

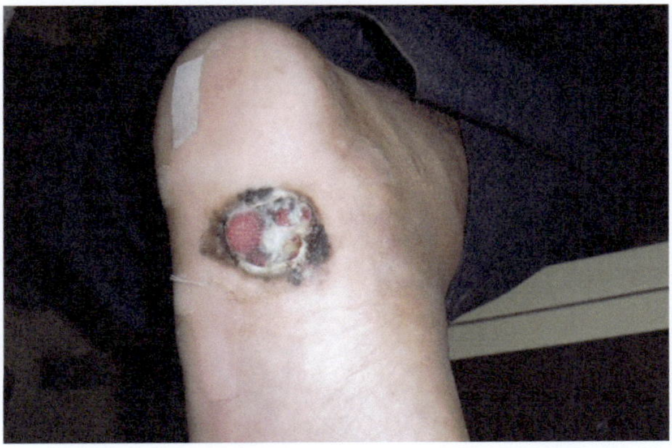

Fig. 23.1 Ulcer over the sole in malignant melanoma

23.5 Diagnostic Dictums (ABCDE)

Melanoma features are frequently referred to by the abbreviation ABCDE and comprise the following:

- A—Asymmetry
- B—Irregular border (Fig. 23.2)
- C—Color changes, particularly red, white, and blue tones in a brown or black lesion
- D—Diameter >6 mm
- E—Elevated surface

Melanomas can also itch, bleed, ulcerate, or form satellites. The examination includes a local inspection of the lesion (Fig. 23.3) as well as in-transit (Fig. 23.4) and satellite nodule evaluation (Fig. 23.5). Patients with metastatic disease or primary sites other than the skin frequently experience signs and symptoms that are related to the organ system in question. It is also crucial to check all of the body's lymph node groups.

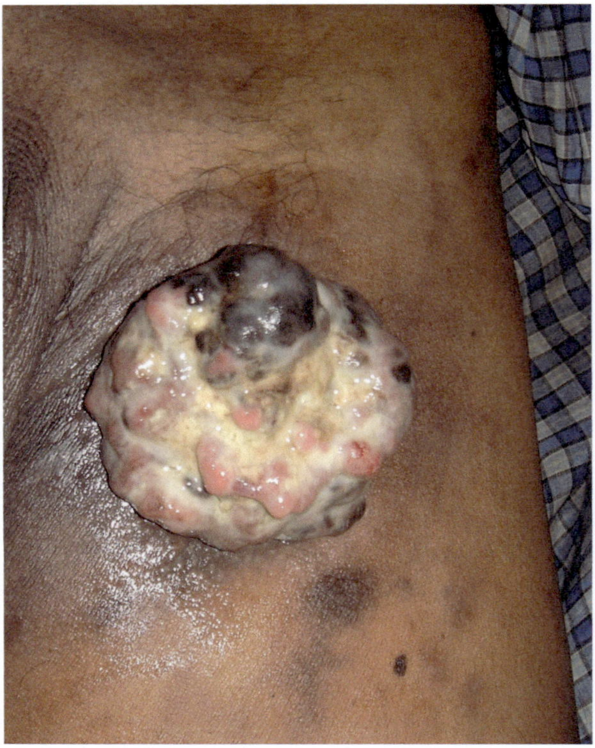

Fig. 23.2 Melanoma of left inguinal region with ulceration in a 65-year-old male

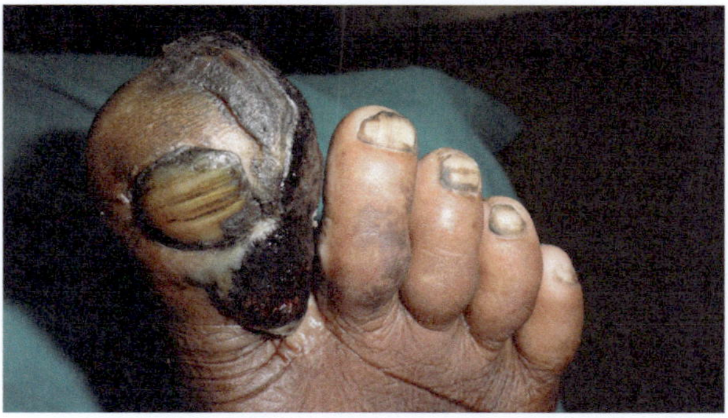

Fig. 23.3 Ulceration with pigmentation of left big toe in a 72-year-old male

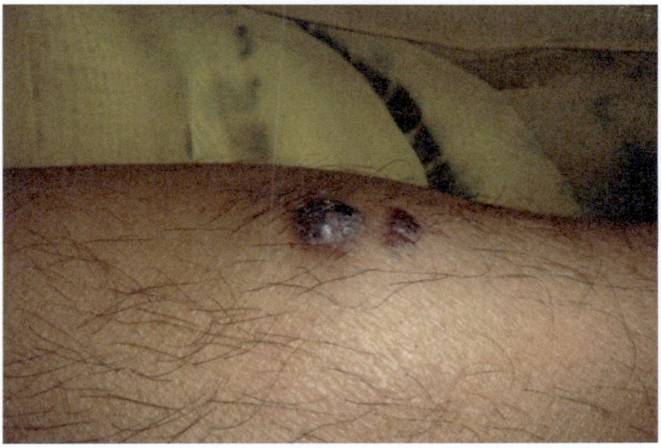

Fig. 23.4 Malignant melanoma of left leg with in-transit nodule

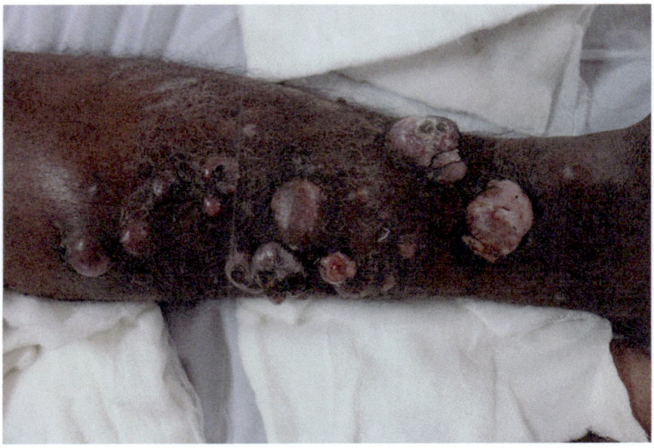

Fig. 23.5 Ulceration, pigmentation, and multiple satellite nodules in malignant melanoma of right lower limb

23.6 History and Physical Examination

23.6.1 Family History

First a careful and complete family history of melanoma or skin cancer in any member of family is taken [8]. A family history of irregular, conspicuous moles is also essential. Around 10% of all melanoma patients have a family history of the disease. These people are more likely to acquire melanoma at a younger age, have more aggressive behavior, a worse prognosis, and have many dysplastic nevi and primary. Patients having a family history of pancreatic cancer or astrocytoma should be evaluated for the presence of a familial melanoma syndrome. Mutations in the CDKN2A tumor suppressor gene are the most prevalent genetic aberration (p16).

23.6.2 Patient History

Patients' previous melanoma history must be elicited. Patients with multiple dysplastic nevi are more likely to have multiple primaries. This inherited tendency to develop multiple dysplastic nevi and melanoma is known as family atypical mole or melanoma (FAMM) syndrome.

23.6.3 Sun Exposure

It is crucial to have a history of previous sun exposure, especially if you have had severe sunburns as a child. The ability to tan is important because those who tan readily have a lower risk of developing melanoma than people who burn easily.

23.6.4 Moles

Any changes in size, color, or symmetry of the lesion (Fig. 23.6), as well as the development of bleeding or ulceration (Fig. 23.7), must be documented.

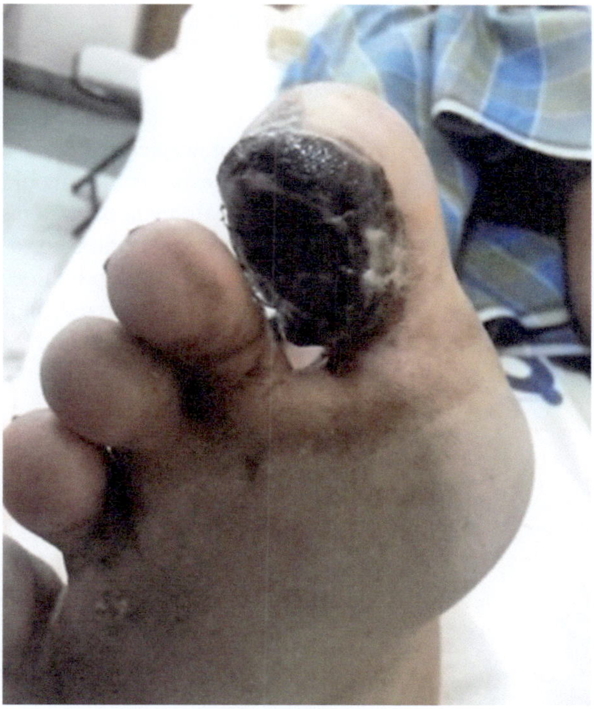

Fig. 23.6 Right great toe malignant melanoma with pigmentation and ulceration in a 60-year-old male

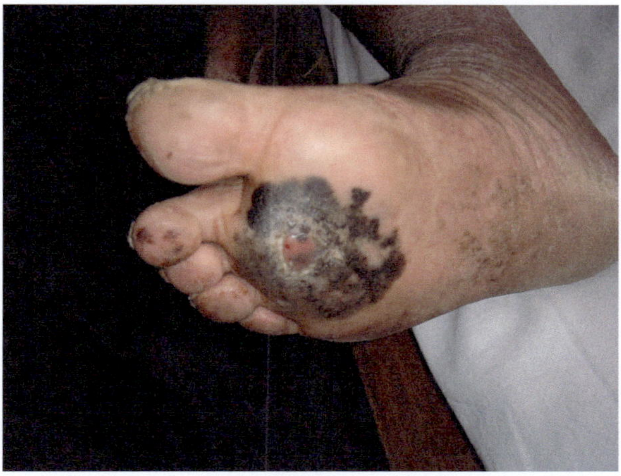

Fig. 23.7 Malignant melanoma of right sole

23.7 Physical Examination

23.7.1 Total Body Examination

When examining a patient with an atypical nevus or melanoma, a full-body skin examination is essential. The skin examination should be done at the time of the patient's initial evaluation and at all future appointments. A well-lit examining room and a completely undressed patient are essential for a thorough skin examination. Serial photography and new techniques like epiluminescence microscopy and digital image analysis can be helpful. Computerized image analysis saves images of lesions and allows them to be compared across time [8].

23.7.2 Compete Skin Examination

Assessment of the total number of nevi on the patient's skin during examination and an effort to distinguish between typical and atypical lesions are essential. The ABCDE diagnostic dictums (Asymmetry, B-Border irregularity, C-Color, D-Diameter >6 mm, E-Elevated) are used to distinguish early melanomas from benign nevi.

23.7.3 Lymph Node Examination

Examine all lymph node groups if a patient has been diagnosed with melanoma. Melanoma can spread through the lymphatic system, causing regional lymph node involvement, or hematogenously, causing involvement of any nodal basin in the body.

23.8 Workup

23.8.1 Approach Considerations

An excisional biopsy confirms the diagnosis of melanoma. In some individuals, a sentinel lymph node biopsy or a gene profile assay may be useful as a predictive tool; however, there is little evidence that they have an impact on survival. Laboratory and imaging tests are rarely needed in the early stages of illness. When triggered by signs or symptoms at any time, they are often suitable. In most melanoma patients, preoperative imaging investigations are expensive and provide little benefit [9]. The best imaging study for diagnosing lymph node involvement is ultrasonography, while the best imaging study for looking for further metastatic locations is positron emission tomography, computed tomography scanning (PET/CT) [10].

23.8.2 Histologic Findings

Although no single histologic finding is pathognomonic for melanoma, there are several common characteristics. Large, pleomorphic, hyperchromic nuclei with prominent nucleoli are almost usually present, as are expanded cells with large, pleomorphic, hyperchromic nuclei. Several mitotic figures are frequently observed. Immunohistochemical stains are rarely required for diagnosis; nevertheless, they may be required in cases of ambiguous histology. In melanocytes, the S-100 and HMB 45 stains are both positive. The junctional component of benign nevi can be stained with PRAME (preferentially expressed antigen in melanoma), but dermal staining indicates malignancy. Other malignancies, such as testicular tumors and cellular neurothekeoma, are stained by it, but it is not totally selective. It is especially useful for telling the difference between nevus remnants and melanoma [11–13]. The use of fluorescent in situ hybridization (FISH) assays is growing, and molecular predictors of biologic response to targeted immunotherapy are becoming more widespread, with BRAF testing being the most popular [14–16].

23.8.3 Complete Chemistry Panel (CCP)

The chemistry panel suggests metastatic disease as well as general condition. An elevated alkaline phosphatase level is indicative of metastasis to the bone or liver, while impaired liver function suggests metastasis to the liver. Nutritional status assessed by total protein and albumin while Creatinine level a must prior to chemotherapy as nephrotoxicity in impaired kidney may be catastrophic.

23.8.4 Lactate Dehydrogenase Assay (LDH)

The level of lactate dehydrogenase (LDH) is high in a variety of situations, although it is not particular to any of them. It could be effective in the follow-up management of some melanoma patients. The level of LDH, which has been shown to be an independent predictor of poor prognosis, is included in the melanoma staging system.

23.8.5 Radiography of the Chest (CXR)

A normal chest radiograph at diagnosis, however, provides a baseline for future comparison. Because the lungs are generally the first location of metastatic illness, patients with stage III disease, in-transit disease, or local recurrence should obtain a chest radiograph or computed tomography (CT) scan of the chest.

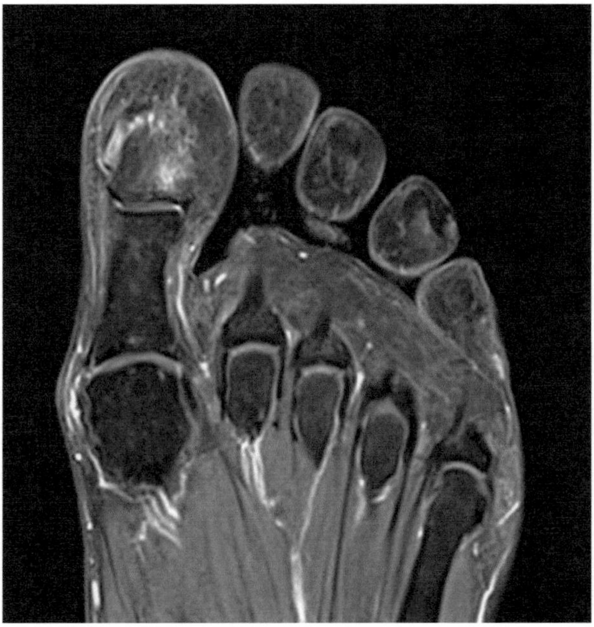

Fig. 23.8 MRI image of malignant melanoma right big toe

23.8.6 Magnetic Resonance Imaging (MRI)

To define the lesion with dimension and effect on adjoining structures MRI (Fig. 23.8) is of help but important role is to detect further asymptomatic cerebral metastatic illness during the workup of a patient with known distant metastases. This is especially true for patients who are being treated with high-dose interleukin-2. Only patients with neurologic symptoms should receive a brain MRI if they have no known metastatic illness.

23.9 Computed Tomography (CT)

23.9.1 Chest Computed Tomography (CT) Scan

To detect asymptomatic metastatic lesions, a chest CT scan should be included in the staging workup of a patient with stage IV disease (i.e. a patient with known distant metastases). A chest CT scan should be conducted only if clinically justified in individuals with stage I, II, or III illness.

23.9.2 CT Scan of the Abdomen

When examining a patient with stage III, locally recurrent, or in-transit illness, a CT scan of the abdomen is frequently performed. A negative CT scan provides a baseline study for future comparison, despite the low yield.

23.9.3 CT Scan of Pelvis

Only if a patient has local regional recurrence below the waist, is symptomatic, or has known metastatic illness with a history of primary tumors below the waist should be recommended for CT scan of pelvis.

23.10 Positron Emission Tomography (PET)

PET/CT is the most sensitive technology for diagnosing metastatic illness right now. PET scans are not indicated in early stage disease (stage I or II), but a PET scan may aid in staging patients with known node involvement or in-transit or satellite lesions. Fluorodeoxyglucose (FDG) PET/CT scans, in particular, are a useful technique for detecting further metastases in patients with advanced and metastatic melanoma as part of the preoperative examination [17].

23.11 Biopsy of a Suggestive Lesion

It is preferable to perform a thorough excisional biopsy. The sample should have a healthy skin margin of 1–3 mm and include all layers of skin as well as some subcutaneous fat.

Fascia is no longer considered standard. If the suggestive lesion is large or located in a cosmetically sensitive area, an incisional or punch biopsy may be required. The source of the incisional biopsy samples should be the most abnormal site of the lesion. In situations of lentigo maligna melanoma in situ, a broad shave biopsy may help improve diagnostic sampling when the index of suspicion is low [18].

23.12 Surgical Excision or Re-excision After Biopsy

Excision or re-excision after biopsy should be done always with safe margins as per recent guidelines:

- 0.5–1 cm margin for in situ lesions.
- Lesions with a thickness of less than 1 mm have a 1 cm border.
- Lesions with a thickness of 1.01–2 mm and a border of 1–2 cm.
- Lesions with a thickness of 2.01–4 mm and a margin of 2 cm.
- Lesions with a thickness of more than 4 mm—at least a 2 cm border [19].

23.13 Elective Lymph Node Dissection

A lymph node dissection should be performed on patients who have clinically enlarged lymph nodes but no signs of distant illness. However, studies show that in patients with melanomas that are 1–4 mm thick, LND may not yield a significant survival advantage. The only patients who seem to benefit from LND are those with lesions 1.1–2 mm thick and who are younger than 60 years.

23.14 Sentinel Lymph Node Biopsy

To determine which node is the sentinel node, the following two techniques, often in combination, are used. The first method includes injecting a blue dye at the original melanoma site and establishing the location of the sentinel node through a tiny incision above the nodal basin. The second method includes injecting a radiolabeled solution into the primary site and determining the position of the sentinel node with a hand-held gamma detector. After that, the node is removed for pathologic examination. Prior to performing a large excision of the primary, the node should be removed [20]. Sentinel lymph node biopsy (SLNB) is now widely recognized as a valuable source of prognostic, diagnostic, and therapeutic data [21]. Patients with thick melanomas (T4; Breslow thickness >4 mm) have less evidence, although sentinel lymph node biopsy is advised for staging and regional disease control. Although there is insufficient evidence to support routine sentinel lymph node biopsy in individuals with thin melanomas (T1; Breslow thickness 1 mm), it may be an option in some patients with high-risk features.

23.15 Staging

The American Joint Committee on Cancer (AJCC) tumor/node/metastasis (TNM) classification and staging systems for cutaneous melanoma are provided below [22]. The TNM system has incorporated the older Breslow classification of melanoma thickness, whose four classes of lesion depth correspond with levels T1–4. Clark levels, another older classification of melanoma, are now largely used for historical reference.

23.15.1 T Classification

- TX: It is impossible to assess the primary tumor (shave biopsy)
- T0: No sign of original tumor
- T1: 1.0 mm Melanoma in situ (ulceration unknown or unspecified)
- T1a: 0.8 mm without ulceration; 0.8–1.0 mm with or without ulceration
- T1b: 0.8 mm with ulceration
- T2a: >1.0–2.0 mm without ulceration

- T2b: >1.0–2.0 mm with ulceration
- T3: >2.0–4.0 mm (ulceration unknown or unspecified)
- T4: >4.0 mm (ulceration unknown or undetermined)
- T4a: >4.0 mm without ulceration
- T4b: >4.0 mm with ulceration

23.15.2 N Classification

- N0: No regional metastases found
- N1: One tumor-involved node; or in-transit, satellite, and/or microsatellite metastases with no tumor-involved nodes
- N1a: One clinically occult (i.e. not discovered by sentinel lymph node biopsy); no in-transit, satellite, or microsatellite metastases
- N1b: One clinically detected; no in-transit, satellite, or microsatellite metastases
- N2: Two or three tumor-involved nodes; or in-transit, satellite, or microsatellite metastases
- N2a: Two or three clinically occult (i.e. not detected by sentinel lymph node biopsy); no in-transit, satellite, or microsatellite metastases
- N2b: Two or three clinically detected; no in-transit, satellite, or microsatellite metastases
- N2c: One occult or clinically diagnosed metastasis; in-transit, satellite, and/or microsatellite metastases discovered
- N3: 2 tumor-involved nodes or any number of matted nodes without or with in-transit, satellite, and/or microsatellite metastases with 4 tumor-involved nodes or in-transit, satellite, and/or microsatellite metastases.
- N3a: 4 clinically occult (i.e. identified by sentinel lymph node biopsy); no in-transit, satellite, or microsatellite metastases
- N3b: 4 clinically detectable (i.e. detected by sentinel lymph node biopsy); no in-transit, satellite, or microsatellite metastases
- N3c: 2 clinically occult or clinically detectable nodes, with in-transit, satellite, and/or microsatellite metastases

23.15.3 M Classification

- M0: There are no signs of distant metastases.
- M1a: Skin, subcutaneous, or non-regional nodal metastases that are far away.
- M1b: Lung metastases, whether or not M1a is involved.
- M1c: Distant metastases to visceral locations outside the central nervous system (CNS), with or without M1a or M1b involvement.
- M1d: Long-distance CNS metastases, with or without M1a-c involvement.

Cases where the lactate dehydrogenase (LDH) level is known (beyond M0) are given the suffix (0) for normal LDH level or (1) for high LDH level.

23.16 Surgical Management

For primary cutaneous melanoma of any thickness, as well as melanoma in situ, surgical excision with histologically negative margins is the preferred and first-line treatment. The depth of excision should be up to the fascia [23–26], with margins based on tumor thickness. Sentinel lymph node biopsy should be conducted before broad excision of the primary tumor, if possible, and in the same operating environment. For lentigo maligna type melanoma in situ on the face, ears, or scalp, Mohs micrographic surgery (MMS) or phased excision with paraffin-embedded permanent sections may be used for tissue-sparing excision and extensive histologic examination of peripheral borders.

23.16.1 Wide Local Excision

Primary melanomas should be excised with clear margins in the setting of resectable clinical stage III illness to ensure local control. When possible, wide local excision (WLE) with a clinical 1 cm margin is recommended, with primary closure to avoid reconstruction. There is no need to resect the original tumor in clinical stage IV illness if there are no symptoms or diagnostic tissue is required. If excision of the original lesion is indicated, it should be done with clean margins and no additional safety margins.

23.16.2 Radical Lymph Node Dissection

After pathological examination (cytology or histology of the lesion preoperatively) and proper staging [27], radial lymph node dissection is advised for cases of clinically diagnosed lymph node metastases in resectable stage III illness. When it comes to lymph node surgery, radical node dissection is preferred over "node picking."

23.16.3 Treatment of Satellite or In-Transit Metastases

Resection with clear margins is indicated for resectable in-transit metastases that can consist of few, tiny, and non-rapidly recurring lesions. Resections and reconstructions that are extensive and recurrent should be avoided. Loco-regional treatments (e.g. isolated limb perfusion or infusion, talimogene laherparepvec [TVEC], electrochemotherapy, 10% rose Bengal solution [PV-10]) may be used to treat unresectable satellite/in-transit metastases or inoperable primary tumors of the limbs without additional metastases.

23.16.4 Adjuvant Radiotherapy After Lymphadenectomy

The basic prescription for patients with advanced stage III disease who have had lymphadenectomy is adjuvant systemic therapy and surveillance, with additional surgery and radiotherapy (RT) reserved for any recurring disease. Adjuvant RT, however, could be beneficial for high-risk individuals in whom regional control is a key concern and/or systemic therapy is not an option.

23.16.5 Neoadjuvant Therapy

Neoadjuvant methods should only be evaluated in the context of a clinical trial for easily resectable stage III illness with tolerable surgical morbidity. Outside of a clinical trial, neoadjuvant treatments should be considered for technically resectable but bulky nodal and/or in-transit disease where surgery is expected to result in positive resection margin status or necessitate postoperative RT.

23.16.6 Mohs Micrographic Surgery (MMS)

The primary treatment option for melanoma in situ is Mohs micrographic surgery (MMS), which is augmented by immunohistochemistry staining. Antibodies to a melanoma antigen identified by T cells were used in the stain (MART-1). All recurrent melanoma in situ and lentigo maligna, as well as primary lesions in the following sites: head and neck, hands, feet, pretibial surface, nails, and ankles, should be treated with MMS [28].

23.16.7 Radiation Therapy

- Primary disease: As an adjuvant treatment in individuals with deep desmoplastic melanoma with narrow margins, significant neurotropism, or locally recurrent cancer, among other criteria.
- Regional disease: Adjuvant treatment after excision of category 2B nodes and LDH 1.5 times upper limit of normal, as well as extra-nodal tumor extension; palliative treatment for unresectable illness.
- Metastatic disease: Used to treat brain metastases as an adjuvant or primary treatment.

For localized or solitary distant metastatic illness, stereotactic radiotherapy has been advised.

23.17 Treatment for Advanced Melanoma

Resection is indicated in cases of restricted illness; alternatively, observation or systemic medication may be used.

Systemic therapy is used to treat individuals with unresectable cancer who do not have brain metastases; patients with brain metastases require treatment for the central nervous system [29–33].

Immunotherapy regimens for systemic therapy that are first-line (category 1)

- Nivolumab/ipilimumab
- Pembrolizumab or nivolumab as anti–programmed cell death protein 1 (PD-1) monotherapy

The following are second-line or follow-up therapy recommendations:

- **Targeted therapy if a BRAF V600 activating mutation is present: Pembrolizumab/Nivolumab/Ipilimumab**
  - Anti-PD-1 monotherapy: Pembrolizumab/nivolumab/ipilimumab
  - High-dose interleukin-2
  - Dabrafenib/trametinib or vemurafenib/cobimetinib (IL-2)
  - Imatinib, a cytotoxic drug, is used to treat cancers with KIT activating mutations.

23.18 Follow-Up for Melanoma Cancer Survivors

Melanoma survivors should have the following follow-up:

History and physical examination every 3–6 months for 2 years, then every 3–12 months for 2 years, then annually as clinically recommended. Blood tests on a regular basis are not advised.

To screen for recurrence or metastatic disease, consider imaging every 3–12 months for 2 years, then every 6–12 months for another 3 years (unless otherwise compelled by clinical trial participation). After 5 years, routine imaging to check for asymptomatic recurrence or metastatic illness is not advised.

23.19 Prognosis

The following factors have a poor prognosis [34]:

- Measurement of thickness (worse prognosis in thicker lesions)
- Ulceration (ulcers indicate advanced lesion and poor prognosis)
- Lymph nodes involvement (stage III disease)
- Number of positive lymph nodes (more positive nodes, poor prognosis)
- Distant metastasis (stage IV disease)

- Anatomic site (extremity lesions better prognosis than face or trunk)
- Male sex (worse prognosis)

Prognosis depends on the disease stage at the time of diagnosis with 5-year survival for stage I disease (>90%), stage II disease (45–77%), stage III disease (27–70%), metastatic disease-5-year survival rate <20%.

23.20 Complications

Complications are evident in cases of delayed diagnosis and treatment which may be:

- Ulceration: It always indicates advanced stage of the disease.
- Secondary infection: It results from disruption of the normal skin barrier.
- Ugly scar: Either the disease or the treatment with aggressive resection and reconstruction may result in unacceptable or ugly scarring.
- Local recurrence: Advanced cases at the time of diagnosis which included ulceration in melanoma may result in local recurrences often.
- Metastases: Local recurrences, metastases are more common with advanced cases and malignant melanoma is notorious.
- Lymphedema: Lymphatic invasion by the disease or removal of the lymph nodes leads to lymphedema.
- Stress, depression, and anxiety: Fear of the disease considering aggressive nature and cosmesis issues connected with the treatment and disease leads to a lot of psychological issues.

23.21 Conclusion

Multi-etiological causes, misdiagnosis, and multimodal approach in the management must be considered malignant ulcers which stands true for malignant melanoma. Atypical presentation, abnormal location, arrest in healing are alarming bells for malignant ulcers which stands true for malignant melanoma. Consider the surgical margins first before doing a wide local excision. Skin grafting or tissue transfers may be required if the closure is not possible. Adjuvant therapy for patients with advanced melanoma is reserved for medical management. The prognosis for isolated lesions is good with surgery, but the prognosis for advanced melanoma after ulcerations develop is gloomy, but the interprofessional team approach to care will optimize the patient's chances for a better outcome.

References

1. Kahle B, Hermanns HJ, Gallenkemper G. Evidence-based treatment of chronic leg ulcers. Dtsch Arztebl Int. 2011;108(14):231–7. https://doi.org/10.3238/arztebl.2011.0231.

2. Senet P, Combemale P, Debure C, Baudot N, Machet L, Aout M, Lok C. Malignancy and chronic leg ulcers: the value of systematic wound biopsies: a prospective multicentre, cross-sectional study. Arch Dermatol. 2012;148:704–8.
3. Heistein JB, Acharya U. Malignant melanoma. In: Stat Pearls. Treasure Island (FL): Stat Pearls Publishing; 2021.
4. American Cancer Society. Cancer facts & figures 2021. American Cancer Society. https://www.cancer.org/content/dam/cancer-org/research/cancer-facts-and-statistics/annual-cancer-facts-and-figures/2021/cancer-facts-and-figures-2021.pdf. Accessed 20 Mar 2022.
5. Donley GM, Liu WT, Pfeiffer RM, McDonald EC, Peters KO, Tucker MA, Cahoon EK. Reproductive factors, exogenous hormone use and incidence of melanoma among women in the United States. Br J Cancer. 2019;120(7):754–60.
6. Dalvin LA, Damento GM, Yawn BP, Abbott BA, Hodge DO, Pulido JS. Parkinson disease and melanoma: confirming and reexamining an association. Mayo Clin Proc. 2017;92(7):1070–9.
7. Amber TL, Bruce HL. The Washington manual of surgery. 6th ed. St Luis: Wolters-Kluwer-Lippincott Williams and Wilkins; 2012.
8. Kantor J, Kantor DE. Routine dermatologist-performed full-body skin examination and early melanoma detection. Arch Dermatol. 2009;145(8):873–6.
9. Sabel MS, Wong SL. Review of evidence-based support for pretreatment imaging in melanoma. J Natl Compr Cancer Netw. 2009;7(3):281–9.
10. Xing Y, Bronstein Y, Ross MI, Askew RL, Lee JE, Gershenwald JE, et al. Contemporary diagnostic imaging modalities for the staging and surveillance of melanoma patients: a meta-analysis. J Natl Cancer Inst. 2011;103(2):129–42.
11. Farah M, Chung HJ. Diagnostic utility of preferentially expressed antigen in melanoma immunohistochemistry in the evaluation of melanomas with a co-existent nevoid melanocytic population: a single-center retrospective cohort study. J Am Acad Dermatol. 2021;87:486.
12. Cesinaro AM, Piana S, Paganelli A, Pedroni G, Santandrea G, Maiorana A. PRAME expression in cellular neurothekeoma: a study of 11 cases. J Cutan Pathol. 2021;49:338.
13. Hu J, Cai X, Lv JJ, Wan XC, Zeng XY, Feng ML, et al. PRAME immunohistochemistry as an adjunct for differential diagnosis in acral lentiginous melanoma and acral nevi. Hum Pathol. 2021;120:9.
14. Rashid S, Tsao H. Recognition, staging, and management of melanoma. Med Clin North Am. 2021;105(4):643–61.
15. Wilson ML. Histopathologic and molecular diagnosis of melanoma. Clin Plast Surg. 2021;48(4):587–98.
16. Revythis A, Shah S, Kutka M, Moschetta M, Ozturk MA, Pappas-Gogos G, et al. Unraveling the wide spectrum of melanoma biomarkers. Diagnostics (Basel). 2021;11(8).
17. Bronstein Y, Ng CS, Rohren E, Ross MI, Lee JE, Cormier J, et al. PET/CT in the management of patients with stage IIIC and IV metastatic melanoma considered candidates for surgery: evaluation of the additive value after conventional imaging. AJR Am J Roentgenol. 2012;198(4):902–8.
18. National Comprehensive Cancer Network. NCCN clinical practice guidelines in oncology: melanoma: cutaneous. NCCN. http://www.nccn.org/professionals/physician_gls/pdf/melanoma.pdf. Version 1.2022–3 Dec 2021; Accessed 6 Dec 2021.
19. Gillgren P, Drzewiecki KT, Niin M, et al. 2-cm versus 4-cm surgical excision margins for primary cutaneous melanoma thicker than 2 mm: a randomised, multicentre trial. Lancet. 2011;378(9803):1635–42.
20. Melanoma Treatment (PDQ®)–Health professional version. National Cancer Institute. https://www.cancer.gov/types/skin/hp/melanoma-treatment-pdq#link/_25_toc. 2021. Accessed 25 Apr 2022.
21. Bachter D, Michl C, Buchels H, Vogt H, Balda BR. The predictive value of the sentinel lymph node in malignant melanomas. Recent Results Cancer Res. 2001;158:129–36.
22. American Joint Committee on Cancer. Melanoma of the skin. In: Amin MB, Edge S, Greene F, Byrd DR, Brookland RK, et al., editors. AJCC staging manual. 8th ed. New York: Springer; 2016.

23. Swetter SM, Tsao H, Bichakjian CK, Curiel-Lewandrowski C, Elder DE, Gershenwald JE, et al. Guidelines of care for the management of primary cutaneous melanoma. J Am Acad Dermatol. 2019;80(1):208–50.
24. Michielin O, van Akkooi A, Lorigan P, et al. ESMO consensus conference recommendations on the management of locoregional melanoma: the ESMO guidelines committee. Ann Oncol. 2020;31:1449.
25. Garbe C, et al. European Dermatology Forum (EDF), the European Association of Dermato-Oncology (EADO), and the European Organization for Research and Treatment of Cancer (EORTC). European consensus-based inter-disciplinary guideline for melanoma. Part 1: diagnostics—update 2019. Eur J Cancer. 2020;126:141–58.
26. Bichakjian CK, Halpern AC, Johnson TM, Foote Hood A, Grichnik JM, Swetter SM, et al. Guidelines of care for the management of primary cutaneous melanoma. American Academy of Dermatology. J Am Acad Dermatol. 2011;65:1032.
27. Faries MB, Thompson JF, Cochran AJ, Andtbacka RH, Mozzillo N, et al. Completion dissection or observation for sentinel-node metastasis in melanoma. N Engl J Med. 2017;376(23):2211–22.
28. Kunishige JH, Brodland DG, Zitelli JA. Surgical margins for melanoma in situ. J Am Acad Dermatol. 2012;66(3):438–44.
29. Saberian C, Sperduto P, Davies MA. Targeted therapy strategies for melanoma brain metastasis. Neurooncol Adv. 2021;3(Suppl 5):v75–85.
30. Khaddour K, Maahs L, Avila-Rodriguez AM, Maamar Y, Samaan S, Ansstas G. Melanoma targeted therapies beyond BRAF-mutant melanoma: potential druggable mutations and novel treatment approaches. Cancers (Basel). 2021;13(22).
31. Zeng H, Liu F, Zhou H, Zeng C. Individualized treatment strategy for cutaneous melanoma: where are we now and where are we going? Front Oncol. 2021;11:775100.
32. Teixido C, Castillo P, Martinez-Vila C, Arance A, Alos L. Molecular markers and targets in melanoma. Cell. 2021;10(9).
33. Ferrucci PF, Lens M, Cocorocchio E. Combined BRAF-targeted therapy with immunotherapy in BRAF-mutated advanced melanoma patients. Curr Oncol Rep. 2021;23(12):138.
34. Murali R, Desilva C, Thompson JF, Scolyer RA. Factors predicting recurrence and survival in sentinel lymph node-positive melanoma patients. Ann Surg. 2011;253(6):1155–64.

Squamous Cell Carcinoma

24

Sandeep Agarwal

Squamous cell carcinoma (SCC) is one of the most encountered types of cancers worldwide. It is an aggressive disease that affects the majority of the human body organs including the lungs, head and neck, esophagus, skin, genitourinary tract, thyroid, and other parts. SCC is a highly metastasizing disease with a relatively low overall survival rate.

24.1 Pathogenesis

The pathogenesis of squamous cell carcinoma is multifactorial and includes many extrinsic and intrinsic factors. The most important extrinsic factor is generally recognized as UV sunlight exposure. As lifetime UV exposure increases, so does the incidence of squamous cell carcinoma. The human papillomavirus type 16 is present in many of the genital and periungual forms of squamous cell, but human papillomavirus types 5, 8, 9, 18, 31, 33, 35, 39, 40, and 51–60 have all been isolated from squamous cell tumors. Other extrinsic factors that are related to the development of squamous cell carcinoma are industrial carcinogens, such as pitch, tar, crude paraffin oil, fuel oil, creosote, lubricating oils, arsenic, and nitrosoureas.

Intrinsic factors associated with squamous cell carcinoma include age, lighter skin pigmentation, scars, and dermatoses associated with photosensitivity (chronic cutaneous lupus), ulcerations, and lichen planus. There are two hereditary conditions that increase the risk of developing squamous cell carcinoma. Xeroderma pigmentosa is an autosomal recessive condition leading to an inability to repair UV-induced DNA damage. Oculocutaneous albinism results in insufficient melanin production, thereby decreasing the body's defense against UV damage.

S. Agarwal (✉)
Institute of Vascular and Endovascular Sciences, Sir Ganga Ram Hospital, New Delhi, India

A. K. Khanna, S. K. Tiwary (eds.), *Uncommon Ulcers of the Extremities*, https://doi.org/10.1007/978-981-99-1782-2_24

Immunosuppressed individuals, whether by AIDS or organ transplant, have shown not only an increased incidence of squamous cell carcinoma but also a tendency to develop more aggressive tumors [1].

24.2 Squamous Cell Carcinoma: Development and Variants

The prototypical invasive squamous cell lesion can be identified with relative ease by its appearance. Most commonly, they are indurated papules, plaques, or nodules, with thick adherent scale or hyperkeratosis. Fortunately, many squamous cell carcinomas move through multiple stages before reaching the invasive presentation. If these precursors are identified, more conservative treatments can be utilized.

24.2.1 Actinic Keratosis

The actinic keratosis is the first observable precursor to an invasive squamous cell carcinoma. Histologically, an actinic keratosis is defined by atypical keratinocytes, arising in the stratum spinosum, which extend up to but do not involve the stratum corneum (Fig. 24.1). These keratinocytes are enlarged and crowded and show loss of polarity. Clinically, actinic keratoses present as less than 1 cm, tan-brown, red, or skin-colored, rough, sandpaper-like patches. Cutaneous horns can develop in lesions that produce excess keratin. The most common sites of occurrence are the face, ears, and dorsum of the hands and arms. These precancerous lesions can be treated conservatively and successfully with cryosurgery, electrodessication and curettage, chemotherapeutic creams, or topical immune modulators. Without treatment, it is generally believed that a percentage of these lesions will spontaneously resolve, but some can continue to mutate and form squamous cell carcinoma in situ [2].

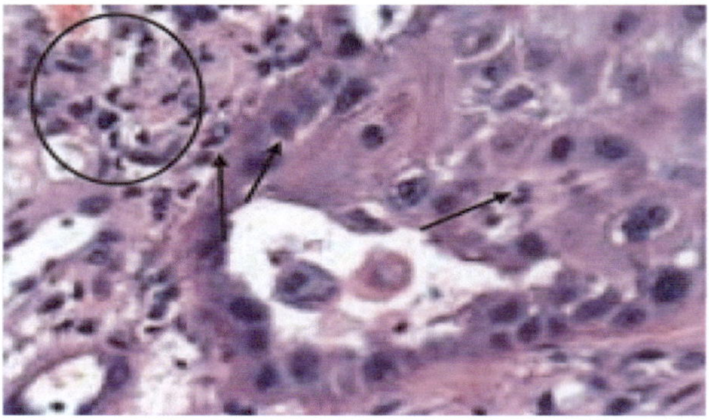

Fig. 24.1 Actinic keratosis. Note the irregular nuclei of varying size

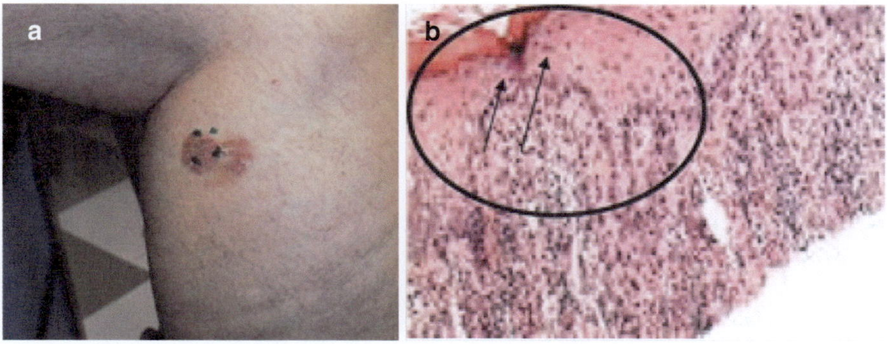

Fig. 24.2 (**a**) Squamous cell carcinoma in situ on medial aspect of upper calf. (**b**) Squamous cell carcinoma in situ showing atypical keratinocytes approaching the stratum lucidum

24.2.2 Squamous Cell Carcinoma In Situ

Clinically, squamous cell carcinoma in situ presents as a well-demarcated, scaling, or hyperkeratotic macule, papule, or plaque (Fig. 24.2a). They can be nearly indistinguishable from actinic keratoses to the naked eye. Evidence of erosion and, at times, evidence of bleeding should increase clinical suspicion. Histopathologically (Fig. 24.2b), squamous cell carcinoma in situ involves the entire thickness of the epidermis with pleomorphic (multiple sizes and shapes) keratinocytes and involves the adnexal epithelium. No evidence of invasion into the dermis is observed. Like their precursors, squamous cell carcinoma in situ may be treated with cryosurgery, electrodessication and curettage, chemotherapeutic creams, excision, and topical immune modulators. Without timely and appropriate treatment, these lesions can advance to form invasive squamous cell carcinoma.

24.2.3 Invasive Squamous Cell Carcinoma

The common invasive squamous cell carcinoma is a malignancy of the keratinocytes from the epidermis that invade the dermis. Having transversed the basement membrane, these malignancies have the potential to invade fat, muscle, bone, and cartilage and to metastasize to regional lymph nodes and distant sites. The cells of an invasive squamous cell carcinoma resemble those of an actinic keratosis. They have enlarged and irregularly contoured nuclei, increased numbers of nucleoli, and irregular mitotic figures. The important clinical distinction is that there is invasion into the dermis, which necessitates more aggressive treatment to prevent further damage to the surrounding cutaneous and underlying structures and metastasis (Figs. 24.3 and 24.4). Surgical excision is the treatment of choice for all invasive tumors. Usually, treatment is performed under local anesthesia with a 3- to 4-mm margin taken. For high-risk lesions, such as those on the face, ears, and lips, as well

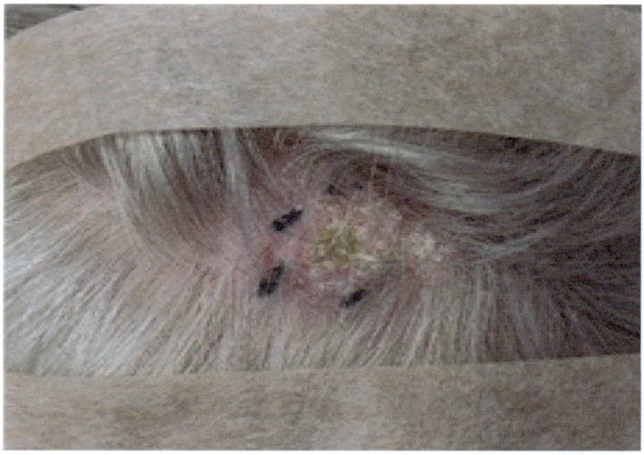

Fig. 24.3 Invasive squamous cell carcinoma on the scalp

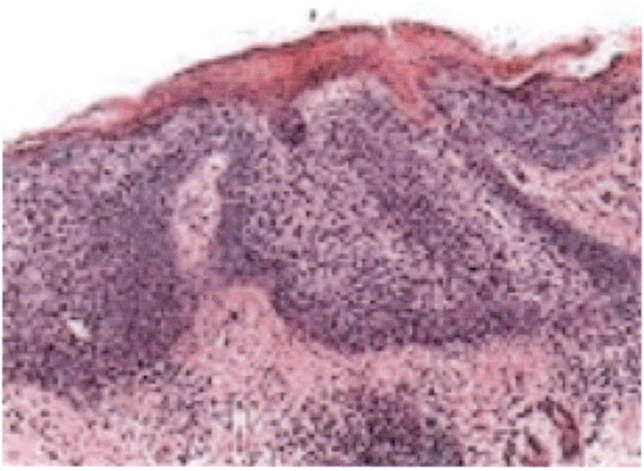

Fig. 24.4 Full thickness atypia, extending into the dermis (dermis is not shown)

as recurrent tumors and tumors larger than 2 cm, Mohs micrographic surgery should be employed to ensure the highest possible cure rate. Failure to treat or insufficient treatment can lead to recurrence and metastasis.

There are many factors that contribute to the aggressiveness, recurrence rate, and metastatic potential of squamous cell carcinomas. Tumor size is a major determinant. For lesions larger than 2 cm, the recurrence rate doubles and the metastatic rate triples to 30%. Tumors with rapid growth rates also have a higher metastatic potential. Tumors originating in burn scars have a 30% metastasis rate. The rate for metastatic disease increases the closer a tumor is to the oral cavity. Recurrent tumors also have a greater metastatic rate, especially on the lips and ears, where the rate is 32% and 45%, respectively. Metastasis from squamous cell carcinoma appears most commonly in the regional lymph nodes, followed by the lungs and liver [3, 4].

Rare varieties of the squamous cell carcinoma are difficult to diagnose and treat if the common variety were all that existed. There are, however, multiple variants of this disease, including spindle cell, acantholytic, verrucous, lymphoepithelioma-like, desmoplastic, adenosquamous, cystic, and keratoacanthoma. Each of these variants differs in histology and prognosis, but the treatment is identical to the more common form.

Spindle cell carcinoma is a rare variant in which the neoplastic keratinocytes infiltrate the dermis as single cells with elongated nuclei.

Verrucous squamous cell carcinoma (Fig. 24.5) is a low-grade variant that is typified by well-differentiated keratinocytes lacking significant atypia. These are not believed to have a metastatic risk and are identified by their location. The three main forms are oral, plantar, and Buschke-Loewenstein tumors.

Lymphoepithelioma-like carcinoma is a rare form of squamous cell carcinoma, recently classified by the World Health Organization. Its histogenesis is as yet uncertain. Due to the presence of sebaceous, eccrine, and trichilemmal differentiation within these neoplasms, it is widely believed that they originate in adnexal structures.

Desmoplastic squamous cell carcinomas are another subtype that has an increased risk of recurrence and metastasis. The most common site for these tumors is the ear. Histologically, these tumors are characterized by infiltrating cords of neoplastic keratinocytes with a dense sclerotic stroma that comprises at least one-third of the tumor. Perineural invasion and cytological atypia are often present.

Adenosquamous carcinoma is a form of squamous cell carcinoma that has the cytological features of both a keratinocyte-derived epidermal tumor and a

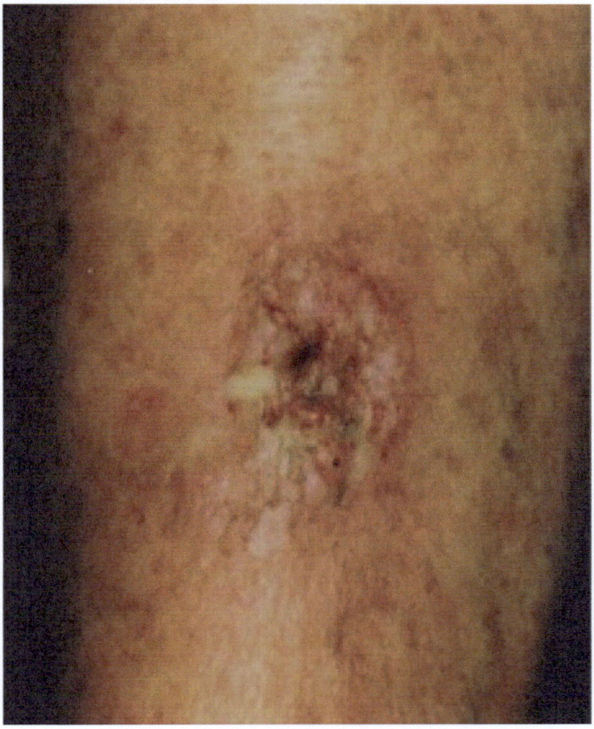

Fig. 24.5 Verrucous squamous cell carcinoma on the lower leg

gland-derived epithelial tumor. Its architecture is identical to the common squamous cell carcinoma except for the presence of deeply invasive nests and gland-like cystic spaces with areas of mucin production.

Keratoacanthomas are a distinct and interesting subtype of squamous cell carcinoma (Fig. 24.6). The debate still rages as to whether this is a form of squamous cell and if it should be treated as a malignancy at all. Histologically (Fig. 24.7), these tumors resemble the common squamous cell carcinoma and at the early stages are nearly indistinguishable. In the mature tumor, there is a crateriform squamous

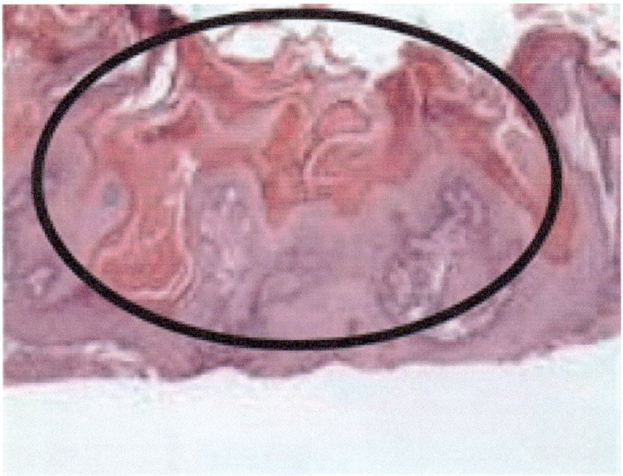

Fig. 24.6 Keratoacanthoma on the lower leg

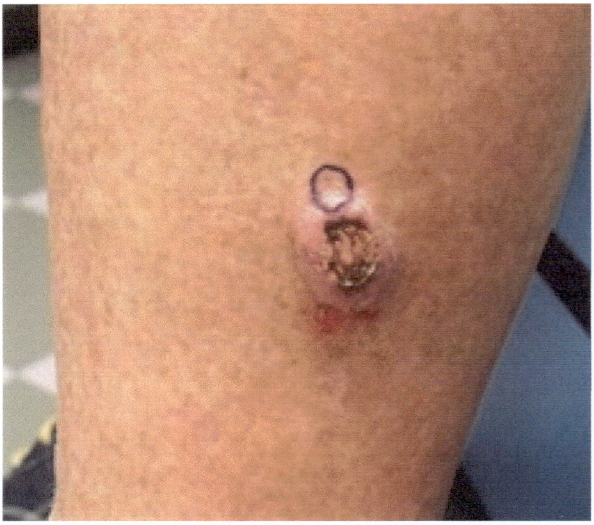

Fig. 24.7 Keratoacanthoma. Note the crateriform morphology

proliferation with a central core of compact hyperkeratosis. These tumors evolve rapidly over weeks to months, and then many will spontaneously resolve. There are many factors associated with the development of these lesions, including solar radiation, trauma, genetics, and possible viral etiologies. There are various forms of keratoacanthomas including Grzybowski, Ferguson-Smith, and Witten and Zak.

24.3 Clinical and Dermoscopic Presentation [5, 6]

A presumptive diagnosis of SCC is based on the physician's interpretation of clinical information, including appearance and morphology, anatomic location, and patient-reported history. While the most frequent clinical presentation of SCC in situ is an erythematous scaly patch or slightly elevated plaque, which is barely noticed by the patients, invasive SCC is often ulcerated and can be patchy, papulonodular (Fig. 24.8), papillomatous, or exophytic.

Although histopathology remains the gold standard for the diagnosis of SCC, some noninvasive optical technologies such as dermoscopy and RCM have recently been applied in an attempt to enhance clinical diagnosis accuracy and to obtain an in vivo characterization of the tumor [7–9].

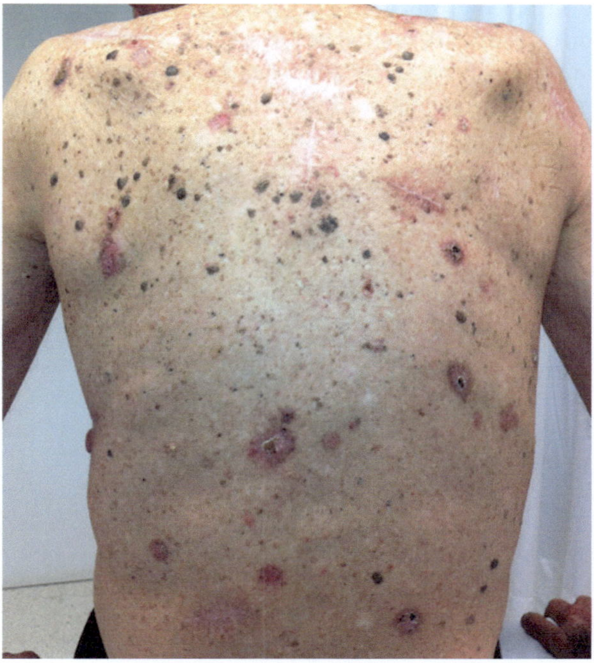

Fig. 24.8 Papulonodular

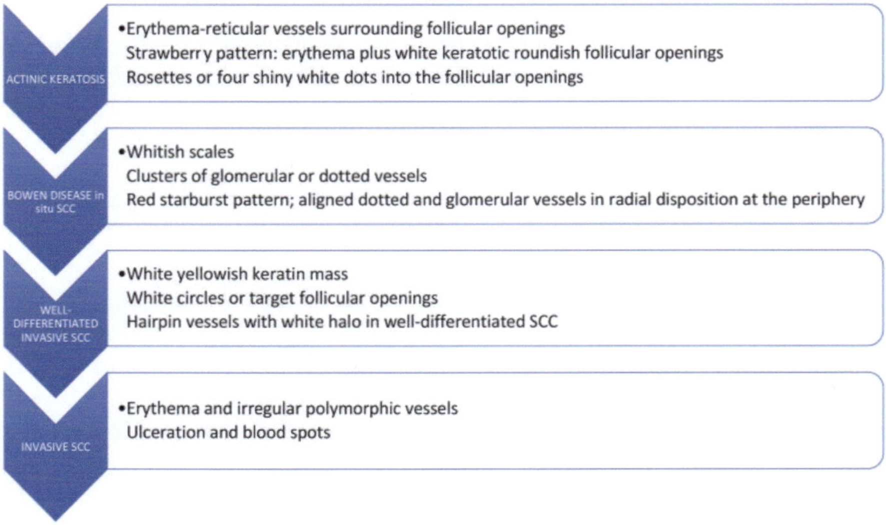

In situ SCC (Bowen disease) is characterized by yellowish white opaque scales and clusters of 2 types of roundish vascular pattern: small dotted vessels and glomerular or coiled vessels. Both patterns often appear within the same lesion and are distributed in small, densely packed clusters or groups [10]. In pigmented Bowen disease, other dermoscopic features are represented by small brown globules, which are regularly packed or aligned in a patchy distribution, and by gray to brown homogeneous pigmentation. White circles are a specific feature of early SCC and actinic keratosis. They are white structures within the hair follicle that might present a ring-like or targetoid appearance due to the white yellowish keratotic plug in the center of the follicular opening and white halo surrounding it [11].

When in situ SCC progresses to microinvasive SCC, the lesion thickens clinically, and hairpin and/or linear-irregular vessels appear in dermoscopy examination, occasionally giving a red starburst-like image on dermoscopy. In addition to typical vessel morphology, a keratotic center and ulceration might be seen. Invasive SCC presents more polymorphic vessels such as linear irregular, hairpin, and grouped glomerular/dotted vessels over a whitish background with a central mass of keratin or ulceration. Such dermoscopic features reflect a "vertical" growth phase (dermal invasion).

24.4 Other In Vivo Imaging Techniques

24.4.1 Reflectance Confocal Microscopy

RCM is a noninvasive technique for in vivo imaging of the skin with a cellular-level resolution (0.5–1.0 mm in the lateral dimension and 4–5 mm the axial) that uses near-infrared laser light at 830 nm. This technique reproduces horizontal images of the skin in shades of gray, with a resolution comparable with that of conventional histology. It is painless and harmless; it allows the evaluation of a larger area of skin, the mapping of a whole tumor and margins, and the imaging of exactly the same location over time, and it does not induce any kind of skin damage or inflammatory response. However, there is a clear limitation to the ability of the microscope to evaluate the thickest components of the tumors, as occurs in some cases of SCC in which hyperkeratosis predominates. The presence of hyperkeratotic surface on the lesion can make the RCM examination challenging, as the epidermal layers might be poorly visualized due to limited RCM laser penetration [12, 13].

24.4.2 High-Frequency Ultrasonography and Doppler Mode [10, 14]

High-frequency ultrasonography (HFUS) is a fast and accessible, noninvasive, convenient, practical, and safe dermatological diagnostic imaging examination that is now widely used in skin cancer. It allows real-time visual information with high diagnostic value and provides the physician with an extra hand in everyday practice. HFUS uses frequencies of approximately 20 MHz, which are dedicated to depicting the skin and allow scanning of the whole skin (epidermis, papillary, reticular dermis, blood vessels, and upper parts of subcutaneous tissue—depending on the localization).

In HFUS, tumor depth is ascertained with B-mode, and Doppler blood flow technologies permit the measurement of tumor neovascularity and the mapping of vascular structures. SCC is usually seen as a hypoechogenic mass in relation to the surrounding tissue, without clear specific features that allow the differential diagnosis from other nonmelanoma skin cancer or other skin lesions. However, HFUS is useful for determining the local aggressiveness of the tumor [15, 16].

24.4.3 Optical Coherence Tomography

Optical coherence tomography (OCT) is an emerging technology that uses infrared light for performing high-resolution, cross-sectional imaging. OCT is analogous to ultrasound imaging, except that it uses light instead of sound [10] and it magnifies the surface of a skin lesion using near-infrared light. Used in conjunction with clinical or dermoscopic examination of suspected skin cancer, or both, OCT may offer additional diagnostic information. As occurs in HFUS, the method is useful for preoperative evaluation of the tumor size in patients with SCC, as it provides a real-time imaging of nonmelanoma skin cancer to a depth of approximately 1.5 mm. However, its specificity is low and there are no pathognomonic features of SCC under OCT examination [17].

24.4.3.1 Diagnosis Confirmation [18]

Diagnosis is routinely confirmed by biopsy, and histological examination will differentiate between in situ and invasive SCC and detect aggressive histopathological growth patterns. However, conventional histopathological examination is also undergoing some changes, as new imaging techniques are emerging and beginning to replace the typical fixation, processing, and staining methods. This is the case of ex vivo fluorescence and RCM, which allows a rapid microscopic examination of freshly excised unfixed tissue directly in the surgery room during Mohs surgery after a few seconds of immersion in a fluorescence media. This optical imaging modality uses the inherent light-scattering properties of the different components of the tissue and generates optical images similar to H&E-stained tissue sections obtained by cutting frozen or fixed tissues.

Under conventional histopathology or ex vivo RCM, features such as the degree of differentiation, aggressive histological subtypes (acantholytic, adenosquamous, and carcinosarcomatous), depth greater than 2 mm (measured from the granular layer of the adjacent intact epidermis), Clark level IV or greater, and presence of perineural and/or angiolymphatic invasion classify the lesion as high risk. The differential diagnosis between SCC subtypes is mandatory, as it will further determine the therapeutic approach and follow-up of the tumor.

Once an invasive/aggressive SCC is diagnosed, it must be staged as the risk for metastasis is reported to be approximately 4%, and even two to three times higher in immunosuppressed individuals. Locoregional invasion can be assessed by HFUS or OCT in some cases as mentioned above. However, additional imaging techniques such as computed tomography (CT) or magnetic resonance imaging (MRI) are frequently required to assess the depth of invasion in critical areas such as the face or the scalp, as SCC is more likely to invade soft tissues, cartilage, and adjacent bone than other nonmelanoma skin cancer. Cutaneous in-transit regional lymph node metastases are the most common metastatic presentation; therefore, clinical assessment of regional lymph nodes must be always included in the physical examination and supported by complementary imaging techniques such as ultrasonography and positron emission computed tomography (PET/CT).

Staging of the tumor is classically performed according to the TNM (tumor, node, and metastasis) American Joint Committee on Cancer (AJCC) criteria.

TNM staging—For Staging visit = AJCC official website

https://www.facs.org/quality-programs/cancer-programs/american-joint-committee-on-cancer/

In all the staging scales there are several clinical-pathological markers of high-risk SCC such as tumor size (which can vary depending on the location), Breslow or tumor depth, perineural and lymph/vascular invasion, histological differentiation of the tumor (despite not being included in the latest AJCC classification), and the immune status of the patient (worse prognosis is seen in immunocompromised patients). When the patient fulfills two or more high-risk markers, further staging by sentinel lymph node biopsy (SLNB) is recommended, as about 20% of these patients will present positive SLNB. However, the impact on the overall survival or disease-free survival has still not been established.

Follow-up of patients must be individualized and determined both by the clinical history of the individual and the subtype of the SCC; however, screening for new primary skin cancers should be performed at least once per year, adjusting frequency on the basis of individual patient risk.

24.5 Surgical Treatment

Surgical excision is still the gold standard and includes conventional and Mohs surgery [18]. Conventional excision must ensure complete removal and therefore include a margin of clinically normal-appearing skin around the tumor and surrounding erythema. Clinical margins can be assessed prior to surgery by imaging techniques such as dermoscopy, RCM, HFUS, or OCT, which decrease the rates of incomplete excision and affected margins. NCCN guidelines recommend 4- to 6-mm clinical margins for standard excision of low-risk SCC, whereas Mohs surgery is recommended in high-risk SCC, SCC in immunocompromised patients, or "special-site SCC" such as head and neck, where tissue conservation is important [19, 20].

24.6 Nonsurgical Treatment

24.6.1 Low-Risk SCC

If surgical therapy is not feasible or elected, nonsurgical local approaches may be considered [2]. For in situ or low-risk SCC, the physician can choose photodynamic therapy (a 2-step method consisting of topical application of a photosensitizer, either 5-aminolevulinic acid or methylaminolevulinate, followed by 1 to several hours of incubation by light irradiation, typically with a blue, red, or broadband light source), or topical therapy with imiquimod (3.75–5%), or 5-fluorouracil. These modalities not only treat the tumor but also have an effect on the cancerization field if applied in a larger area.

Nonsurgical ablative modalities are also accepted in some cases in which surgery is not feasible, contraindicated, or not preferred by the patient. These include laser ablation (CO_2, erbium), electrocoagulation, and cryosurgery. However, given the lack of histological margin control with these approaches, the recurrence rate of SCC is higher. Primary local radiation can also be used in special situations when other therapies are contraindicated or impractical.

24.6.2 High-Risk SCC and Metastatic Disease

High-risk SCC should always be surgically excised, preferably by Mohs technique; however, adjuvant radiation therapy to the local tumor site following surgical treatment may be considered in primary SCC concerning perineural invasion or at high risk for regional or distant metastasis.

Regarding locally advanced and metastatic SCC, treatment is based on the extent of disease. If lymph nodes are involved, dissection must be performed whenever possible, and adjuvant radiation with or without concurrent systemic therapy must be considered. Systemic therapies such as capecitabine or epidermal growth factor receptor inhibitors (cetuximab, panitumumab) have demonstrated efficacy in patients with advanced, unresectable SCC. Based on the high mutational loads of SCC, the well-known infiltration with lymphocytes, and programmed death ligand 1 (PD-L1) expression, there is a promising utility in treating SCC with the immune checkpoint inhibitors such as pembrolizumab [21, 22].

Recently the first anti-PD1 drug cemiplimab was approved by the US Food and Drug Administration (September 2018) and by the European Medicines Agency (July 2019) after having demonstrated responses in about 50% of advanced or metastatic SCC.

References

1. Kim C, Cheng J, Colegio OR. Cutaneous squamous cell carcinomas in solid organ transplant recipients: emerging strategies for surveillance, staging, and treatment. Semin Oncol. 2016;43(3):390–4.
2. Alam M, Armstrong A, Baum C, et al. Guidelines of care for the management of cutaneous squamous cell carcinoma. J Am Acad Dermatol. 2018;78(3):560–78.
3. Malvehy J, Hanke-Martinez M, Costa J, Salerni G, Carrera C, Puig S. Semiology and pattern analysis in nonmelanocytic lesions. In: Hofmann-Wellenhof R, Pellacani G, Malvehy J, Soyer HP, editors. Reflectance confocal microscopy for skin diseases. Berlin: Springer; 2012. p. 237–52.
4. Pellacani G, Ulrich M, Casari A, et al. Grading keratinocyte atypia in actinic keratosis: a correlation of reflectance confocal microscopy and histopathology. J Eur Acad Dermatol Venereol. 2015;29(11):2216–21.
5. Zalaudek I, Giacomel J, Argenziano G, et al. Dermoscopy of facial nonpigmented actinic keratosis. Br J Dermatol. 2006;155(5):951–6.
6. Pan Y, Chamberlain AJ, Bailey M, Chong AH, Haskett M, Kelly JW. Dermatoscopy aids in the diagnosis of the solitary red scaly patch or plaque-features distinguishing superficial basal cell carcinoma, intraepidermal carcinoma, and psoriasis. J Am Acad Dermatol. 2008;59(2):268–74.
7. Seyed Jafari SM, Timchik T, Hunger RE. In vivo confocal microscopy efficacy assessment of daylight photodynamic therapy in actinic keratosis patients. Br J Dermatol. 2016;175(2):375–81.
8. Moscarella E, Rabinovitz H, Zalaudek I, et al. Dermoscopy and reflectance confocal microscopy of pigmented actinic keratoses: a morphological study. J Eur Acad Dermatol Venereol. 2015;29(2):307–14.
9. Peppelman M, Nguyen KP, Hoogedoorn L, van Erp PE, Gerritsen MJ. Reflectance confocal microscopy: non-invasive distinction between actinic keratosis and squamous cell carcinoma. J Eur Acad Dermatol Venereol. 2015;29(7):1302–9.
10. Warszawik-Hendzel O, Olszewska M, Maj M, Rakowska A, Czuwara J, Rudnicka L. Non-invasive diagnostic techniques in the diagnosis of squamous cell carcinoma. J Dermatol Case Rep. 2015;9(4):89–97.
11. Rishpon A, Kim N, Scope A, et al. Reflectance confocal microscopy criteria for squamous cell carcinomas and actinic keratoses. Arch Dermatol. 2009;145(7):766–72.
12. Carrera C, Puig S, Malvehy J. In vivo confocal reflectance microscopy in melanoma. Dermatol Ther. 2012;25(5):410–22.

13. Pellacani G, Scope A, Ferrari B, et al. New insights into nevogenesis: in vivo characterization and follow-up of melanocytic nevi by reflectance confocal microscopy. J Am Acad Dermatol. 2009;61(6):1001–13.
14. Ulrich M, Stockfleth E, Roewert-Huber J, Astner S. Noninvasive diagnostic tools for nonmelanoma skin cancer. Br J Dermatol. 2007;157(Suppl 2):56–8.
15. Wortsman X, Wortsman J. Clinical usefulness of variable-frequency ultrasound in localized lesions of the skin. J Am Acad Dermatol. 2010;62(2):247–56.
16. Marmur ES, Berkowitz EZ, Fuchs BS, Singer GK, Yoo JY. Use of high-frequency, high-resolution ultrasound before Mohs surgery. Dermatol Surg. 2010;36(6):841–7.
17. Fujimoto JG, Pitris C, Boppart SA, Brezinski ME. Optical coherence tomography: an emerging technology for biomedical imaging and optical biopsy. Neoplasia. 2000;2(1–2):9–25.
18. National Comprehensive Cancer Center. NCCN clinical practice guidelines in oncology; squamous cell carcinoma (V1.2017). Accessed Dec 2019.
19. Mohs FE. Chemosurgery for the microscopically controlled excision of skin cancer. J Surg Oncol. 1978;1(2):150–66.
20. Grossi Marconi D, Da Costa Resende B, Rauber E, et al. Head and neck non-melanoma skin cancer treated by superficial X-ray therapy: an analysis of 1021 cases. PLoS One. 2016;11(7):e0156544.
21. Maubec E, Petrow P, Scheer-Senyarich I, et al. Phase II study of cetuximab as first-line single-drug therapy in patients with unresectable squamous cell carcinoma of the skin. J Clin Oncol. 2011;29(25):3419–26.
22. Foote MC, McGrath M, Guminski A, et al. Phase II study of single-agent panitumumab in patients with incurable cutaneous squamous cell carcinoma. Ann Oncol. 2014;25(10):2047–52.

Basal Cell Carcinoma of the Extremity

25

Sanjeev Kumar Gupta

25.1 Introduction

Chronic ulcers affecting the extremities have diverse etiology. These ulcers are more common in the lower extremity than in the upper extremity. The prevalence of lower extremity ulcers ranges from 0.18% to 2% but increases to 5% in patients older than 65 years [1]. Some of the common extremity ulcers include diabetic foot ulcers, ulcers of chronic venous disease, ischemic ulcers, chronic infections such as tuberculosis, autoimmune diseases, and malignant ulcers. Of the various types of ulcers mentioned above, malignant ulcers are relatively uncommon. These ulcers can be either primary or result from malignant transformation in a chronic ulcer. The prevalence of malignancy in chronic leg ulcers ranges from 2.0% to 4%. Squamous cell cancer (SCC) and basal cell cancer (BCC) are the most common ulcerating skin tumors. Cutaneous lymphoma, Kaposi's sarcoma, and angiosarcoma are some of the rarer types of malignant ulcerative lesions of the lower extremity [2]. Since the prevalence of malignant extremity ulcers is quite low, their diagnosis requires a high degree of suspicion. Inability in instituting appropriate treatment due to delayed diagnosis or misdiagnosis results in poor outcome. Basal cell cancer which was earlier known as basal epithelioma was first described by Jacob in 1824 [3]. It is a slow growing tumor which tends to be locally infiltrative and rarely causes distant metastases. It is seldom fatal but can cause local tissue destruction resulting in disfigurement.

S. K. Gupta (✉)
Department of General Surgery, Institute of Medical Sciences, Banaras Hindu University, Varanasi, India

A. K. Khanna, S. K. Tiwary (eds.), *Uncommon Ulcers of the Extremities*,
https://doi.org/10.1007/978-981-99-1782-2_25

25.2 Epidemiology

Basal cell carcinoma is the commonest skin cancer in humans which usually affects fair skinned individuals. The incidence of BCC worldwide is showing an increasing trend but since it is not consistently recorded in cancer registries, the exact incidence is difficult to determine [4]. There are wide geographical variations with the highest incidence being reported from Australia (up to 1000/100,000 population per year) followed by the USA (212–407/100,000 population per year). In USA nearly 3 out of 10 white people will develop basal cell cancer during their lifetime. The lowest incidence has been reported in Africa (<1/100,000 population per year). In India too, even though exact data is not available, the incidence is similar to that seen in Africa [5, 6]. The incidence of basal cell cancer increases with increasing age with the median age at diagnosis being 68 years. Males are generally more commonly affected than females.

25.3 Etiology and Molecular Pathways

The most common environmental factor implicated in causation of BCC is chronic exposure to ultraviolet radiation particularly the UVB wavelengths and to a smaller degree to the UVA wavelengths. This is responsible for its predilection to the sun exposed parts of the body. Classically more than 80% of BCCs occur in the head and neck region with truncal and extremity lesions being uncommon. Ultraviolet rays can not only cause direct as well as indirect DNA damage but can also cause dose dependent immune suppression. Ultraviolet B rays cause direct DNA damage by causing C/T or CC/TT transition resulting in formation of mutagenic cyclodipyrimidine dimers. Melanin absorbs UVA and indirectly damages DNA through generation of cytotoxic and mutagenic free radicals [6]. Typically, there is a time lag of 15–20 years between UV exposure induced DNA damage and development of BCC. Hence exposure duration and intensity particularly in childhood and adolescence play an important role in the causation of BCC. In addition to the environmental factors, certain genetic mutations also play an important role. The most commonly affected gene is the PTCH1 gene and the second most commonly affected is the p53 gene. PTCH1 gene mutations leading to activation of the hedgehog pathway (Hh) occur in 70–80% of individuals with sporadic BCC [7, 8]. Exposure to UV rays is not the only risk factor because nearly 10–20% of BCCs occur in areas not exposed to the sunlight. The other factors implicated include exposure to ionizing radiation, arsenic exposure, immunosuppression, and genetic predisposition. Increased risk of BCC has been seen in patients with xeroderma pigmentosum, basal cell nevus syndrome (Gorlin syndrome), and Rombo syndrome. Furthermore, a previous history of BCC causes a ten-fold increase in the risk of developing a second BCC.

25.4 Clinical Features

Basal cell cancers arise in the basal layer of the epidermis from the follicular and interfollicular pluripotent stem cells related to the hair follicles (pilo-sebaceous unit). These cancers are heterogeneous with different morphological subtypes which have distinct biological behavior. The most recognized clinical variants of BCC are superficial, nodular, and morphea-like BCC. Nodular BCC is the most common clinical type accounting for 60–70% of all basal cell cancers [9, 10]. They appear as shiny, pink or flesh colored papule or nodule with telangiectasia. Patients often give a history of crusting and repeated bleeding. These lesions tend to enlarge and ulcerate. These ulcers which typically have rolled-up borders infiltrate into adjacent tissues hence the name rodent ulcer. In dark skinned individuals, pigmented nodular BCCs are common and have to be distinguished from melanoma. The commonest site for nodular BCC is the face, typically above a line joining the angle of the mouth to the ear lobule. Superficial BCC, the second commonest clinical subtype, appears as a well circumscribed pink-red scaly macular lesion which may have telangiectasia. These are usually multiple and occur more frequently on upper back, chest, or shoulders. Pigmented variants of superficial BCC can occur and they can evolve into the nodular type over time. The morphea form or sclerosing clinical subtype frequently presents as white or flesh colored lesion with ill-defined borders and surrounding induration. The surface of the lesion is smooth but crusts with underlying erosion or ulceration may also be present. These account for 5–10% of all basal cell cancers. BCCs invade locally and cause tissue destruction but involvement of regional lymph nodes is not seen [11, 12] (Figs. 25.1, 25.2, 25.3, and 25.4).

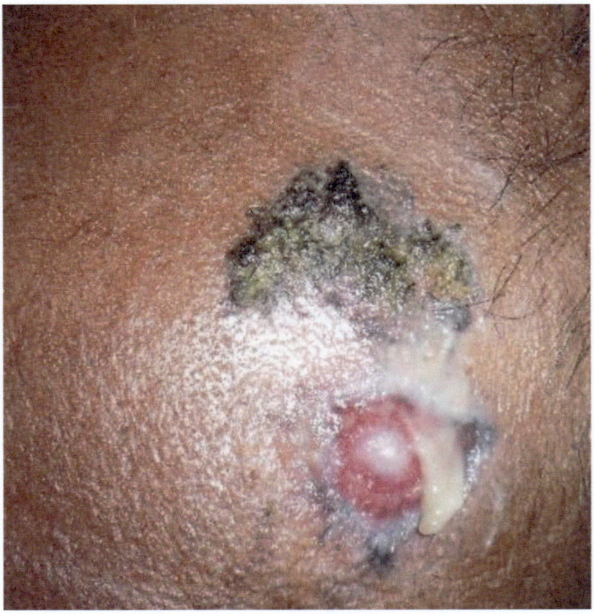

Fig. 25.1 Basal cell carcinoma of thigh. Blackish color may be mistaken for melanoma

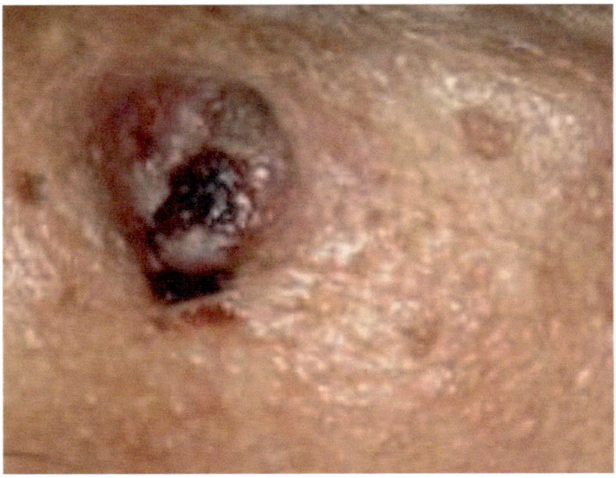

Fig. 25.2 Typical BCC with everted rolled out edges

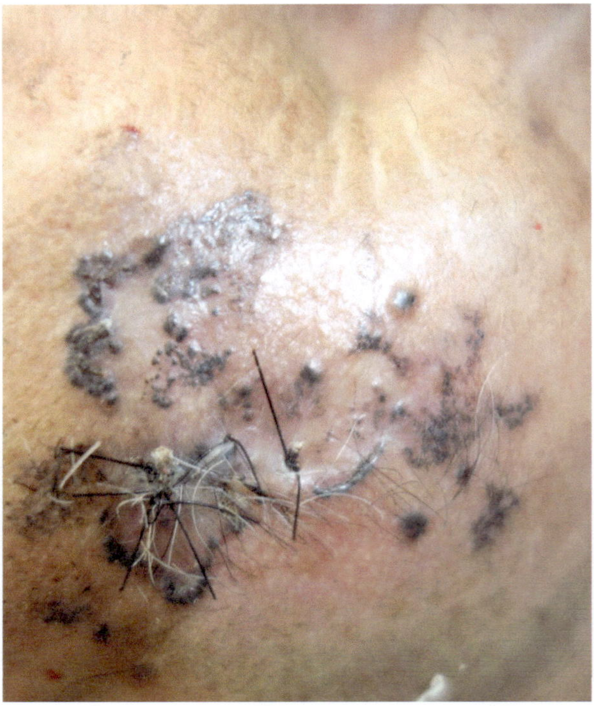

Fig. 25.3 Typical basal cell carcinoma with field fire BCC where concomitant crusting, ulceration, and scarring spread peripherally with a central area of regression

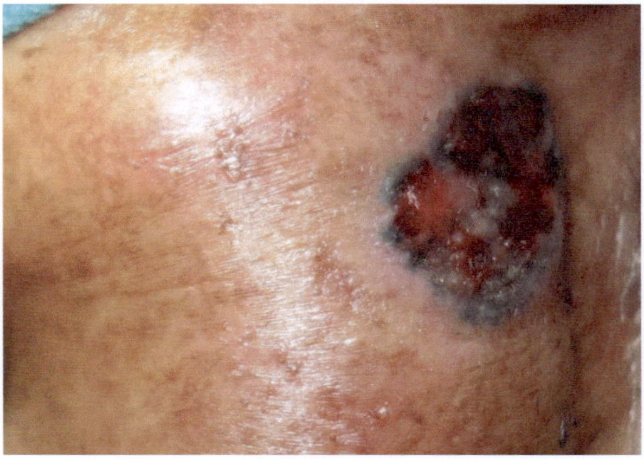

Fig. 25.4 BCC with blackish discoloration

25.5 Investigations

The diagnosis of BCC can be confirmed by skin biopsy which could either be a shave biopsy, a punch biopsy, or an excision biopsy. It is important to include the dermis in the biopsy to differentiate between superficial and other histological subtypes of BCC. Imaging studies are required only if there is a suspicion of bony involvement in which case magnetic resonance imaging is the modality of choice to delineate the extent and the depth of the lesion [13].

25.6 Treatment

Treatment of basal cell cancer is primarily surgical but there are other options such as medical treatment or radiation therapy depending on the patients' age and gender and also the site, size, and type of lesion. The aim of treatment is complete excision of tumor to prevent future recurrence, to provide good cosmesis, and to correct any functional impairment. Various types of therapeutic interventions for BCC include Mohs micrographic surgery (MMS), standard surgical excision, radiotherapy, photodynamic therapy, cryosurgery, topical therapies, and systemic medications [14].

25.6.1 Surgery

Mohs micrographic surgery is preferred in high-risk BCC, recurrent BCC, and lesions in critical areas. MMS entails serial excisions of the lesion with examination of 100% tissue margins. Since thin slices of the tissue are removed sequentially, the wound size is minimized, thereby leading to better cosmetic outcomes. It also ensures complete removal of the tumor tissue. In a prospective randomized controlled trial comparing standard excision and Mohs micrographic surgery, the 10-year probability of recurrence was 12.2% versus 4.4% for primary BCC and 13.5% versus 3.9% for recurrent BCC [15]. Mohs surgery is therefore considered to be the gold standard because of its high long-term cure rate and tissue sparing effect.

In a standard surgical excision (SE) a 4 mm margin is considered adequate if the lesion is well circumscribed and less than 2 cm in diameter and is situated in a low-risk area. Wider lateral margins ranging from 5 to 15 mm may be required in ulcerated lesions larger than 2 cm situated in high-risk areas [16]. The depth of excision is up to the subdermal fat or to the level of deep fascia, perichondrium, or periosteum in the face. Postoperative histopathology is essential to ensure complete excision of the lesion as recurrences are fairly common. However, there is no specific recommendation for re-excision in cases with narrow margins. Incomplete excision is associated with recurrence rates of up to 40% after 2–5 years of follow-up. Re-excision with wider margins is recommended for such cases.

25.6.2 Radiotherapy

Radiotherapy is an alternative modality of treatment in elderly patients with co-morbidities or in those who refuse surgery. It can be administered as external beam radiotherapy, brachytherapy, or contact therapy. Recurrence rates are similar to those as reported for surgery. Its use as an adjuvant treatment in patient with incomplete excision has not been studied and hence there are no specific recommendations. It is contraindicated in patients with BCC nevus syndrome.

25.6.3 Chemotherapy

The role of chemotherapy in BCC has not been evaluated. Most of the regimens used are platinum based and the response rate is approximately 20–30%. However, since the duration of response is only 2–3 months chemotherapy is generally not considered as a useful modality for treatment. For superficial or small nodular BCCs, certain medical treatments have been used. One such agent is Imiquimod which is an immune response modifier and is applied topically. Another agent for topical application is 5-fluorouracil 5%. However, there are limited indications for their usage in superficial, low-risk lesions <2 cm in diameter. The long-term results of these agents have not been evaluated. Certain destructive treatments such as photodynamic therapy (PDT) with 5-aminolaevulinic acid (ALA) or its methyl ester (MAL) have been used for superficial and small nodular BCC less than 2 mm thick. PDT is an option for patients with multiple lesions [17].

25.6.4 Newer Agents

The systemic treatment of difficult to treat or advanced basal cell cancer has to be discussed in a multidisciplinary committee. The agents which have been approved for systemic therapy include Hedgehog inhibitors Vismodegib and Sonidegib. These are still under evaluation and their routine use outside clinical trials is not recommended. The prognosis of BCC depends upon its location and size. Extremities are considered to be a low-risk location in contrast to the centrofacial areas, nose, etc. which are high-risk areas. Primary superficial BCC or nodular BCC <2 cm in diameter in the extremity has a good prognosis as compared to primary nodular lesions >2 cm or recurrent basal cell cancers [18].

25.7 Conclusions

Basal cell cancers even though being the commonest skin cancers are relatively much less common in Indian patients. The most common site of occurrence is the head and neck and extremity involvement is uncommon. They are slow growing tumors which cause local tissue destruction. Metastases to distant sites is extremely rare. Surgical excision is the treatment of choice. A better understanding of molecular pathways has led to the development of systemic therapies for difficult to treat locally advanced or metastatic basal cell carcinoma.

References

1. Spentzouris G, Labropoulos N. The evaluation of lower extremity ulcers. Semin Intervent Radiol. 2009;26:286–95.
2. Toussaint F, Erdmann M, Berking C, Erfurt-Berge C. Malignant ulcers presenting as chronic leg or foot ulcers. J Clin Med. 2021;10:2252. https://doi.org/10.3390/jcm1012251.
3. Jacob A. Observations respecting an ulcer of peculiar character, which attacks the eyelids and other parts of the face. Dublin Hosp Represent. 1824;4:232–9.
4. Asgari MM, Moffet HH, Ray GT, Quesenbery CP. Trends in basal cell carcinoma incidence and identification of high-risk subgroups, 1998-2012. JAMA Dermatol. 2015;151:976–81.
5. Lear W, Dahlke E, Murray CA. Basal cell carcinoma: review of epidemiology, pathogenesis and associated risk factors. J Cutan Med Surg. 2007;11:19–30.
6. Kasumagic-Halilovic E, Hasic M, Ovcina-Kurtoviv N. A clinical study of Basal cell carcinoma. Med Arch. 2019;73:394–8.
7. Skoda AM, Simovic D, Karin V, Kardum V, Vranic S, Serman L. The role of the Hedgehog signaling pathway in cancer: a comprehensive review. Bosn J Basic Med Sci. 2018;18:8–20.
8. Hanna A, Shevde LA. Hedgehog signaling: modulation of cancer properties and tumor microenvironment. Mol Cancer. 2016;15:24.
9. Cameron MC, Lee E, Hibler BP, et al. Basal cell carcinoma: epidemiology; pathophysiology; clinical and histological subtypes; and disease associations. J Am Acad Dermatol. 2019;80:303–17.

10. Basset-Seguin N, Herms F. Update on management of basal cell carcinoma. Acta Derm Venereol. 2020;100:adv00140. https://doi.org/10.2340/00015555-3495.
11. Rubin AI, Chen EH, Ratner D. Basal-cell carcinoma. N Engl J Med. 2005;353:2262–9.
12. Madan V, Lear JT, Szeimies RM. Non-melanoma skin cancer. Lancet. 2010;375:673–85.
13. Peris K, Fargnoli MC, Garbe C, et al. Diagnosis and treatment of basal cell carcinoma; European consensus based interdisciplinary guidelines. Eur J Cancer. 2019;118:10–34.
14. Drucker AM, Adam GP, Rofeberg V, et al. Treatment of primary basal cell carcinoma of the skin: a systematic review and network meta-analysis. Ann Intern Med. 2018;169:456–66.
15. Van Loo E, Mosterd K, Krekels GM, et al. Surgical excision versus Mohs' micrographic surgery for basal cell carcinoma of the face: a randomized clinical trial with 10 years follow-up. Eur J Cancer. 2014;50:3011–20.
16. Nahhas AF, Scarborough CA, Trotter S. A review of the global guidelines on surgical margins for non-melanoma skin cancers. J Clin Aesthet Dermatol. 2017;10:37–46.
17. Trakatelli M, Morton C, Nagore M, et al. Update of the European guidelines for basal cell carcinoma management. Eur J Dermatol. 2014;24:312–29.
18. Telfer NR, Colver GB, Morton CA. Guidelines for the management of basal cell carcinoma. Br J Dermatol. 2008;159:35–48.

Kaposi Sarcoma

26

Divya Khanna and Ajay K. Khanna

Moritz Kaposi, an Austro-Hungarian physician and dermatologist, first described Kaposi sarcoma (KS) in 1872, when he documented five patients with multifocal pigmented cutaneous and extra-cutaneous tumour in elderly European males, all of whom died within 2 years [1]. Since then, other varieties of this tumour have been identified, each with its own epidemiologic characteristics and clinical history but with similar histology. The cause of KS was unknown until 1994. Late epidemiologic investigations suggested that KS was caused by an infectious agent other than Human Immunodeficincy Virus (HIV), leading to the discovery that KS is caused by the KS herpesvirus (KSHV; also known as Human herpesvirus 8 (HHV8)) and decreased host immunity [2, 3]. In addition KSHV causes Primary Effusion Lymphoma (PEL) [4], Multicentric Castleman Disease (MCD) [5]—two lymphoproliferative diseases and KSHV inflammatory cytokine syndrome [3].

26.1 Epidemiology of Kaposi Sarcoma

Before the Acquired Immunodeficiency Syndrome (AIDS) crisis in the early 1980s, KS was a rare disease that was regularly documented in males who had sex with men (MSM) [6, 7]. AIDS patients in the USA reported KS 20,000 times higher than the general population and 300 times more than other immune-suppressed patient groups [8]. Australia [9] and Europe [10] both reported similar trends. Since the onset of the AIDS epidemic in sub-Saharan Africa (SSA), the incidence of KS has

D. Khanna (✉)
Department of Preventive Oncology, Mahamana Pandit Madan Mohan Malaviya Cancer Centre, Tata Memorial Centre, Varanasi, India

A. K. Khanna
Department of Surgery, Institute of Medical Sciences, Banaras Hindu University, Varanasi, Uttar Pradesh, India

A. K. Khanna, S. K. Tiwary (eds.), *Uncommon Ulcers of the Extremities*,
https://doi.org/10.1007/978-981-99-1782-2_26

increased by roughly 20-fold. In several SSA nations, such as Uganda, Malawi, Zimbabwe, and Swaziland, KS is the most prevalent cancer in males and the second most frequent cancer in women [11, 12]. GLOBOCAN 2020 estimated that 34, 270 KS cases were diagnosed globally [13].

The heterogenity in the population prevalence of two main infectious risk factors, namely the KSHV, along with HIV, which severely worsens the carcinogenic outcome of KSHV infection through impaired immune functioning, is guiding these disproportionately high KS cases, with nearly three quarters of global KS cases occurring in SSA [3].

However, the classic form of KS that was first described in elderly men of Mediterranean/Jewish/ Eastern European ancestry, and more recently in HIV-negative MSM, the endemic form in parts of Central and Eastern Africa, and the iatrogenic form in immunosuppressed organ transplant recipients are all recognised to occur in the absence of HIV infection [2, 14–20].

After the introduction of combination antiretroviral therapy (cART) in 1996, the incidence of AIDS-related KS decreased dramatically [21]. Between 1997 and 1999, prospective studies from the USA, Europe, and Australia revealed a decrease in the incidence rate of KS from 15.2 per 1000 person-years in 1992 to 4.9 per 1000 person-years, owing mostly to a decrease in AIDS-related KS cases [22]. However, KS continues to occur among HIV-positive people, despite a decline in global prevalence.

26.2 Variants of Kaposi Sarcoma

There are four forms of KS, each with its own demographic and clinical course, but all with very similar histological alterations.

26.2.1 Epidemic (AIDS-associated) Kaposi Sarcoma

Epidemic or AIDS-associated KS is the most common kind of KS and is regarded as an AIDS-defining illness [8]. Multiple cutaneous lesions on the limbs, trunk, and face are seen clinically. In 20% of cases there is a mucosal lesion, and in 15% of cases there is visceral involvement. Oedema caused by the tumour is frequently seen. Improving CD4 cell counts and the use of cART reduce the risk of developing KS [3]. When comparing patients with CD4 counts of 200, 200–349, and 350–499 cells/mm to those with patients having counts of 500 cells/mm, the rate ratio for developing KS was 18.9, 3.6, and 4.1, respectively [23].

The majority of cases are indolent; however, visceral involvement is not uncommon and with effective cART, it may regress. According to a recent systematic review, HIV is responsible for around 80% of KS in SSA, compared to 50% in the rest of the globe. Southern Africa (6.0 cases per 100,000) and Eastern Africa (3.4 cases per 100,000) have the highest rates of HIV-attributable KS [24].

26.2.2 Classic (Mediterranean/Sporadic) Kaposi Sarcoma

Classic KS primarily affects the elderly and middle-aged of Mediterranean, Eastern European, and Middle Eastern descent. Men are more likely to have it than women. Usually observed as fewer lesions limited to the lower limbs that do not grow as quickly or as frequently. The gastrointestinal system is the most common site of visceral and mucosal involvement. It is rarely aggressive or widespread [3]. There is some evidence that the risk groups of people who appear with classic KS are shifting. A retrospective cohort study on classic KS patients in Paris between 2006 to 2015, reported that less than 40% of patients were of Mediterranean background and 28% were MSM [25].

26.2.3 Endemic (African) Kaposi Sarcoma

Endemic KS, often known as African KS, affects people living in equatorial Africa. Because KSHV infection is far more common in Africa than it is in other parts of the world, the risk of Endemic KS is much higher. Other conditions that impair the immune system, such as malnutrition, chronic infections, and malaria, are likely to contribute to the development of KS. Children and women are both affected by the disease. Younger persons are more likely to have endemic KS (usually less than 40 years) [2, 26]. In children before puberty, a more aggressive type of endemic KS is occasionally encountered, which frequently involves lymph nodes and other organs and advances rapidly [27]. The distribution of HHV-8 seropositivity in endemic KS is similar to that of HHV-8 seropositivity in the paediatric population [28]. In paediatric patients, rates of HHV-8 seropositivity range from 2% in Eritrea to over 100% in the Central African Republic [29].

26.2.4 Iatrogenic (Transplant-related) Kaposi Sarcoma

Iatrogenic, or transplant-related KS, occurs when persons develop KS as a result of iatrogenic immunodeficiency, as seen in organ transplant recipients. When compared to the general population, transplant patients have a 400- to 500-fold higher risk of getting KS. For iatrogenic KS, the male-to-female ratio is 3:1. Patients who get a bone marrow or peripheral blood stem cell transplant have a considerable lower risk of developing KS than those who receive a solid organ transplant [30]. Immunosuppressive medicines are used by the majority of transplant recipients to prevent new organ rejection. This immunosuppression raises the likelihood of infection with KSHV. Immunosuppressive medicines can be stopped or reduced, which can cause KS lesions to disappear or shrink [3].

Finally, many cases of KS have been observed in MSM who are not HIV-positive, and KS in MSM who are not HIV-positive is becoming widely recognised as a unique fifth form of KS [3, 25].

26.3 Clinical Signs and Symptoms

Cutaneous manifestations: Cutaneous lesions in all variants of KS usually appear as numerous, pigmented, raised or flat, painless lesions that do not blanch when pressure is applied. Patch, plaque, and nodule are the three clinical stages of skin lesions [31]. Asymptomatic pigmented macules or tiny papules ranging in colour from pale pink to vivid purple are the most common cutaneous lesions. The characteristic features of the lesions are often used to diagnose KS. Even skilled clinicians sometimes misdiagnose KS; hence, the diagnosis should be confirmed histologically. On the trunk, larger oblong plaques follow the skin folds. Exophytic, ulcerated, and bleeding nodules are occasionally found, and they are associated with uncomfortable oedema [3] (Figs. 26.1, 26.2, 26.3, and 26.4).

Visceral manifestations: Noncutaneous disease most commonly affects the oral cavity, gastrointestinal tract, and respiratory system. Visceral signs are uncommon, thanks to the widespread use of antiretroviral medication and a variety of therapeutic options [32]. In around one-third of KS patients, the oral cavity is afflicted, and in about 15% of instances, it is the first site of involvement. A biopsy should be utilised to confirm the diagnosis of KS whenever possible [33]. The most common intraoral location is the palate, followed by the gingiva. Pain, bleeding, ulceration, and secondary infections are all possible complications of intraoral lesions. Dysphagia is a symptom of advanced lesions [34]. Patients with AIDS-related KS are more likely to develop visceral lesions in the lungs and gastrointestinal tract. Weight loss, stomach pain, nausea and vomiting, upper or lower gastrointestinal haemorrhage, malabsorption, intestinal blockage, and/or diarrhoea are common symptoms of gastrointestinal lesions, which are confirmed by endoscopy [35, 36]. Pulmonary lesions are potentially fatal. Shortness of breath, fever, cough,

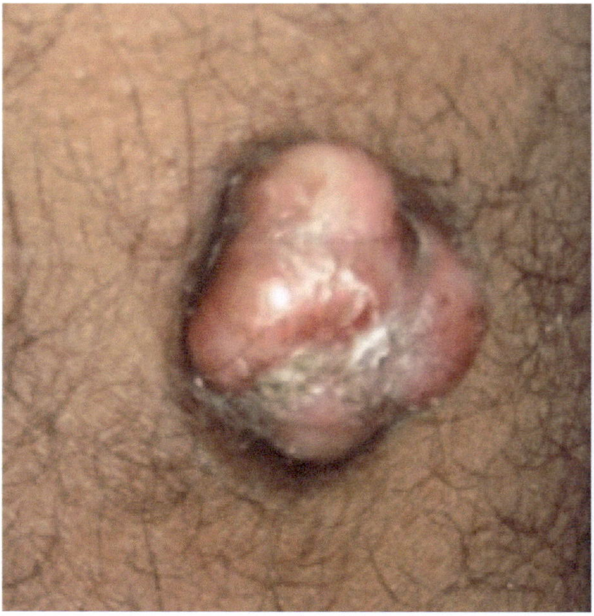

Fig. 26.1 Nodule seen on thigh

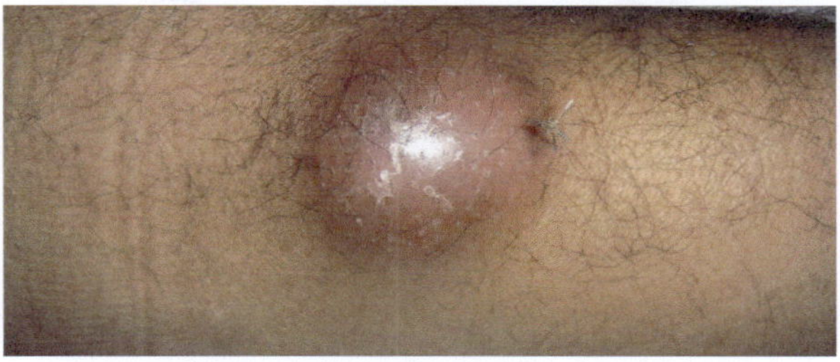

Fig. 26.2 Nodule seen on arm as inflamed swelling

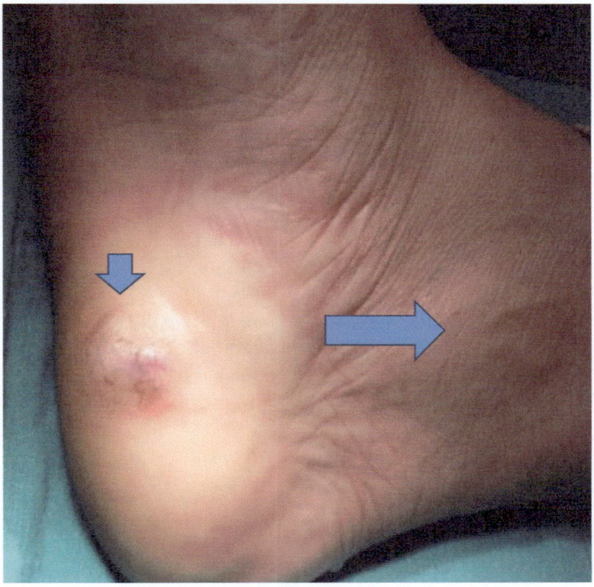

Fig. 26.3 Multiple lesions seen round ankle and sole

hemoptysis, and chest pain are all symptoms of pulmonary involvement. Radiographs can reveal nodular, interstitial, and alveolar infiltrates, pleural effusion, and hilar and/or mediastinal adenopathy [3, 37]. In African children and young adults, endemic KS is commonly linked with lymphoedema and is difficult to manage [4]. However, visceral lesions associated with KS are infrequent. Only 15% of 469 AIDS-related KS patients had visceral lesions, according to one study [32]. As a result, CT scans, bronchoscopy, and endoscopy are not indicated in patients who do not have symptoms that indicate visceral lesions [3].

26.4 Staging of Kaposi Sarcoma

To date, the American Joint Committee on Cancer (AJCC) tumour, node, and metastasis (TNM) staging approach has not been incorporated into the staging of KS. AIDS-related KS is staged using the Modified AIDS Clinical Trials Group (ACTG) staging criteria, based on tumour, immunological state, and systemic

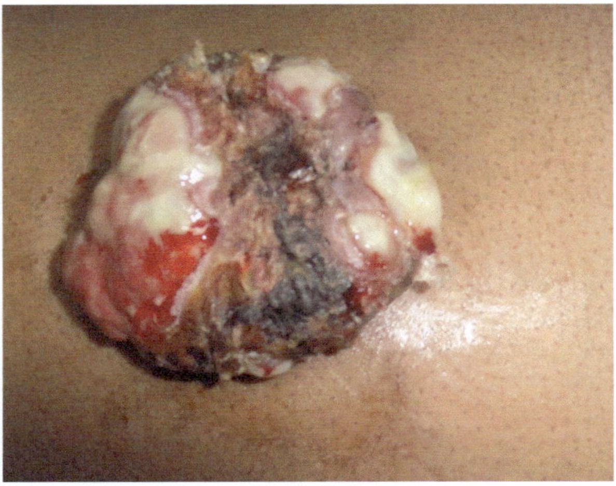

Fig. 26.4 Ulcerated big nodule on arm

Table 26.1 Staging classification for AIDS-related KS by the AIDS Clinical Trial Group (ACTG) of the National Institute of Health [38]

	Good risk (all of the following)	Poor risk (any of the following)
Tumor, T	T0: Confined to skin and/or lymph nodes and/or minimal oral disease (non-nodular KS confined to palate)*	T1: Tumour-associated oedema or ulceration, extensive oral KS, gastrointestinal KS, KS in other non-nodal viscera
Immune system, I	I0: CD4 cell count >200/μL	I1: CD4 cell count <200/μL
Systemic illness, S	S0: No history of opportunistic infection or thrush No unexplained fever, night sweats, >10% involuntary weight loss, or diarrhoea persisting more than 2 weeks Karnofsky performance status ≥70	S1: History of opportunistic infection and/or thrush Unexplained fever, night sweats, >10% involuntary weight loss, or diarrhoea persisting more than 2 weeks present Karnofsky performance status <70 Other HIV-related illness (e.g., neurological disease, lymphoma)

* Minimal oral disease is nonnodular KS confined to the palate

sickness (TIS) (Table 26.1). There are no defined staging systems for endemic or iatrogenic KS, and classic KS classification focuses solely on the tumour [3].

26.5 Diagnosis

26.5.1 Histopathology

In settings with appropriate resources, a biopsy is conducted for clinically questionable KS cases to histologically confirm the diagnosis. However, in resource-limited countries, such as Africa, where KS is most prevalent, and clinical visualisation is often the sole means for diagnosing KS, this procedure can be difficult [3]. According to one study from Eastern Africa, visual diagnosis showed only an 80% positive predictive value for KS. Incorrect diagnosis of KS results in the unnecessary administration of chemotherapy [39]. Task-shifting, teledermatology, and telepathology are some of the strategies under evaluation to improve the histologic diagnosis of KS [3].

The histopathological diagnosis of the patch stage is performed by traditional haematoxylin and eosin (H&E) staining, which is characterised by spindle cell proliferation. Vascular proliferation in the dermis, resulting in slitlike spaces not lined by endothelium, an increase in the number of vessels without an endothelial cell lining, the presence of extravasated blood resulting in hyaline globules and haemosiderin accumulation, and an inflammatory infiltrate are all common features of spindle cell [31, 40].

Pleomorphism, nuclear atypia, and mitotic figures may be seen in advanced nodule lesions with the enhancement of the slit-like lumens. Significant inflammatory infiltrates consisting of lymphocytes, histiocytes, plasma cells, and, rarely, neutrophils are present in all phases of KS [31, 40].

KS in situ, anaplastic KS, lymphangiectatic KS, bullous KS, ecchymotic KS, glomeruloid KS, and hyperkeratotic KS are the histologic variations of KS [31].

26.5.2 Immunohistochemistry

Because KS lesions have varied cellular compositions, they express a variety of markers. The presence of endothelial markers such as CD34, podoplanin, LYVE1, and VEGF receptor 3 suggests lymphatic endothelial cell origin [41, 42]. Vimentin and other mesenchymal markers are also expressed [43]. Based on the immunohistochemistry (IHC), gene expression, and experimental data, spindle cells appear to be reprogrammed lymphatic endothelial, vascular endothelial, and/or mesenchymal cells that create cells with an abnormal immunophenotype. In KS lesions, lymphocytes, plasma cells, and histiocytes are abundant [3].

The identification and localisation of HHV8 within KS lesional cells using LANA (latency-associated nuclear antigen) is the most diagnostically valuable immunostaining approach for separating KS from its imitators [31]. LANA immunoreactivity in KS cells appears as a stippled nuclear staining that is separate from cytoplasmic haemosiderin or melanin [3, 31]. Every infected cell is thought to express LANA; nevertheless, the proportion of infected cells varies from less than 10% to more than 90% of the overall cell population in the lesion. As a result, a negative stain does not necessarily rule out KS because sampling errors or false negatives might occur due to poor tissue preservation or other technical artefacts [3].

26.5.3 Molecular Diagnosis

KSHV DNA is virtually always found in nucleic acid amplification techniques (NAAT) of KS lesions (>95% of all epidemiologic types of KS) [44]. KSHV DNA detection by PCR is very sensitive, if not ideal for KS diagnosis, the lack of KSHV DNA in a well-prepared sample effectively rules out the diagnosis of KS. PCR for KSHV DNA is currently available in only highly specialised clinical and research molecular pathology labs [3].

26.6 Etiopathogenesis

KS is causally linked to HHV8/KSHV. HHV8 belongs to the Herpesviridae subfamily and the Rhadinovirus genus [45]. Gamma herpesviruses play a critical role in cellular proliferation and malignancies. The HHV8 viral genome can be found in all phases and clinical variations of KS lesions. KSHV is a linear double-stranded DNA virus with an icosahedral capsid and a tegument that is encased (space between the envelopes and nucleocapsid containing proteins and RNAs). Endothelial cells are assumed to be the KSHV-infected cell type in KS because endothelial cell markers are expressed [46].

The time it takes from HHV8 infection to the onset of KS varies depending on the clinical type. Immunosuppression has a significant role in illness progression and presentation. According to limited evidence, 50% of HIV-positive people acquire KS within 3.5 years of KSHV discovery in their blood. The typical time it takes for KS to emerge after transplantation is 13–21 months [47]. For classic KS, the duration is longer and the other contributors are not yet established [3].

26.6.1 Transmission

The exact mode(s) of transmission for HHV-8 remains unclear.

26.6.1.1 Sexual Transmission

The high reported incidence of KS in homosexual and bisexual patients and those with certain sexual practices originally suggested a role in the sexual transmission of the virus. In later epidemiological studies, sexual activities were confirmed as a route for HHV8 transmission and the risk increases with the number of sexual partners and with certain practices such as oral/genital and oral/anal sex [48–50].

26.6.1.2 Nonsexual Transmission

The virus is also widespread in Mediterranean countries and Africa, strongly suggesting nonsexual transmission among family members [51]. The oropharynx is a vigorous site for viral replication. High HHV8 copy numbers are present in saliva [50]. Based on this, nonsexual transmission via saliva is widely assumed to play the most important role in childhood transmission in endemic areas [50]. Vertical transmission from mother to child during pregnancy or birth does not seem to play an important role [52].

26.6.1.3 Iatrogenic Transmission

It is crucial to emphasise for medical professionals that HHV8 can be transferred by blood, blood products, and donor organs [53–55].

26.6.2 HHV8/KSHV Epidemiology

Although the seroprevalence of HHV8/KSHV infection is less than 10% in regions like northern Europe, Asia, and the USA, it is greater than 40% in most of Sub-Saharan Africa. Adult seroprevalence in SSA ranges from 22% to 71%. Seroprevalence rates in the Mediterranean region (Italy, Sicily, and Sardinia) are moderate (10–30%). The causes for these geographic differences in HHV8/KSHV incidence are unknown; however, there is some evidence that environmental factors, such as coinfection with malaria and other parasite illnesses, may increase viral shedding in saliva, resulting in higher transmission rates. However, the impact of these coinfections on saliva shedding has yet to be proven [3, 45].

26.6.3 Life Cycle of HHV8/KSHV

Endothelial cells, B cells, epithelial cells, dendritic cells, monocytes, and fibroblasts are all susceptible to HHV8/KSHV infection [56]. The viral envelope contains glycoproteins that engage with cell type-specific cellular entry receptors. HHV8/KSHV enters endothelial cells by attaching to integrins, the cystine–glutamate transporter xCT, heparan sulphate, and the EPHA2 tyrosine-protein kinase receptor. This binding triggers a signalling cascade that causes cellular modifications that allow the virus to enter the cell and travel through the cytoplasm. Viral entrance causes the virion capsid to be delivered into the cytoplasm, followed by the uncoating of the virion capsid and the transport of the viral genome into the nucleus. The genome survives as an episome in the nucleus. During the lifespan, the virus either goes into latency or has irregular lytic reactivation episodes [56–59].

26.6.3.1 Virus Latency Phase

Because of the latency, infection with HHV8/KSHV is life-long, as it is with other herpesviruses. ORF71 (also known as ORFK13; encoding viral FLICE inhibitory protein), ORF72 (encoding vCyclin), ORF73 (encoding LANA), ORFK12 (encoding the kaposins), and various microRNAs (miRNAs) are all expressed by the virus. They are seen in the majority of KSHV-infected tumour cells and are thought to stimulate tumour growth. The HHV8/KSHV LANA tethers the latent viral genome to the host chromosome, allowing the viral genome to replicate alongside the host genome during normal cell division. Other latent genes' protein products aid infected cell survival by boosting the nuclear factor $_{\kappa}$B (NF-$_{\kappa}$B) pathway (increases cell survival), blocking apoptosis, increasing endothelial cell reprogramming, driving endothelial cell migration and invasion, and avoiding latency reactivation [60–68].

26.6.3.2 Virus Lytic Phase

HHV8/KSHV experiences periodic spontaneous lytic reactivation throughout the host's lifetime, while the physiological triggers are unknown. The lytic phase permits the viral genome to replicate and infectious viral progeny to be produced. Immediate early (IE) genes are the first to be expressed, and they encode RTA, a transcription factor that assures the expression of viral genes necessary for viral replication. After IE genes, delayed early (DE) genes and late genes are expressed. They code for proteins that regulate the replication of viral DNA. The late lytic phase produces the infectious virus by expressing all of the viral structural proteins [60, 69–74].

26.6.4 Modulating Host Signalling Pathways

HHV8/KSHV has evolved to modify multiple host cell signalling pathways, including the phosphoinositide 3kinase (PI3K)–AKT–mTOR pathway, the mitogen-activated protein kinase (MAPK) system, and the NFB route, to allow virus-infected cells to survive. As a result, the virus encodes a slew of proteins that influence host cell signalling pathways, allowing for cell survival and proliferation as well as viral replication. Their expression results in the secretion of cytokines and growth factors that might influence neighbouring cells, causing angiogenesis and inflammation, and thereby contributing to the pathogenesis of KS [3, 60].

26.6.5 Immune System and HHV8/KSHV

HHV8/KSHV, like other herpesviruses, strikes a delicate balance with the host's immune system to create a long-lasting latent infection. The substantially higher incidence of HHV8/KSHV infection in patients with immunodeficiency than in people with a healthy immune system demonstrates this regulation [75].

LANA appears to be the most immunogenic of the latent viral proteins, whereas K8.1 appears to be the most immunogenic of the lytic proteins. ORF38, ORF61, ORF59, and K5 all produced detectable responses in people with KSHV-related illnesses, according to a systemic study of antibodies to all KSHV proteins [76]. Though, antibodies against KSHV are rarely neutralising [77].

Despite the host mounting an immunological response to KSHV via Toll-like receptors (TLRs), a retinoic acid-inducible gene I protein (RIGI) like receptors (RLRs), and type I interferon induction, KSHV persists in the infected host for a lifetime by expressing both lytic and latent proteins [3].

KSHV K3 and K5 are lytic genes that encode MIR1 and MIR2, respectively, which hinder the immune system from identifying KSHV-infected cells by inhibiting MHC class I antigen presentation [78]. MIR1 inhibits all four alleles or allotypes of the human leukocyte antigen (HLA) gene (HLA-A, HLA-B, HLA-C, and HLA-E), while MIR2 inhibits HLA-A and HLA-B [79]. Interferon regulatory factors (viral IRFs; vIRFs) are lytic proteins that inhibit type I interferons in KSHV homologues. vIRF1, vIRF2, vIRF3, and vIRF4 are the four vIRFs encoded by the KSHV genome [80]. These work by preventing IRF from transactivating interferon gene promoters by binding to STING and blocking cGAS–STING signalling as well as IFN induction [81, 82]. KSHV ORF52 and LANA both block the cGAS–STING pathway, but they do so by targeting cGAS rather than STING [83, 84]. KSHV encodes three CCchemokine ligands (CCLs) that inhibit inflammation: vCCL1 (encoded by ORFK6), vCCL2 (encoded by ORFK4), and vCCL3 (encoded by ORFK4.1) [85].

The KSHV K14 gene generates a viral OX2 (vOX2), a member of the immunoglobulin superfamily that interacts with the CD200R receptor and is comparable to the cellular OX2 membrane glycoprotein (OX2) [86]. In neutrophils induced to perform phagocytosis, KSHV vOX2 fused to a crystallisable fragment (Fc) antibody domain lowered neutrophil activation, decreased CCL2 (also known as MCP1) and IL-8 production, and inhibited oxidative burst [87]. Purified glycosylated vOX2 protein, however, stimulated primary monocytes, macrophages, and dendritic cells to produce inflammatory cytokines such as IL-1, IL-6, monocyte chemoattractant protein 1, and TNF [88]. If vOX2 is produced in cells undergoing lytic replication in the lesions, this activation of inflammatory cytokines may contribute to the inflammatory infiltrates found in KS [3].

26.7 Management of Kaposi Sarcoma

KS often requires multi-modality management (Table 26.2). The first-line strategy in patients with forms of KS in which immunosuppression is possibly reversible is to boost the immune system; for example, treating HIV with cART in patients with AIDS-related KS may produce T0 tumour regression. Similarly, patients with iatrogenic KS may be treated by lowering immunosuppression or switching immunosuppressive drugs while assessing the risks and benefits, as lowering immunosuppression may increase the chance of transplant rejection. High-quality data for the clinical care of KS is restricted to AIDS-related KS, while the strategy for treating other types of KS is based on small retrospective case series and physician experience.

The current therapeutic options for classic KS include monitoring of patients with a small number of asymptomatic lesions, elastic compression stockings for lower extremity oedema, and several local and systemic tumour-directed medications similar to those used for AIDS-related KS [3].

Clinical staging plays a significant role in the treatment of AIDS-related KS. Patients with T0 stage disease should start cART (if they are not already on it), to which KS frequently responds (i.e., lesions diminish by 50% in size and/or number) within 6–12 months. Nearly 80% of patients with T0 stage who have not previously been treated with cART will only require ongoing cART for the next 10 years [32].

In randomised controlled trials conducted in the USA and the UK, single-agent liposomal anthracyclines were found to be superior to conventional combination

Table 26.2 Treatment modalities for Kaposi's sarcoma [88, 89]

<table>
<tr><th colspan="2">Localised disease: local therapy</th></tr>
<tr><td colspan="2">Surgical excision
Cryotherapy
Topical 9-ci retinoic acid
Radiation therapy
Intralesional chemotherapy (vinblastine, vincristine, bleomycin)
Laser
Sclerotherapy
Photodynamic therapy</td></tr>
<tr><th colspan="2">Disseminated disease with internal organ involvement: systemic therapy</th></tr>
<tr><td>AIDS-related KS</td><td>cART</td></tr>
<tr><td>For AIDS patients not responding to cART alone-systemic cytotoxic chemotherapy</td><td>Liposomal anthracyclines (e.g., liposomal doxorubicin 20–40 mg/m^2 every 2–4 weeks)
Paclitaxel (100 mg/m^2 given every 2 weeks)</td></tr>
<tr><td>Classical KS</td><td>Liposomal anthracyclines
Interferonα</td></tr>
<tr><td>For patients on immunosuppressive therapy</td><td>Reevaluation of drug regimen</td></tr>
</table>

chemotherapy for treating patients with advanced-stage or progressive AIDS-related KS [90–92]. Safety and tolerability of liposomal anthracyclines in cART patients have now been proven, and they are now considered the standard first-line treatment for advanced AIDS-related KS [93, 94]. Several phase II studies suggest paclitaxel's efficacy in treating AIDS-related KS [95, 96]. In the only head-to-head comparison of pegylated liposomal doxorubicin and paclitaxel for advanced AIDS-related KS, there were no significant differences in response rate, progression-free survival, or overall survival. Paclitaxel produced greater neurotoxicity ($P = 0.045$) and baldness (P 0.001) than pegylated liposomal doxorubicin [96].

IFN and alitretinoin (a retinoid receptor panagonist) are two pathogenesis-directed therapies for AIDS-related KS, although their use has been limited. Several pathogenesis-targeted therapies are in the early phases of development and have not yet been authorised for patient use [3].

26.8 Prevention and Early Detection

Early detection of KS is associated with a better clinical outcome. The availability of cART has significantly improved the prognosis of KS patients. During the cART era, one of the largest studies of prognosis found that T1 disease at diagnosis had a 2.6-fold higher rate of death than T0 disease at diagnosis [97]. Another study of AIDS-related KS patients in Switzerland found that those with T1 disease at diagnosis had a 5.2-fold higher death rate than those with T0 disease at diagnosis [98]. Similarly, T1 disease had a 2.4-fold higher fatality rate than T0 disease in South Africa [99]. These advantages have not been proven in randomised trials, and doing so would be expensive and time-consuming, especially in resource-constrained SSA regions [3].

KS does not have a pre-cancer stage. Furthermore, KS usually manifests itself first on the skin and/or mucous membranes that are visible. As a result, patients are the ones who first notice it. Thus, except for lesions in the oral cavity, which are frequently the initial anatomic site of involvement in AIDS-related KS, traditional screening by healthcare practitioners for established KS before the onset of clinical symptoms is of poor utility. Because visceral organ involvement is uncommon in KS, screening of the lower respiratory tract and gastrointestinal tract is not advised [3, 100].

KS can be prevented by interventions targeted at preventing HIV infection (including preexposure prophylaxis) [101], reducing HIV replication, and maintaining patients' immune systems [102]. Interventions to prevent KSHV infection are not clearly characterised, owing to a lack of understanding of the exact routes of KSHV transmission. MSM's use of saliva in sexual practises has the potential to spread KHSV infection, necessitating health education and counselling [103]. However, there is currently no place in the general population for a wide recommendation to avoid saliva exposure [3].

26.9 Quality of Life of Patients with Kaposi Sarcoma

KS-related physical and emotional disorders affect QOL. Pain, oedema, and ulcerated skin sores can make walking difficult. External genital oedema can also impede urination. In severe cases, facial and periorbital oedema might impair eyesight. Dyspnoea, cough, and haemoptysis can be distressing pulmonary symptoms. Gastrointestinal lesions can cause discomfort, bleeding, eating issues, diarrhoea, obstruction, malabsorption, and weight loss. Lesions on the face, chest, and limbs can cause social and psychological isolation. Because current KS therapies are not curative, symptom reduction is a major goal.

Chemotherapy for KS increases the quality of life despite its downsides. Chemotherapy reduces KS discomfort and swelling. Although improved QOL are sometimes connected with a quantifiable objective response of KS to treatment (e.g., 50% tumour shrinkage), symptom palliation occurred in many people without the objective response [97, 104]. These data suggest evaluating KS therapy based on QOL and patient benefit, especially in resource-constrained settings [3].

References

1. Kaposi M. Idiopatisches multiples pigmentsarkom der haut [German]. Arch Dermatol Syph. 1872;4:265–73.
2. Chang Y, et al. Identification of herpesvirus-like DNA sequences in AIDS-associated Kaposi's sarcoma. Science. 1994;266:1865–9.
3. Cesarman E, Damania B, Krown SE, Martin J, Bower M, Whitby D. Kaposi sarcoma. Nat Rev Dis Primers. 2019;5(1):1–21.

4. Cesarman E, Chang Y, Moore PS, Said JW, Knowles DM. Kaposi's Sarcoma-associated herpesvirus-like DNA sequences in AIDS-related body cavity-based lymphomas. N Engl J Med. 1995;332:1186–91.
5. Soulier J, et al. Kaposi's sarcoma-associated herpesvirus-like DNA sequences in multicentric Castleman's disease. Blood. 1995;86:1275–80.
6. Gottlieb GJ, et al. A preliminary communication on extensively disseminated Kaposi's sarcoma in young homosexual men. Am J Dermatopathol. 1981;3:111–4.
7. Hymes KB, et al. Kaposi's sarcoma in homosexual men—a report of eight cases. Lancet. 1981;2:598–600.
8. Beral V, Peterman TA, Berkelman RL, Jaffe HW. Kaposi's sarcoma among persons with AIDS: a sexually transmitted infection? Lancet. 1990;335:123–8.
9. Elford J, McDonald A, Kaldor J. Kaposi's sarcoma as a sexually transmissible infection: an analysis of Australian AIDS surveillance data. The National HIV Surveillance Committee. AIDS. 1993;7:1667–71.
10. Hermans P, et al. Epidemiology of AIDS-related Kaposi's sarcoma in Europe over 10 years. AIDS in Europe Study Group. AIDS. 1996;10:911–7.
11. Wabinga HR, Parkin DM, Wabwire-Mangen F, Mugerwa JW. Cancer in Kampala, Uganda, in 1989-91: changes in incidence in the era of AIDS. Int J Cancer. 1993;54:26–36.
12. Parkin DM, et al. Part I: cancer in indigenous Africans—burden, distribution, and trends. Lancet Oncol. 2008;9:683–92.
13. Ferlay J, Ervik M, Lam F, et al. Global cancer observatory: cancer today. Lyon: International Agency for Research on Cancer; 2020.
14. Moore PS, Chang Y. Detection of herpesvirus-like DNA sequences in Kaposi's sarcoma in patients with and those without HIV infection. N Engl J Med. 1995;332(18):1181–5.
15. Chuck S, Grant RM, Katongole-Mbidde E, Conant M, Ganem D. Frequent presence of a novel herpesvirus genome in lesions of human immunodeficiency virus-negative Kaposi's sarcoma. J Infect Dis. 1996;173(1):248–51.
16. Buonaguro FM, Tornesello ML, Beth-Giraldo E, Hatzakis A, Mueller N, Downing R, Biryamwaho B, Sempala SD, Giraldo G. Herpesvirus-like DNA sequences detected in endemic, classic, iatrogenic and epidemic Kaposi's sarcoma (KS) biopsies. Int J Cancer. 1996;65(1):25–8.
17. Sitas F, Carrara H, Beral V, Newton R, Reeves G, Bull D, Jentsch U, Pacella-Norman R, Bourboulia D, Whitby D, Boshoff C. Antibodies against human herpesvirus 8 in black South African patients with cancer. N Engl J Med. 1999;340(24):1863–71.
18. Purvis SF, Katongole-Mbidde E, Johnson JL, Leonard DG, Byabazaire N, Luckey C, Schick HE, Wallis R, Elmets CA, Giam CZ. High incidence of Kaposi's sarcoma-associated herpesvirus and Epstein-Barr virus in tumor lesions and peripheral blood mononuclear cells from patients with Kaposi's sarcoma in Uganda. J Infect Dis. 1997;175(4):947–50.
19. Dupin N, Grandadam M, Calvez V, Aubin JT, Huraux JM, Agut H, Gorin I, Havard S, Lamy F, Leibowitch M, Escande JP. Herpesvirus-like DNA sequences in patients with Mediterranean Kaposi's sarcoma. Lancet. 1995;345(8952):761–2.
20. Gao SJ, Kingsley L, Hoover DR, Spira TJ, Rinaldo CR, Saah A, Phair J, Detels R, Parry P, Chang Y, Moore PS. Seroconversion to antibodies against Kaposi's sarcoma–associated herpesvirus–related latent nuclear antigens before the development of Kaposi's sarcoma. N Engl J Med. 1996;335(4):233–41.
21. Roshan R, et al. T-cell responses to KSHV infection: a systematic approach. Oncotarget. 2017;8:109402–16.
22. International Collaboration on HIV and Cancer. Highly active antiretroviral therapy and incidence of cancer in human immunodeficiency virus-infected adults. J Natl Cancer Inst. 2000;92:1823–30.
23. Lodi S, Guiguet M, Costagliola D, Fisher M, de Luca A, Porter K. Kaposi sarcoma incidence and survival among HIV-infected homosexual men after HIV seroconversion. J Natl Cancer Inst. 2010;102:784–92.

24. Ibrahim Khalil A, Franceschi S, de Martel C, Bray F, Clifford GM. Burden of Kaposi sarcoma according to HIV status: a systematic review and global analysis. Int J Cancer. 2022;150(12):1948–57.
25. Denis D, et al. A fifth subtype of Kaposi's sarcoma, classic Kaposi's sarcoma in men who have sex with men: a cohort study in Paris. J Eur Acad Dermatol Venereol. 2018;32:1377–84.
26. What is Kaposi sarcoma? www.cancer.org, https://www.cancer.org/cancer/kaposi-sarcoma/about/what-is-kaposi-sarcoma.html. Accessed 29 May 2022.
27. El-Mallawany NK, Villiera J, Kamiyango W, Peckham-Gregory EC, Scheurer ME, Allen CE, McAtee CL, Legarreta A, Dittmer DP, Kovarik CL, Chiao EY. Endemic Kaposi sarcoma in HIV-negative children and adolescents: an evaluation of overlapping and distinct clinical features in comparison with HIV-related disease. Infect Agents Cancer. 2018;13(1):1–7.
28. Fatahzadeh M. Kaposi sarcoma: review and medical management update. Oral Surg Oral Med Oral Pathol Oral Radiol. 2012;113(1):2–16.
29. Etta EM, Alayande DP, Mavhandu-Ramarumo LG, Gachara G, Bessong PO. HHV-8 seroprevalence and genotype distribution in Africa, 1998−2017: a systematic review. Viruses. 2018;10(9).
30. Bishop BN, Lynch DT. Kaposi sarcoma. In: StatPearls. StatPearls Publishing; 2021.
31. Radu O, Pantanowitz L. Kaposi sarcoma. Arch Pathol Lab Med. 2013;137(2):289–94.
32. Bower M, DallaPria A, Coyle C, Andrews E, Tittle V, Dhoot S, Nelson M. Prospective stage-stratified approach to AIDS-related Kaposi's sarcoma. J Clin Oncol. 2014;32(5):409–14.
33. Zeichner SB, Ruiz AL, Suciu GP, Zeichner RL, Rodriguez E. Trends in Kaposi's sarcoma in Miami Beach from 1987 to 2007. ISRN Oncol. 2012;2012.
34. Nichols CM, Flaitz CM, Hicks MJ. Treating Kaposi's lesions in the HIV-infected patient. J Am Dent Assoc. 1993;124(11):78–84.
35. Danzig JB, Brandt LJ, Reinus JF, Klein RS. Gastrointestinal malignancy in patients with AIDS. Am J Gastroenterol. 1991;86(6).
36. Laine L, Amerian J, Rarick M, Harb M, Gill PS. The response of symptomatic gastrointestinal Kaposi's sarcoma to chemotherapy: a prospective evaluation using an endoscopic method of disease quantification. Am J Gastroenterol. 1990;85(8).
37. Joshi M, Markelova N, Palacio D, Schapira RM. A patient with HIV, dyspnea, and multiple pulmonary nodules. Chest. 2006;130(6):1924–8.
38. Krown SE, Metroka C, Wernz JC. Kaposi's sarcoma in the acquired immune deficiency syndrome: a proposal for uniform evaluation, response, and staging criteria. AIDS Clinical Trials Group Oncology Committee. J Clin Oncol. 1989;7:1201.
39. Amerson E, et al. Accuracy of clinical suspicion and pathologic diagnosis of Kaposi sarcoma in East Africa. J Acquir Immune Defic Syndr. 2016;71:295–301.
40. Marušić Z, Billings SD. Histopathology of spindle cell vascular tumors. Surg Pathol Clin. 2017;10(2):345–66.
41. Kahn HJ, Bailey D, Marks A. Monoclonal antibody D2-40, a new marker of lymphatic endothelium, reacts with Kaposi's sarcoma and a subset of angiosarcomas. Mod Pathol. 2002;15:434–40.
42. Pyakurel P, et al. Lymphatic and vascular origin of Kaposi's sarcoma spindle cells during tumor development. Int J Cancer. 2006;119:1262–7.
43. Massarelli G, Scott CA, Ibba M, Tanda F, Cossu A. Immunocytochemical profile of Kaposi's sarcoma cells: their reactivity to a panel of antibodies directed against different tissue cell markers. Appl Pathol. 1989;7:34–41.
44. International Agency for Research on Cancer. In: IARC monographs on the evaluation of carcinogenic risks to humans, vol. 100B. International Agency for Research on Cancer; 2012.
45. Mesri EA, Cesarman E, Boshoff C. Kaposi's sarcoma and its associated herpesvirus. Nat Rev Cancer. 2010;10(10):707–19.
46. Jha HC, Banerjee S, Robertson ES. The role of gammaherpesviruses in cancer pathogenesis. Pathogens. 2016;5(1):18.
47. Euvrard S, Kanitakis J, Claudy A. Skin cancers after organ transplantation. N Engl J Med. 2003;348(17):1681–91.

48. Martin JN, Ganem DE, Osmond DH, Page-Shafer KA, Macrae D, Kedes DH. Sexual transmission and the natural history of human herpesvirus 8 infection. N Engl J Med. 1998;338(14):948–54.
49. Butler LM, Osmond DH, Jones AG, Martin JN. Use of saliva as a lubricant in anal sexual practices among homosexual men. J Acquir Immune Defic Syndr. 2009;50:162–7.
50. Dukers NH, Rezza G. Human herpesvirus 8 epidemiology: what we do and do not know. AIDS. 2003;17(12):1717–30.
51. Plancoulaine S, Abel L, van Beveren M, Trégouët DA, Joubert M, Tortevoye P, de Thé G, Gessain A. Human herpesvirus 8 transmission from mother to child and between siblings in an endemic population. Lancet. 2000;356(9235):1062–5.
52. Mantina H, Kankasa C, Klaskala W, Brayfield B, Campbell J, Du Q, Bhat G, Kasolo F, Mitchell C, Wood C. Vertical transmission of Kaposi's sarcoma-associated herpesvirus. Int J Cancer. 2001;94(5):749–52.
53. Hladik W, Dollard SC, Mermin J, Fowlkes AL, Downing R, Amin MM, Banage F, Nzaro E, Kataaha P, Dondero TJ, Pellett PE. Transmission of human herpesvirus 8 by blood transfusion. N Engl J Med. 2006;355(13):1331–8.
54. Barozzi P, Luppi M, Facchetti F, Mecucci C, Alù M, Sarid R, Rasini V, Ravazzini L, Rossi E, Festa S, Crescenzi B. Post-transplant Kaposi sarcoma originates from the seeding of donor-derived progenitors. Nat Med. 2003;9(5):554–61.
55. Luppi M, Barozzi P, Schulz TF, Setti G, Staskus K, Trovato R, Narni F, Donelli A, Maiorana A, Marasca R, Sandrini S. Bone marrow failure associated with human herpesvirus 8 infection after transplantation. N Engl J Med. 2000;343(19):1378–85.
56. Bechtel JT, Liang Y, Hvidding J, Ganem D. Host range of Kaposi's sarcoma-associated herpesvirus in cultured cells. J Virol. 2003;77:6474–81.
57. Kumar B, Roy A, Veettil MV, Chandran B. Insight into the roles of E3 ubiquitin ligase c-Cbl, ESCRT machinery, and host cell signaling in Kaposi's sarcoma-associated herpesvirus entry and trafficking. J Virol. 2018;92:e01376–17.
58. Damania B, Cesarman E. In: Knipe DM, et al., editors. Field's virology, vol. 2. Lippincott Williams & Wilkins; 2013. p. 2080–128.
59. Kumar B, Chandran B. KSHV entry and trafficking in target cells-hijacking of cell signal pathways, actin and membrane dynamics. Viruses. 2016;8:305.
60. Karabajakian A, Ray-Coquard I, Blay JY. Molecular mechanisms of Kaposi sarcoma development. Cancers. 2022;14(8):1869.
61. Zhu Q, Ding L, Zi Z, Gao S, Wang C, Wang Y, Zhu C, Yuan Z, Wei F, Cai Q. Viral-mediated AURKB cleavage promotes cell segregation and tumorigenesis. Cell Rep. 2019;26:3657–71.
62. Kim YJ, Kim Y, Kumar A, Kim CW, Toth Z, Cho NH, Lee H-R. Kaposi's sarcoma-associated herpesvirus latency associated nuclear antigen dysregulates expression of MCL-1 by targeting FBW7. PLoS Pathog. 2021;17:e1009179.
63. Tagawa T, Serquiña A, Kook I, Ziegelbauer J. Viral non-coding RNAs: stealth strategies in the tug-of-war between humans and herpesviruses. Semin Cell Dev Biol. 2021;111:135–47.
64. Withers JB, Mondol V, Pawlica P, Rosa-Mercado NA, Tycowski KT, Ghasempur S, Torabi SF, Steitz JA. Idiosyncrasies of viral noncoding RNAs provide insights into host cell biology. Annu Rev Virol. 2019;6:297–317.
65. Suffert G, Malterer G, Hausser J, Viiliäinen J, Fender A, Contrant M, Ivacevic T, Benes V, Gros F, Voinnet O, et al. Kaposi's sarcoma herpesvirus microRNAs target caspase 3 and regulate apoptosis. PLoS Pathog. 2011;7:e1002405.
66. Li T, Ju E, Gao SJ. Kaposi sarcoma-associated herpesvirus miRNAs suppress CASTOR1-mediated mTORC1 inhibition to promote tumorigenesis. J Clin Invest. 2019;129:3310–23.
67. Abend JR, Uldrick T, Ziegelbauer JM. Regulation of tumor necrosis factor-like weak inducer of apoptosis receptor protein (TWEAKR) expression by Kaposi's sarcoma-associated herpesvirus microRNA prevents TWEAK-induced apoptosis and inflammatory cytokine expression. J Virol. 2010;84:12139–51.

68. Tagawa T, Gao S, Koparde VN, Gonzalez M, Spouge JL, Serquiña AP, Lurain K, Ramaswami R, Uldrick TS, Yarchoan R, et al. Discovery of Kaposi's sarcoma herpesvirus-encoded circular RNAs and a human antiviral circular RNA. Proc Natl Acad Sci U S A. 2018;115:12805–10.
69. Wakeham K, Johnston WT, Nalwoga A, Nalwoga A, Webb EL, Mayanja BN, Miley W, Elliott AM, Whitby D, Newton R. Trends in Kaposi's sarcoma-associated Herpesvirus antibodies prior to the development of HIV-associated Kaposi's sarcoma: a nested case-control study. Int J Cancer. 2015;136:2822–30.
70. Yang TY, Chen SC, Leach MW, Manfra D, Homey B, Wiekowski M, Sullivan L, Jenh C-H, Narula SK, Chensue SW, et al. Transgenic expression of the chemokine receptor encoded by human herpesvirus 8 induces an angioproliferative disease resembling Kaposi's sarcoma. J Exp Med. 2000;191:445–54.
71. Zhang Z, Chen W, Sanders M, Brulois KF, Dittmer DP, Damania B. The K1 protein of Kaposi's sarcoma associated herpesvirus augments viral lytic replication. J Virol. 2016;90:7657–66. Cancers 2022, 14, 1869 11 of 13.
72. Gramolelli S, Weidner-Glunde M, Abere B, Viejo-Borbolla A, Bala K, Rückert J, Kremmer E, Schulz TF. Inhibiting the recruitment of PLCγ1 to Kaposi's sarcoma herpesvirus K15 protein reduces the invasiveness and angiogenesis of infected endothelial cells. PLoS Pathog. 2015;11:e1005105.
73. Gaglia MM. Kaposi's sarcoma-associated herpesvirus at 27. Tumour Virus Res. 2021;12:200223. https://doi.org/10.1016/j.tvr.2021.200223.
74. Parsons CH, Szomju B, Kedes DH. Susceptibility of human fetal mesenchymal stem cells to Kaposi sarcoma-associated herpesvirus. Blood. 2004;104:2736–8.
75. Adler B, Sattler C, Adler H. Herpesviruses and their host cells: a successful liaison. Trends Microbiol. 2017;25(3):229–41.
76. Labo N, et al. Heterogeneity and breadth of host antibody response to KSHV infection demonstrated by systematic analysis of the KSHV proteome. PLoS Pathog. 2014;10:e1004046.
77. Olp LN, et al. Longitudinal analysis of the humoral response to Kaposi's sarcoma-associated herpesvirus after primary infection in children. J Med Virol. 2016;88:1973–81.
78. Coscoy L, Ganem D. Kaposi's sarcoma-associated herpesvirus encodes two proteins that block cell surface display of MHC class I chains by enhancing their endocytosis. Proc Natl Acad Sci U S A. 2000;97:8051–6.
79. Ishido S, Wang C, Lee BS, Cohen GB, Jung JU. Downregulation of major histocompatibility complex class I molecules by Kaposi's sarcoma-associated herpesvirus K3 and K5 proteins. J Virol. 2000;74:5300–9.
80. Jacobs SR, et al. The viral interferon regulatory factors of Kaposi's sarcoma-associated herpesvirus differ in their inhibition of interferon activation mediated by toll-like receptor 3. J Virol. 2013;87:798–806.
81. Burysek L, et al. Functional analysis of human herpesvirus 8-encoded viral interferon regulatory factor 1 and its association with cellular interferon regulatory factors and p300. J Virol. 1999;73:7334–42.
82. Ma Z, et al. Modulation of the cGAS-STING DNA sensing pathway by gammaherpesviruses. Proc Natl Acad Sci U S A. 2015;112:E4306–15.
83. Wu JJ, et al. Inhibition of cGAS DNA sensing by a herpesvirusvirion protein. Cell Host Microbe. 2015;18:333–44.
84. Zhang G, et al. Cytoplasmic isoforms of Kaposi sarcoma herpesvirus LANA recruit and antagonize the innate immune DNA sensor cGAS. Proc Natl Acad Sci U S A. 2016;113:E1034–43.
85. Nicholas J, et al. Kaposi's sarcoma-associated human herpesvirus-8 encodes homologues of macrophage inflammatory protein-1 and interleukin-6. Nat Med. 1997;3:287–92.
86. Foster-Cuevas M, Wright GJ, Puklavec MJ, Brown MH, Barclay AN. Human herpesvirus 8 K14 protein mimics CD200 in down-regulating macrophage activation through CD200 receptor. J Virol. 2004;78:7667–76.
87. Rezaee SA, Gracie JA, McInnes IB, Blackbourn DJ. Inhibition of neutrophil function by the Kaposi's sarcoma-associated herpesvirus vOX2 protein. AIDS. 2005;19:1907–10.

88. Chung YH, Means RE, Choi JK, Lee BS, Jung JU. Kaposi's sarcoma-associated herpesvirus OX2 glycoprotein activates myeloid-lineage cells to induce inflammatory cytokine production. J Virol. 2002;76:4688–98.
89. Writing Group, Bower M, Palfreeman A, Alfa-Wali M, Bunker C, Burns F, Churchill D, Collins S, Cwynarski K, Edwards S, Fields P. British HIV Association guidelines for HIV-associated malignancies 2014. HIV Med. 2014;15:1–92.
90. Stewart S, et al. Randomized comparative trial of pegylated liposomal doxorubicin versus bleomycin and vincristine in the treatment of AIDS-related Kaposi's sarcoma. International Pegylated Liposomal Doxorubicin Study Group. J Clin Oncol. 1998;16:683–91.
91. Northfelt DW, et al. Pegylated-liposomal doxorubicin versus doxorubicin, bleomycin, and vincristine in the treatment of AIDS-related Kaposi's sarcoma: results of a randomized phase III clinical trial. J Clin Oncol. 1998;16:2445–51.
92. Gill PS, et al. Randomized phase III trial of liposomal daunorubicin versus doxorubicin, bleomycin, and vincristine in AIDS-related Kaposi's sarcoma. J Clin Oncol. 1996;14:2353–64.
93. Esdaile B, et al. The immunological effects of concomitant highly active antiretroviral therapy and liposomal anthracycline treatment of HIV-1-associated Kaposi's sarcoma. AIDS. 2002;16:2344–7.
94. Lichterfeld M, et al. Treatment of HIV-1-associated Kaposi's sarcoma with pegylated liposomal doxorubicin and HAART simultaneously induces effective tumor remission and $CD4^+$ T cell recovery. Infection. 2005;33:140–7.
95. Stebbing J, et al. Paclitaxel for anthracycline-resistant AIDS-related Kaposi's sarcoma: clinical and angiogenic correlations. Ann Oncol. 2003;14:1660–6.
96. Tulpule A, et al. Multicenter trial of low-dose paclitaxel in patients with advanced AIDS-related Kaposi sarcoma. Cancer. 2002;95:147–54.
97. Cianfrocca M, et al. Randomized trial of paclitaxel versus pegylated liposomal doxorubicin for advanced human immunodeficiency virus-associated Kaposi sarcoma. Cancer. 2010;116:3969–77.
98. Nasti G, et al. AIDS-related Kaposi's sarcoma: evaluation of potential new prognostic factors and assessment of the AIDS Clinical Trial Group staging system in the Haart Era—the Italian Cooperative Group on AIDS and Tumors and the Italian Cohort of Patients Naive From Antiretrovirals. J Clin Oncol. 2003;21:2876–82.
99. El Amari EB, et al. Predicting the evolution of Kaposi sarcoma, in the highly active antiretroviral therapy era. AIDS. 2008;22:1019–28.
100. Chu KM, et al. AIDS-associated Kaposi's sarcoma is linked to advanced disease and high mortality in a primary care HIV programme in South Africa. J Int AIDS Soc. 2010;13:23.
101. Stebbing J, et al. The presentation and survival of patients with non-cutaneous AIDS-associated Kaposi's sarcoma. Ann Oncol. 2006;17:503–6.
102. World Health Organization. Consolidated guidelines on HIV prevention, diagnosis, treatment, and care for key populations: policy brief—2016 update. WHO; 2017.
103. U.S. Department of Health and Human Services. Guidelines for the use of antiretroviral agents in adults and adolescents living with HIV. AIDSinfo; 2018. https://aidsinfo.nih.gov/guidelines/html/1/adult-and-adolescent-treatment-guidelines.
104. National Cancer Institute, National Institutes of Health. About cancer: infectious agents. National Cancer Institute; 2017. https://www.cancer.gov/about-cancer/causes-prevention/risk/infectious-agents.

Radiation Induced Skin Ulcers

27

Ritusha Mishra, Himanshu Mishra, and Chandraprakash Verma

27.1 Introduction

Skin is the largest organ of the human body. It forms a part of innate immune system and serves as a physical barrier for most of the pathogens and harmful substances. It is made up of three layers: the outermost is epidermis, underneath lies dermis, and the innermost is subcutaneous tissue (hypodermis). The layers of epidermis from superficial to deep are stratum corneum, stratum lucidum, stratum granulosum, stratum spinosum, and stratum basale. The cells in the innermost layer of epidermis are stem cells that regenerate continuously. On infliction of any injury or imbalance in local milieu, these stem cells proliferate, differentiate, and thus restore the integrity of skin.

Rapidly dividing cells such as those of skin, bone marrow, gastrointestinal epithelium are more sensitive to radiation-induced damage [1]. It has been observed that more than 70% patients of malignancy require radiotherapy (RT). More than 95% of patients receiving radiation develop dermatitis of varying degree [2]. The manifestation of skin injury may range from mild desquamation, erythema to frank ulceration or necrosis. It is associated with pain and discomfort affecting the overall quality of life of the patient [3]. Incidence of radiation associated skin toxicity is higher in head and neck cancer with around 25% patients developing severe toxicity [4]. Radiation related skin toxicity can negatively affect patients experience, body image, and overall quality of life [5]. It may lead to unwanted treatment interruptions during RT, thus prolonging treatment duration. This prolongation of overall treatment time (OTT) is associated with inferior oncological outcomes. Therefore, it is imperative to prevent or minimize the severity of skin toxicity.

R. Mishra (✉) · H. Mishra · C. Verma
Department of Radiotherapy and Radiation Medicine, Institute of Medical Sciences, Banaras Hindu University, Varanasi, India

A. K. Khanna, S. K. Tiwary (eds.), *Uncommon Ulcers of the Extremities*,
https://doi.org/10.1007/978-981-99-1782-2_27

A complex interplay of various treatment related and patient related factors determines the degree of skin damage during and after RT. There is a myriad of presentation of skin injury following RT. Acute changes may manifest as mild erythema, hyperpigmentation to frank ulcer, necrosis, or hemorrhage. Chronic skin damage usually presents with fibrosis, atrophy, telangiectasia, altered pigmentation in mild form to chronic nonhealing ulcers in severe forms. Although there has been drastic decrease in more serious skin toxicity with advanced skin sparing RT techniques, simultaneously increased used of chemotherapy, immunotherapy has complicated the situation.

Despite the availability of numerous treatment recommendations there is a variation in practice across various centers [6, 7]. This chapter gives a comprehensive overview of pathophysiology, evaluation, and management of RT induced skin toxicity including ulcers.

27.2 Etiology

The free radicals and reactive oxygen species generated as the result of interaction of radiation with the body tissue cause killing of tumor cells and healthy cells. As cell turnover is rapid in skin the radiation reactions are more early evident here. The severity of skin damage depends upon the self-renewal capacity versus killing of normal skin cells.

27.3 Aggravating Factors

(a) Patient related: Any preexisting skin disease, genetic susceptibility like xeroderma pigmentosa, any associated comorbidity, increased body mass index, nutritional status.
(b) Treatment related: Higher total radiation doses, conventional technique, accelerated RT, use of concurrent chemotherapy, use of chemotherapy drugs causing radiation recall reaction like doxorubicin, and more skin folds in irradiated area.

27.4 Pathophysiology

Hypoxia is considered as a predominant cause of radiation-induced changes in skin. The mechanism of radiation-induced skin reactions includes generation of free radicals consequently a cascade of events leading to cell death. Inflammation may start as early as 24 h after receiving radiotherapy with liberation of free radicals in the actively multiplying cells of the basal layer [8, 9]. The early inflammatory response to radiation is mainly caused by pro-inflammatory cytokines (interleukins and tumor necrosis factor), chemokines (eotaxin and IL-8), receptor tyrosine kinase, and adhesions molecules (intercellular adhesion molecule 1 [ICAM-1], E-selectin, and vascular cell adhesion protein). These factors cause accumulation of eosinophils and neutrophils initiating inflammatory response, leading to self-perpetuating tissue damage and loss of protective barriers. Inflammatory response and oxidative stress interact and promote each other in the cell microenvironment resulting in acute skin reactions [10]. After receiving radiotherapy, cells may die in various forms, predominant mode of cell death being mitotic. In chronic phases, inflammation and oxidative stress lead to changes at level of microcirculation causing telangiectasia, connective tissue causing atrophy, and fibrosis or nonhealing ulcers [11].

The smallest unit of skin that contains microvessel, epidermis, and dermis is known as functional unit of skin. It is to be emphasized that the dose response of functional units defines the dose response of skin as a whole. The functional unit is about 30 pm in diameter and 350 pm in length. The dose response of the skin is like the parallel structures where toxicity is evident only when a significant number of functional subunits are damaged [12]. On histology, acute radiation dermatitis may have epidermal changes, including vacuolar degeneration of basement membrane and necrotic keratinocytes as well as the presence of spongiosis that can lead to subepidermal blister formation. Perivascular inflammatory infiltrates, dilated blood vessels with thrombi, and dermal edema may be observed [13]. Chronic radiation dermatitis shows dermal sclerosis, elastosis, and vascular ectasia; overlying epidermis which is often hyperkeratotic. There may be epidermal spongiosis or basal vacuolar changes. The dermal vessels are typically quite dilated in later stages. Stromal fibroblast and endothelial cells may show some hyperchromasia, enlargement, and atypia. There is often a mixed inflammatory response. Skin may become thin due to atrophic epidermis and loss of the rete pattern. Telangiectatic changes characterized by tortuous vascular pattern, hypocellular dermis with areas of fibrosis, dense collagen, and elastic tissue are commonly observed [14–16].

27.5 Evaluation

27.5.1 History

A complete and meticulous history of hypersensitivity, preexisting skin disease like scleroderma, genetic susceptibility, any drug allergy, contact dermatitis, sun burn should be evaluated. There are some genetic syndromes like Ataxia telangiectasia (mutation in ATM gene) and Fanconi syndrome (autosomal recessive disorder) which are associated with higher probability to develop severe skin reactions [17, 18]. Detailed information of radiation like area receiving radiotherapy, total dose, dose per fraction, overall treatment duration, maximum acute skin toxicity etc. must be obtained. Cumulative total radiation dose and overall treatment time are critically associated with severity of radiation-induced skin reactions. History of comorbidity like diabetes, HIV, tuberculosis, syphilis should be taken as these factors are associated with delayed healing. Details of received chemotherapy also need to be documented, in particular, the type of chemotherapeutic agents used. There are some chemotherapeutic agents that will predispose to radiation recall such as doxorubicin, docetaxel, paclitaxel, etc. Radiation recall is a clinical phenomenon which is characterized by acute inflammatory reactions triggered by the administration of certain systemic agent in previously irradiated area. There are certain chemotherapeutic agents (cisplatin, bleomycin, doxorubicin, etc.) that are considered as relative contraindication to hyperbaric oxygen therapy, a treatment modality to treat radiation-induced late reactions.

27.5.2 Physical Examination

Patient must be examined in a well-lighted area. The area to be examined should be adequately exposed and any changes in skin and under the skin folds are to be noted. The site, size, floor, margin, edge, consistency of any ulcer if present should be noted. Any associated pain, discharge, discoloration, atrophy should also be documented. The grading scales are available from various bodies (Table 27.1), the lesion should be graded accordingly. Radiation-induced skin changes may have following features:

- Redness or darkening of the skin
- Dry desquamation of skin (Image 27.1)
- Swollen skin
- Moist desquamation; patchy or confluent
- Ulceration, hemorrhage, or necrosis (Image 27.2)

Table 27.1 Various toxicity assessment scales

Systems	Grading
Radiation therapy oncology group (RTOG)	0: No change 1: Erythema, dry desquamation, epilation 2: Bright erythema, moist desquamation, edema 3: Confluent moist desquamation, pitting edema 4: Ulceration, hemorrhage, necrosis
World Health Organization (WHO) criteria	0: None 1: Erythema 2: Dry desquamation, vesiculation, pruritus 3: Moist desquamation, ulceration 4: Exfoliative dermatitis, necrosis requiring surgical intervention
Common terminology criteria for adverse events (CTCAE)	0: None 1: Faint erythema or dry desquamation 2: Moderate to brisk erythema 3: Confluent moist desquamation 4: Skin necrosis or ulceration

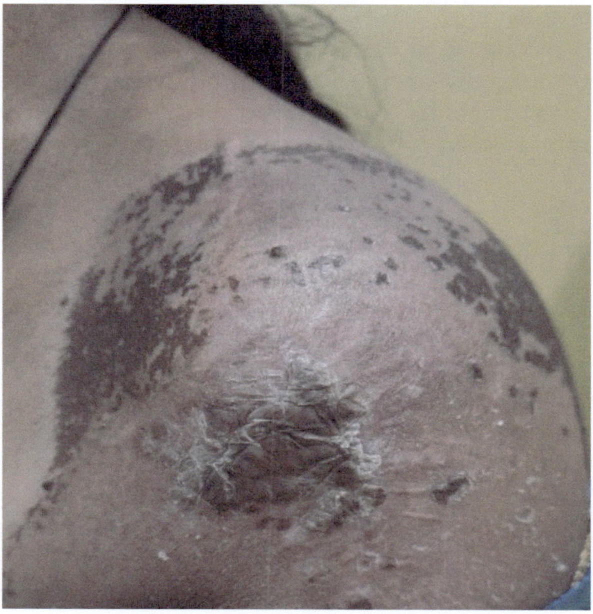

Image 27.1 Post-RT hyperpigmentation and dry desquamation

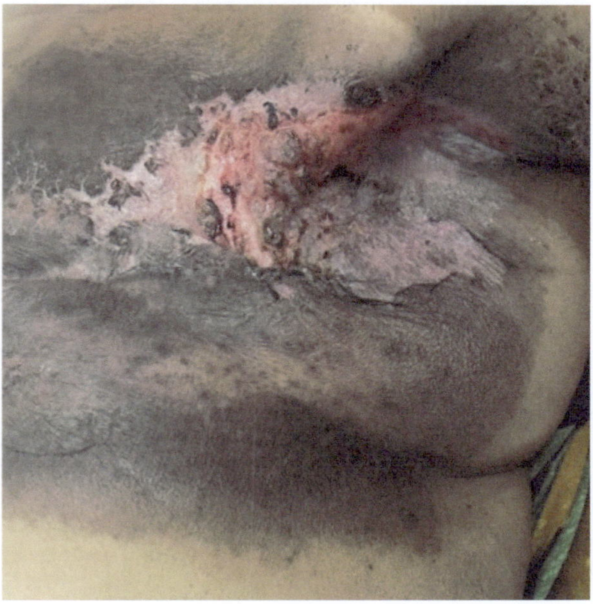

Image 27.2 Post-RT skin ulcer, grade IV toxicity

27.5.3 Investigation

A patient having radiation-induced skin ulcer should be thoroughly investigated to find out probable aggravating factor. Complete blood profile, random blood sugar, erythrocyte sedimentation rate should be routinely performed. Chest X-ray should be performed, if hyperbaric oxygen therapy is chosen as a treatment modality. Culture sensitive of the discharge merits if ulcer is associated with any discharge. For a chronic nonhealing ulcer, a biopsy should be performed to establish the diagnosis as well as to exclude malignant lesion.

27.6 Differential Diagnosis

1. A chronic nonspecific ulcer may have necrotic slough over floor of ulcer, regular margins, and foul smelling discharge.
2. Osteo-radionecrosis also has feature of chronic nonhealing ulcer. On examination, tenderness will be more pronounced. An X-ray may be helpful to reach the diagnosis.
3. Chondronecrosis mimics the osteo-radionecrosis. CECT or MRI may be helpful to rule out and to establish the diagnosis.
4. Acneiform eruptions can be distinguished from acne as there are no comedones (whiteheads or blackheads).
5. Hyperkeratotic reactions are characterized by blackish and leathery appearance of skin.
6. Atypical vascular lesions are pearly, pinkish, and nodular lesion. They may be pulsatile in nature.
7. Primary skin malignant lesion mimics the features of chronic nonhealing ulcer but these ulcers have irregular margins with indurated base and bleeds on touch. Recurrent malignant lesion of skin has history of malignancy and appears as nodular lesion which may ulcerate in due course of time. However, secondary skin metastasis presents with multiple discrete firms to hard nodular lesion may have tenderness.

27.7 Management

27.7.1 Prevention

The effect of ionizing radiation on skin varies from no change to ulceration and necrosis. It depends upon many factors like total EBRT dose, skin folds over irradiated region, use of concurrent chemotherapy, individual care, and patient's intrinsic sensitivity to radiation. However, there are various measures to avoid or reverse radiation-induced skin reactions.

1. **Instructions before EBRT**

   Patients should be given specific instructions regarding skin care before RT. Patients should be advised to maintain good skin hygiene. In a prospective randomized study including 99 patients of breast cancer, Roy et al. demonstrated a trend toward less toxicity while washing skin with water and soap [19].

Although the difference in toxicities was not significant and since the study included patients of breast cancer only, the results may not be generalized to all sites. Instructions should be given to patients to avoid topical irritants, friction, and to wear loose fitted clothing during RT.

2. **Radiation Technique and Doses**

   Apart from total RT dose and dose per fraction, technique also affects the severity of reactions. Patients should be positioned in a manner to minimize skin folds. Use of multiple radiation beams reduces dose to a particular area and thus in turn reduces the severity.

27.7.2 Treatment

27.7.2.1 External Creams

Triethanolamine containing topical agents has been widely used for clinical conditions which affect skin integrity. It enhances wound healing as it provides deep hydration, accelerates fibroblast proliferation, removes necrotic tissue, restores CD34 expression, reduces vascular changes and IL-1 secretion [20]. An oil-in-water topical emulsion containing triethanolamine, Biafine, has been used in management of radiation dermatitis. Szumacher et al. evaluated role of Biafine in patients of carcinoma breast undergoing RT and demonstrated that although majority of patients developed grade 2 skin reactions, there was no treatment delay or interruption because of skin toxicity [21].

Like Biafine, moist exposed burn ointment (MEBO) is also used in the management of radiation dermatitis and subsequent ulcers. It is a mixture of various Chinese medicines. It increases tissue metabolism and causes repair of vascular endothelium. Geara et al. showed that there was no significant difference between MEBO ointment and Biafine in reducing skin dermatitis [22]. Apart from these, Jaungo, a complex herbal medicine has been also shown to be safe and effective in managing radiation dermatitis [23]. However, more elaborate data is required for its routine clinical use.

Since development of radiation associated reaction is associated with inflammatory response, topical corticosteroids are clinically useful. Although the exact mechanism of action is not completely known, the anti-inflammatory effects of corticosteroids are thought to be because of vasoconstriction, reduced capillary permeability and inhibition of leukocyte proliferation and migration [24]. In patients of carcinoma breast receiving adjuvant RT, a randomized study demonstrated that betamethasone was associated with better control of acute radiation dermatitis as compared to two moisturizing creams. Another study by Omidvari et al. demonstrated that preventive and sustained use of 0.1% betamethasone effectively delayed the onset of acute radiation dermatitis in patients of breast cancer undergoing RT [25].

Some other studies have also shown therapeutic efficacy of topical steroids in controlling radiation-induced skin damage [26, 27].

RT induced moist desquamation causes pain, discomfort, and increases risk of infection and subsequent ulcer formation. Gentian violet (GV) paint has been effectively used in management of moist desquamation [28].

27.7.2.2 Dressings

Hydrogel/hydrocolloid dressings, when applied over skin wounds, makes skin surface moist. Moisture promotes cell migration and assists in wound debridement. These dressings are easy to clean, reusable, and effective. In a trial comparing hydrogel dressings with dexpanthenol cream in patients of breast cancer undergoing RT, authors reported that the hydrogel dressing significantly reduced frequency of moist desquamation [29]. Another study comparing hydrogel dressings with GV reported that hydrogel dressings not only cured the RT induced moist desquamation but was more tolerant than GV [30].

Soft silicone dressings adhere to skin, absorb secretions, promote development of granulation tissue, release of growth factors, formation of blood capillaries, and dissolve necrotic tissues. Various studies have shown clinical benefit of soft silicone dressings (Mepilex Lite and Mepitel Film) in management of skin reactions. In a clinical trial by Diggelmann et al., authors demonstrated that Mepitel dressing effectively reduced RT induced erythema [31]. In another study by MacBride et al., it was found that the dressing had no negative effect on wound healing [32]. In a study conducted by University of Toron, Mepitel Film caused decreased radiation dermatitis and significantly favored patient-reported outcomes in patients receiving breast irradiation [33].

27.7.2.3 Hyperbaric Oxygen Therapy (HBOT)

Hyperbaric oxygen is 100% oxygen at two to three times of atmospheric pressure at sea level. Although the definite mechanism is unclear, investigators have proposed that HBOT mainly acts by increasing the oxygen concentration in tissues which in turn can enhance angiogenesis, collagen synthesis, and resist bacterial infections. In a retrospective study, Abdul et al. evaluated the role of HBOT and concluded that considering the efficacy and favorable toxicity profile of HBOT, it should be considered in management of radiation-induced tissue injuries [34]. Regarding HBOT, the existing literature suggests that although it is a safe intervention with promising outcomes, more evidence is required to approve its clinical use in treatment of radiation-induced skin necrosis [35].

27.7.2.4 Mesenchymal Stem Cells (MSCs)

MSCs have strong ability of wound healing owing to its properties of cytokine secretion, immunoregulation, and multipotential differentiation. Many authors have reported that locally injected MSCs are effective in healing radiation-induced ulcerative wounds [36, 37]. A Chinese case study has reported regeneration of radiation-induced skin ulcers in 36 days after combined treatment with MSCs and hematopoietic stem cells [38]. Although the role of MSCs in repairing RISRs has been widely studied in animals, robust clinical data is lacking for humans. Further research may provide a way for widespread clinical use of this promising therapeutic approach.

27.7.2.5 Superoxide Dismutases (SODs)

Being a free-radical scavenger, SODs eliminate free radicals from skin, thus increase tolerance of skin to RT. SODs either ameliorate or avoid the toxicity. In a study of 57 patients, Garcia et al. reported that topical SOD was very effective in treatment of acute radio-dermatitis [39].

27.7.2.6 Low Intensity Laser

Therapy with laser causes normalization of the affected region by promoting acceleration of tissue repair, reduction of edema and analgesia [40, 41]. Schindl et al. evaluated low intensity laser therapy in three patients having RT induced chronic ulcers post-mastectomy and found that the therapy was effective in induction of wound healing in such cases [42]. With further research, this strategy may become one of the advanced methods for treatment of intractable chronic ulcers.

27.7.2.7 Surgery

Surgery is an effective strategy to deal with RT induced ulcers not responding to conservative means. Wide excision of the affected tissue, followed by transplantation of well-vascularized tissue is done. Suitable reconstructive methods vary according to functional and esthetic conditions. The choice of flap varies with the location and size of the wounds. For example, free flap-based transplantation for head and neck, sartorius muscle flaps for groin, fascio-cutaneous and large gluteal musculocutaneous flaps for sacral region can be used [43].

27.7.2.8 Phototherapy

Phototherapy has been used in treatment of many skin diseases. Red light phototherapy increases hemangiectasis and tissue circulation in deep layer of skin. Owing to its property of improved wound healing, it has potential for effective treatment of RISRs and clinical experiments have also demonstrated lower degrees of radiation dermatitis and lower pain scores with its use [44].

27.7.2.9 Plasma

Plasma proteins promote growth of granulation tissue by improving blood circulation and nutrition supply. In a study involving mouse model, Lee et al. reported that platelet-rich plasma accelerates regeneration and wound healing in irradiated skin [45]. Clinical studies have also demonstrated that plasma-based biomaterials were effective at promoting wound closure and mitigating acute radiation toxicity [46].

27.7.2.10 Interleukin (IL)

IL-12 improves cutaneous physical barrier after radiation and accelerates wound healing. It is mainly secreted by dendritic cells, monocytes, and macrophages. It has been identified as a potential mitigator of radiation-induced skin injury; however, more studies are needed to explore its further clinical use [47].

27.7.2.11 Hydrogen

Hydrogen gas can reduce levels of peroxynitrite and hydroxyl radicals that cause radiation-induced damage [48]. It may be used as a novel therapeutic medical gas to prevent radiation-induced adverse effects [49]. A study based on rat model showed that inhalation of hydrogen-containing gas (HCG) prior to the irradiation significantly decreased the delay in wound healing compared with control [50].

References

1. Ryan JL. Ionizing radiation: the good, the bad, and the ugly. J Invest Dermatol. 2012;132:985–93.
2. Singh M, Alavi A, Wong R, et al. Radiodermatitis: a review of our current understanding. Am J Clin Dermatol. 2016;17:277–92.
3. Vaz AF, Pinto-Neto AM, Conde DM, Costa-Paiva L, Morais SS, Esteves SB. Quality of life of women with gynecologic cancer: associated factors. Arch Gynecol Obstet. 2007;276(6):583–9.
4. Ferreira EB, Vasques CI, Gadia R, Chan RJ, Guerra EN, Mezzomo LA, et al. Topical interventions to prevent acute radiation dermatitis in head and neck cancer patients: a systematic review. Support Care Cancer. 2017;25:1001–11.
5. Sutherland AE, Bennett NC, Herst PM. Psychological stress affects the severity of radiation-induced acute skin reactions in breast cancer patients. Eur J Cancer Care. 2017;26.
6. Wong RK, Bensadoun RJ, Boers-Doets CB, et al. Clinical practice guidelines for the prevention and treatment of acute and late radiation reactions from the MASCC Skin Toxicity Study Group. Support Care Cancer. 2013;21:2933–48.
7. Bolderston A, Cashell A, McQuestion M, Cardoso M, Summers C, Harris R. A Canadian survey of the management of radiation-induced skin reactions. J Med Imaging Radiat Sci. 2018;49:164–72.
8. Wei J, Meng L, Hou X, Qu C, Wang B, Xin Y, Jiang X. Radiation-induced skin reactions: mechanism and treatment. Cancer Manag Res. 2018;11:167–77.
9. Hegedus F, Mathew LM, Schwartz RA. Radiation dermatitis: an overview. Int J Dermatol. 2017;56:909–14.
10. Peter RU. Diagnosis and treatment of cutaneous radiation injuries. In: Panizzonand RG, Seegenschmiedt MH, editors. Radiation treatment and radiation reactions in dermatology. Berlin: Springer; 2015. p. 185–8.
11. Bourgeois JF, Gourgou S, Kramar A, et al. Radiation-induced skin fibrosis after treatment of breast cancer: profilometric analysis. Skin Res Technol. 2003;9:39–42.
12. Archambeau JO, Hauser D, Shymko RM. Tissue population configuration as a modifier of organ dose response. Int J Radiat Oncol Biol Phys. 1988;15:727–34.
13. White DC. An atlas of radiation histopathology. Technical Information Center, Office of Public Affairs U.S. Energy Research and Development Administration; 1975.
14. Najafi M, Motevaseli E, Shirazi A, et al. Mechanisms of inflammatory responses to radiation and normal tissues toxicity: clinical implications. Int J Radiat Biol. 2018;94(4):335–56.
15. Zhao W, Robbins ME. Inflammation and chronic oxidative stress in radiation-induced late normal tissue injury: therapeutic implications. Curr Med Chem. 2009;16(2):130–43.
16. Archambeau JO, Pezner R, Wasserman T. Pathophysiology of irradiated skin and breast. Int J Radiat Oncol Biol Phys. 1995;31:1171–85.
17. Savitsky K, Bar-Shira A, Gilad S, et al. A single ataxia telangiectasia gene with a product similar to PI-3 kinase. Science. 1995;268:1749–53.
18. Buchwald M, Moustacchi E. Fanconi anemia caused by a defect in the processing of DNA damage? Mutat Res. 1998;408:75–90.
19. Roy I, Fortin A, Larochelle M. The impact of skin washing with water and soap during breast irradiation: a randomized study. Radiother Oncol. 2001;58(3):333–9.

20. Hymes SR, Strom EA, Fife C. Radiation dermatitis: clinical presentation, pathophysiology, and treatment 2006. J Am Acad Dermatol. 2006;54(1):28–46.
21. Szumacher E, Wighton A, Franssen E, et al. Phase II study assessing the effectiveness of Biafine cream as a prophylactic agent for radiation-induced acute skin toxicity to the breast in women undergoing radiotherapy with concomitant CMF chemotherapy. Int J Radiat Oncol Biol Phys. 2001;51(1):81–6.
22. Geara FB, Eid T, Zouain N, et al. Randomized, prospective, open-label phase III trial comparing Mebo ointment with Biafine cream for the management of acute dermatitis during radiotherapy for breast cancer. Am J Clin Oncol. 2018;41:1257–62.
23. Shin S, Jang BH, Suh HS, et al. Effectiveness, safety, and economic evaluation of topical application of a herbal ointment, Jaungo, for radiation dermatitis after breast conserving surgery in patients with breast cancer (GREEN study): study protocol for a randomized controlled trial. Medicine (Baltimore). 2019;98:e15174.
24. Boström A, Lindman H, Swartling C, Berne B, Bergh J. Potent corticosteroid cream (mometasone furoate) significantly reduces acute radiation dermatitis: results from a double-blind, randomized study. Radiother Oncol. 2001;59(3):257–65.
25. Omidvari S, Saboori H, Mohammadianpanah M, et al. Topical betamethasone for prevention of radiation dermatitis. Indian J Dermatol Venereol Leprol. 2007;73(3):209.
26. Schmuth M, Wimmer MA, Hofer S, et al. Topical corticosteroid therapy for acute radiation dermatitis: a prospective, randomized, double-blind study. Br J Dermatol. 2002;146(6):983–91.
27. Miller RC, Schwartz DJ, Sloan JA, et al. Mometasone furoate effect on acute skin toxicity in breast cancer patients receiving radiotherapy: a phase III double-blind, randomized trial from the North Central Cancer Treatment Group N06C4. Int J Radiat Oncol Biol Phys. 2011;79(5):1460–6.
28. Naylor W, Mallett J. Management of acute radiotherapy induced skin reactions: a literature review. Eur J Oncol Nurs. 2001;5(4):221–33.
29. Censabella S, Claes S, Orlandini M, Braekers R, Thijs H, Bulens P. Retrospective study of radiotherapy-induced skin reactions in breast cancer patients: reduced incidence of moist desquamation with a hydroactive colloid gel versus dexpanthenol. Eur J Oncol Nurs. 2014;18(5):499–504.
30. Gollins S, Gaffney C, Slade S, Swindell R. RCT on gentian violet versus a hydrogel dressing for radiotherapy-induced moist skin desquamation. J Wound Care. 2008;17(6):268–75.
31. Diggelmann KV, Zytkovicz AE, Tuaine JM, et al. Mepilex Lite dressings for the management of radiation-induced erythema: a systematic inpatient controlled clinical trial. Br J Radiol. 2010;83:971–8.
32. MacBride SK, Wells ME, Hornsby C, et al. A case study to evaluate a new soft silicone dressing, Mepilex Lite, for patients with radiation skin reactions. Cancer Nurs. 2008;31:E8–E14.
33. Wan BA, Chan S, Herst P, et al. Mepitel Film and Mepilex Lite for the prophylaxis and treatment of skin toxicities from breast radiation. Breast. 2019;46:87–9.
34. Borab Z, Mirmanesh MD, Gantz M, et al. Systematic review of hyperbaric oxygen therapy for the treatment of radiation-induced skin necrosis. J Plast Reconstr Aesthet Surg. 2017;70:529–38.
35. Tahir AR, Westhuyzen J, Dass J, et al. Hyperbaric oxygen therapy for chronic radiation-induced tissue injuries: Australasia's largest study. Asia Pac J Clin Oncol. 2015;11:68–77.
36. Agay D, Scherthan H, Forcheron F, Grenier N, Hérodin F, Meineke V, Drouet M. Multipotent mesenchymal stem cell grafting to treat cutaneous radiation syndrome: development of a new minipig model. Exp Hematol. 2010;38(10):945–56.
37. Akita S, Akino K, Hirano A, Ohtsuru A, Yamashita S. Mesenchymal stem cell therapy for cutaneous radiation syndrome. Health Phys. 2010;98(6):858–62.
38. Guo M, Dong Z, Qiao J, et al. Severe acute radiation syndrome: treatment of a lethally 60Co-source irradiated accident victim in China with HLA-mismatched peripheral blood stem cell transplantation and mesenchymal stem cells. J Radiat Res. 2014;55(2):205–9.

39. Manzanas Garcia A, Lopez Carrizosa MC, Vallejo Ocana C, et al. Superoxidase dismutase (SOD) topical use in oncologic patients: treatment of acute cutaneous toxicity secondary to radiotherapy. Clin Transl Oncol. 2008;10:163–7.
40. Tumilty S, Munn J, Abbott JH, McDonough S, Hurley DA, Baxter GD. Laser therapy in the treatment of Achilles tendinopathy: a pilot study. Photomed Laser Surg. 2008;26(1):25–30.
41. Yasukawa A, Hrui H, Koyama Y, Nagai M, Takakuda K. The effect of low reactive-level laser therapy (LLLT) with helium-neon laser on operative wound healing in a rat model. J Vet Med Sci. 2007;69(8):799.
42. Schindl A, Schindl M, Pernerstorfer-Schön H, Mossbacher U, Schindl L. Low intensity laser irradiation in the treatment of recalcitrant radiation ulcers in patients with breast cancer—long-term results of 3 cases. Photodermatol Photoimmunol Photomed. 2000;16(1):34–7.
43. Fujioka M. Surgical reconstruction of radiation injuries. Adv Wound Care. 2014;3:25–37.
44. Zhang X, Li H, Li Q, et al. Application of red light phototherapy in the treatment of radioactive dermatitis in patients with head and neck cancer. World J Surg Oncol. 2018;16:222.
45. Lee J, Jang H, Park S, et al. Platelet-rich plasma activates AKT signaling to promote wound healing in a mouse model of radiation-induced skin injury. J Transl Med. 2019;17:295.
46. Miller ED, Song F, Smith JD, et al. Plasma-based biomaterials for the treatment of cutaneous radiation injury. Wound Repair Regen. 2019;27:139–49.
47. Gerber SA, Cummings RJ, Judge JL, et al. Interleukin-12 preserves the cutaneous physical and immunological barrier after radiation exposure. Radiat Res. 2015;183:72–81.
48. Liu C, Cui J, Sun Q, et al. Hydrogen therapy may be an effective and specific novel treatment for acute radiation syndrome. Med Hypotheses. 2010;74:145–6.
49. Schoenfeld MP, Ansari RR, Zakrajsek JF, et al. Hydrogen therapy may reduce the risks related to radiation-induced oxidative stress in space flight. Med Hypotheses. 2011;76:117–8.
50. Watanabe S, Fujita M, Ishihara M, et al. Protective effect of inhalation of hydrogen gas on radiation-induced dermatitis and skin injury in rats. J Radiat Res. 2014;55:1107–13.

28 Extravasation Ulcers Following Chemotherapy

Ajay K. Khanna and Divya Khanna

Intravenous infusion is the principal modality of administration of anti-cancer drugs with numbers exceeding one million infusions each day worldwide [1]. Extravasation is one of the most dreaded complications when administering chemotherapy. It is defined either as the escape of a chemotherapeutic agent from a vessel into the surrounding tissues by leakage or as an involuntary injection of a drug into the tissues. The frequency of extravasation in adults is considered to be between 0.1% and 6% [2]. Extravasation ulcers following chemotherapy is unintended instillation or leakage of drugs into the perivascular space or into the subcutaneous tissue during injection or infusion of chemotherapy in various malignant diseases. The severity of tissue damage can be limited by quick detection of extravasations and swift treatment. A chemotherapeutic extravasation is considered an oncologic emergency. Chemotherapy extravasation is an accidental complication of chemotherapy administration and may result in serious damage to patients leading to severe morbidity, which is defined as the accidental infiltration of chemotherapy into the subcutaneous or sub-dermal tissue at the injection site, and can result in tissue necrosis, ulcerations, limb deformity, and even sometimes septicemia.

A. K. Khanna (✉)
Department of Surgery, Institute of Medical Sciences, Banaras Hindu University, Varanasi, Uttar Pradesh, India

D. Khanna
Department of Preventive Oncology, Mahamana Pandit Madan Mohan Malaviya Cancer Centre, Tata Memorial Centre, Varanasi, India

A. K. Khanna, S. K. Tiwary (eds.), *Uncommon Ulcers of the Extremities*, https://doi.org/10.1007/978-981-99-1782-2_28

28.1 Prevalence

Chemotherapy extravasation can range from 0.1% to 6% when chemotherapeutic drugs are administered through a peripheral intravenous access and from 0.26% to 4.7% when administered through a central venous access device. One of the major unsolved problems is the management of central venous devices after extravasation as drug may accumulate in the mediastinum, pleural space, or in the subcutaneous area of the chest or neck. Although the implantation of a Port-a-Cath® was initially considered safe, extravasation rates up to 4.7% have been reported [3].

28.2 Types of Chemotherapy as per Damage Potential

Intravenously administered drugs can be classified into five categories according to their damage potential: Vesicant, Exfoliants, Irritants, Inflammitants, and Neutrals.

Vesicants can result in tissue necrosis or formation of blisters when accidentally infused into tissue surrounding a vein. Vesicants are drugs that may cause severe and lasting tissue injury and necrosis. Symptoms may arise immediately after extravasation or appear after several days or weeks. Patients may complain of pain or local burning at the infusion site, mild erythema, itching, or swelling. Over time, the symptoms of erythema and pain may increase and a discoloration and induration of the skin, dry desquamation, or blistering may develop. In case of a significant extravasation, necrosis, eschar formation, and ulceration with involvement of underlying tissues may occur. The indolent ulceration lacks granulation tissue formation and there is little peripheral re-epithelization. Vesicant drugs are actinomycin D, dactinomycin, daunorubicin, doxorubicin, epirubicin, idarubicin, mitomycin C, vinblastine, vindesine, vincristine, and vinorelbine.

Exfoliants have low vesicant potential and these drugs cause inflammation and shedding of skin without causing underlying tissue death. Drugs may cause superficial tissue injury, blisters, and desquamation. They include aclacinomycin, cisplatin, docetaxel, liposomal doxorubicin, mitoxantrone, oxaliplatin, and paclitaxel.

Irritants cause inflammation, pain, or irritation at the extravasation site, without any blister formation. Irritants are drugs that can cause an inflammatory reaction, aching, swelling, pain, or phlebitis at the injection site or along the vein. They may cause sclerosis and hyperpigmentation along the vein, burning, local warmth, discomfort, erythema, or tenderness. These symptoms are self-limiting and there are no long-term sequelae. These drugs produce a burning sensation in the vein while being administered: Irritant drugs are: Bendamustine, bleomycin, carboplatin, dexrazoxane, etoposide, teniposide, and topotecan.

Inflammitants cause mild to moderate inflammation, painless skin erythema and elevation (flare reaction) at the extravasation site. They include bortezomib, 5-fluorouracil, methotrexate, and raltitrexed.

Table 28.1 Various types of chemotherapy as per damage potential

Neutrals	Asparaginase, bevacizumab, bleomycin, bortezomib, cetuximab, cyclophosphamide, cytarabarine, eribulin, fludarabine, gemcitabine, ifosfamide, melphenal, rituximab, trastuzumab
Inflammitants	Bortezomib, fluorouracil, methotrexate, raltitrexed
Irritants	Bendamustine, bleomycin, carboplatin, etoposide, teniposide, topotecan
Exfoliants	Aclacinomycin, cisplatin, docetaxel, doxorubicin, mitoxantrone, oxaliplatin, paclitaxel
Vesicants	Actinomycin D, dactinomycin, daunorubicin, doxorubicin, epirubicin, idarubicin, mitomycin C, vinblastine, vindesine, vincristine, vinorelbine

Neutrals neither cause inflammation nor damage upon extravasation. Monoclonal antibodies (rituximab and trastuzumab) are also listed under this category: Asparaginase, bevacizumab, bleomycin, bortezomib, cetuximab, cyclophosphamide, cytarabine, eribulin, fludarabine, gemcitabine, ifosfamide, melphalan, rituximab, and trastuzumab (Table 28.1).

28.3 Various Risk Factors Responsible

Drugs related: Various factors which can increase the vesicant properties of the drug are its concentration, volume, and duration of extravasation of infusion [4]. Factors that determine the extent of tissue damage from chemotherapy extravasation include its pH, osmolarity, vasoconstrictive potential, and duration for which it remains in tissue. Infusion solution whose pH is far from the physiologic pH (7.35–7.40) and/or osmolarity (281–282 mOsm/L) can irritate the venous endothelium and vessel wall and can damage the cell proteins and cause cell death. Hypertonic solutions can further increase tissue injury and lead to necrosis. Vesicants with high vasoconstrictive potential can result in tissue necrosis by severe vasoconstriction of capillary smooth muscles and reducing blood flow. Vesicants that are retained in extravasation tissue area for a long duration lead to a vicious cycle of direct cell injury. Typical examples are anthracyclines which enter the cells and bind to DNA causing immediate and continuous tissue injury. Conversely, vesicants that are easily metabolized and are not retained in tissue include vinca alkaloids and taxanes. Despite their ability to cause direct tissue damage, they cannot bind to DNA and are easily metabolized [5].

Patient related: Small and/or fragile veins, lymphedema, obesity, impaired level of consciousness, and having had previous multiple venipunctures are the various risk factors.

Iatrogenic: Lack of training of nurses, poor cannula size selection, poor location selection, and lack of time. Extravasation can occur upon accidental puncturing of the vein or upon movement of the cannula itself due to movement of the patient or insecure fixing. Prolonged peripheral line infusions of vesicants carry an increased risk of extravasation and vesicants should not be infused as prolonged unsupervised infusions via a peripheral vein.

28.4 Clinical Presentation

The extravasation can present as skin erythema to soft tissue necrosis. Chemotherapy extravasation is manifested by a wide range of symptoms that can be mild and can present as an acute burning pain, swelling at the infusion site, pain and erythema, induration, and skin discoloration which progresses over several days and weeks and may progress to blister formation. Blister formation or necrosis can lead to invasion and destruction of deeper structures. Damage can reach tendons, nerves, and joints depending on the location of the vein where extravasation occurs. Symptoms vary according to the amount and concentration of extravasated drug. Erythema may be associated with associated symptoms edema, pain, induration, phlebitis, ulceration, or necrosis and severe tissue damage [6] (Figs. 28.1, 28.2, 28.3, 28.4, 28.5, 28.6, 28.7, 28.8, and 28.9). **Grade of Damage**: Extravasation injuries can be divided into four grades ranging from 2, which is manifested by erythema with associated edema, pain, induration, and phlebitis, to grade 5, which refers to extravasation that leads to death. There is no grade 1 [7].

Grade of Damage [7]

Grade 1	Not available
Grade 2	Erythema with associated symptoms as oedema, pain, induration, phlebitis
Grade 3	Ulceration or necrosis, severe tissue damage, operative intervention indicated
Grade 4	Life threatening consequences, urgent intervention indicated
Grade 5	Death

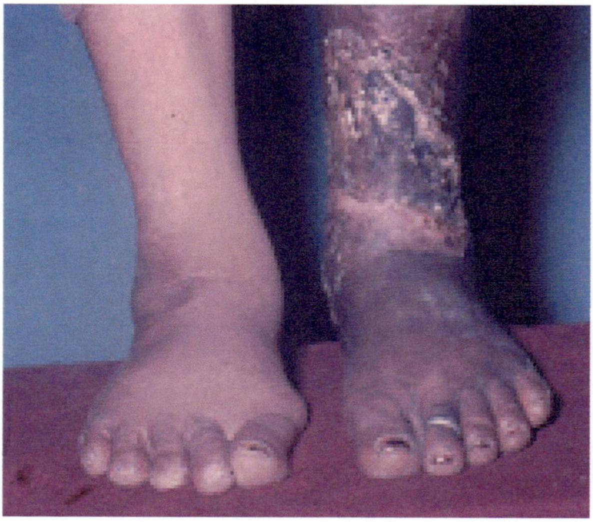

Fig. 28.1 Adriamycin extravasation

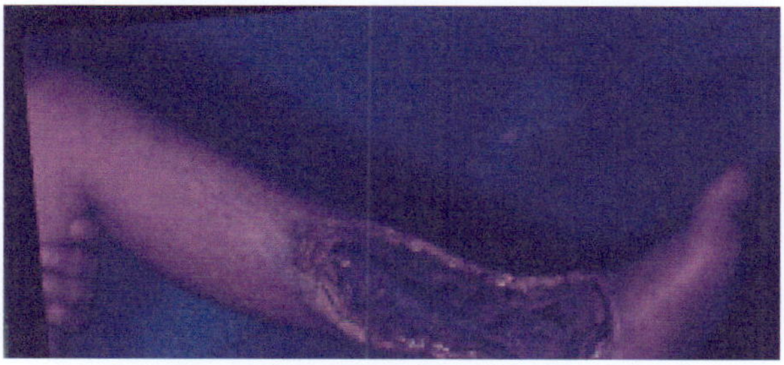

Fig. 28.2 Adriamycin extravasation with gangrenous patches

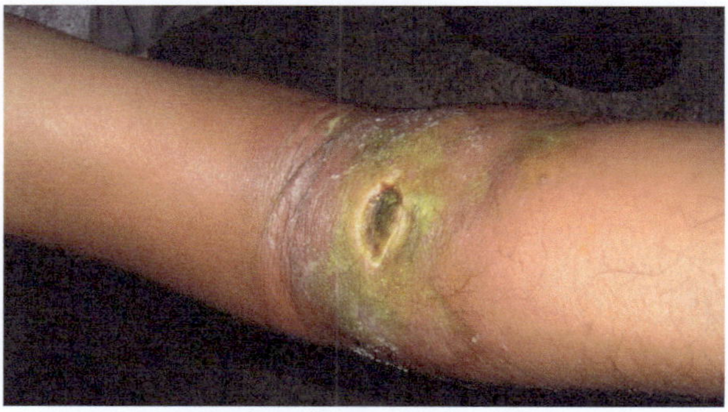

Fig. 28.3 Adriamycin extravasation in cubital fossa

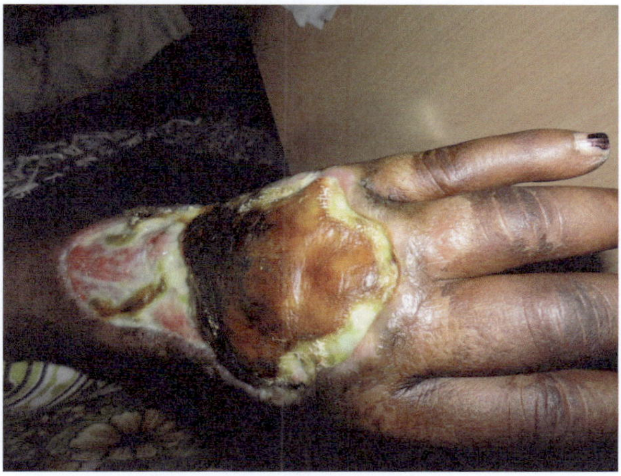

Fig. 28.4 Extravasation ulcer in dorsum of hand

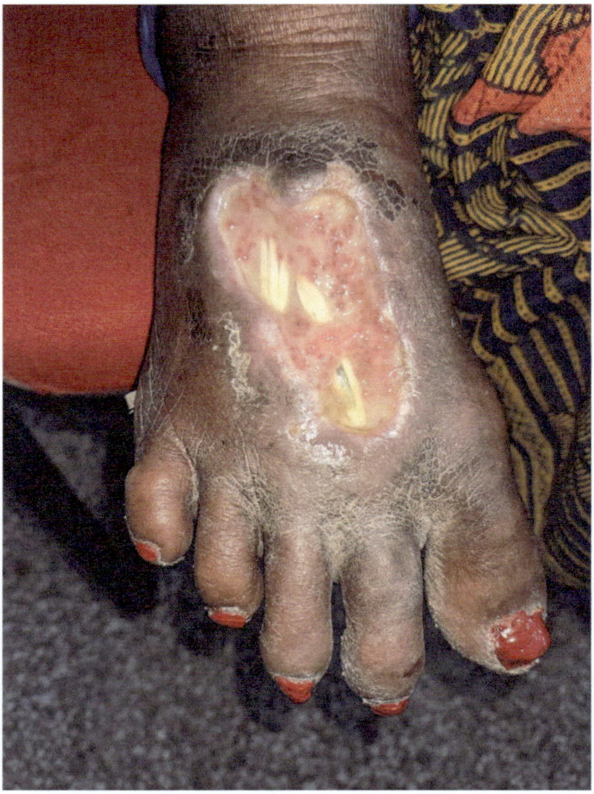

Fig. 28.5 Extravasation ulcer in dorsum of foot exposing tendons

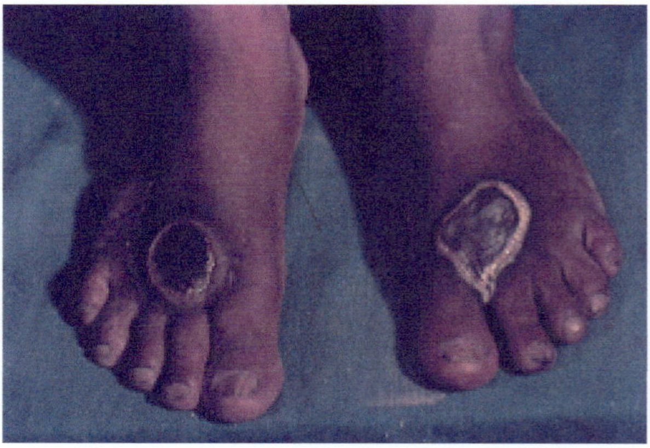

Fig. 28.6 Extravasation in bilateral dorsum of foot with necrosed patches

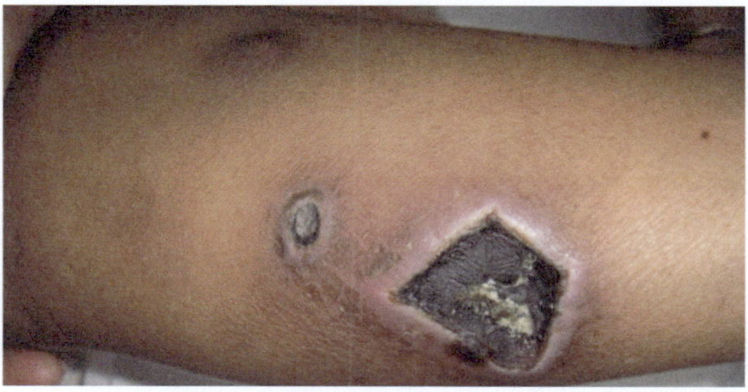

Fig. 28.7 Extravasation ulcer in cubital fossa

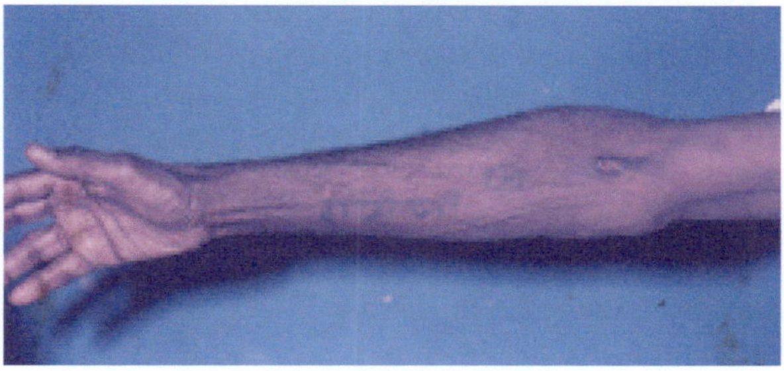

Fig. 28.8 Mitomycin C extravasation in cubital fossa

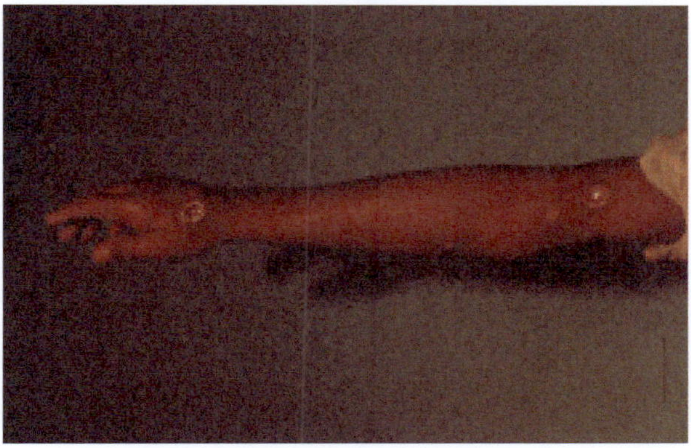

Fig. 28.9 Extravasation ulcer in two places wrist and cubital fossa in same limb

28.5 Prevention

In all departments where cytotoxic drugs are given, written guidelines for handling cytotoxic agents and procedures in case of extravasation should be present. In addition to these guidelines, an extravasation kit, with all the necessary material and drugs to treat extravasation, should be present.

Education and training among nurses and physicians remains the mainstay of safe chemotherapy administration and emphasizes the importance of being preemptive instead of reactive to extravasation.

A cytotoxic agent should not be administered in an extremity if within the previous 48 h there was venopuncture above the place of insertion of the catheter. Consideration of the appropriate vascular access is crucial for the prevention of chemotherapy extravasation. Chemotherapy infusion can be either through a central venous access or through an adequate peripheral vein. Veins that are small and/or fragile should be avoided as they might not withstand the required flow and rate of infusion and may have a lower threshold for extravasation. Locations that are also generally avoided include the dorsum of the hand, the antecubital fossa, and the radial and ulnar aspects of forearm. Patients who do not have adequate peripheral venous access should have a central venous catheter placed.

Peripheral arm assessment consists of: (a) assessing location and fragility of the patient's veins that can be reflected by the inspection and palpation of the vein. Veins that have a small caliber and/or are superficial are generally considered fragile and should be avoided. In addition, assessment also consists of (b) patient's age; (c) presence of diabetes; (d) steroid use; (e) history of previous venipunctures; (f) presence or absence of ecchymosis; (g) prior hospitalization or blood drawing history; (h) lymphedema; (i)vascular accident in an extremity. The level of consciousness of the patient should be also assessed for the purpose of assuring immobility and compliance during catheter insertion [8].

The catheter should never be inserted in a limb that is affected by lymphoedema or has a neurological weakness. Veins adjacent to tendons, nerves, or arteries should be avoided, while areas of high venous pressure should not be used. Selection of the appropriate cannula type and size plays an important role in chemotherapy extravasation prevention. The ideal cannula is one that can remain patent to allow blood flow and that does not dislodge from its place. The recommended choice is to use the smallest size of adequate and appropriate cannula in the largest vein available. Use of 1.2–1.5 cm long small bore plastic cannula and a clear dressing that shows any possible extravasation beneath it are recommended. A butterfly needle should never be used for vesicant chemotherapy administration. Before administering a cytotoxic agent, the catheter is flushed by a free flowing infusion with normal saline 0.9% or glucose 5% solution for at least 5 min. At the end of the administration of a cytotoxic drug, the same procedure is repeated [9].

Patients should be instructed to report any discomfort, pain, redness, or swelling at infusion sites. Nurses and physicians should never underestimate the significance of any patient symptom and check the infusion site and venous patency immediately. Close monitoring of the infusion site every 5–10 min and avoiding infusion of vesicants for more than 30–60 min.

Continuous monitoring at the beginning and during the infusion is essential every 5–10 min. Cancer centers should ensure the availability of "Extravasation Kits" at the treatment units. These kits should contain disposable syringes, cannulas, cold-hot packs, gauze pads, adhesive plaster, gloves, and antidotes that can be used in cases of extravasation [6].

There should also be a form to report the extravasation to the authorities (hospital direction, legal department, nursing department).

28.6 What To Do in Case of Extravasation

28.6.1 General Management of Extravasation

General measures after extravasation of nonvesicants basically include the following:

1. Stop injection/infusion immediately.
2. Get extravasation kit.
3. Put on sterile gloves.
4. Replace infusion lead or syringe with 5 mL disposable syringe and aspirate slowly as much as possible of the extravasated drug.
5. Remove i. v. access while aspirating.
6. Elevate limb and immobilize.
7. Complete extravasation documentation sheet (mention extent of extravasation).
8. Inform and instruct the patient and relatives.
9. Follow the patient regularly until full resolution of symptoms [10].

In case of extravasation, occlusive dressings or moist heat or cold should never be applied, as this increases the risk of skin maceration or necrosis.

Many chemotherapeutic agents do not have known antidotes that are safe to use in order to neutralize their toxic activity. It is important to note that the first goal of treatment is to immediately either localize the extravasated agent or disperse the agent. The choice of localization or dispersion depends on the chemotherapeutic agents. Cold compress will help to constrict local blood vessels and localize tissue damage. Warm compress will act in the opposite, aiding to disperse the chemotherapeutic into surrounding tissues. The second goal of treatment is to neutralize the chemotherapeutic once localized or dilute the agent to allow it to be absorbed and consequently metabolized.

In case of chemotherapy extravasation and as soon as the patient complains of pain or swelling, the first step should be immediate cessation of the infusion while keeping the cannula or port needle in place. This is followed by attempts at aspiration of the chemotherapeutic agent and removing the cannula or port needle.

Aspiration of the drug is usually done by a 10 mL syringe, percutaneous needle aspiration, liposuction, simple squeeze maneuver, or by surgical fenestration and irrigation. Catheter can then be removed if there are no antidotes that need to be infused at the extravasated site. Elevation of the affected limb and thermal application by either cold or hot packs should follow. Elevation of the limb helps in reabsorption of the extravasated agent by decreasing capillary hydrostatic pressure and it is recommended during the first 24–48 h of the incident.

Dexrazoxane is a member of the bisdioxopiperazine family and is an FDA-approved antidote for intravenous anthracycline extravasation. The exact mechanism by which it reduces tissue damage resulting from chemotherapy extravasation is unknown. Dexrazoxane is an iron chelator that prevents anthracycline-iron complexes and free radical formation causing oxidative damage. Furthermore, dexrazoxane has a protective effect on healthy tissue by stabilizing topoisomerase II, thereby preventing damage from anthracycline. This mechanism of action is responsible for its ability to reduce the cardiotoxicity associated with anthracyclines, such as doxorubicin [11, 12].

Hyaluronidase is an enzyme that degrades hyaluronic acid in tissues and promotes diffusion of the extravasated agent. Multiple subcutaneous injections of Hyaluronidase 100–150 units may be injected. Hyaluronidase is an enzyme that degrades hyaluronic acid, improving the absorption of the extravasated drugs into circulation where they can be metabolized. A study with seven human patients with accidental vinca alkaloid extravasation showed no skin necrosis after local treatment with hyaluronidase. Data from this study showed use of a 150 U/mL solution of hyaluronidase injected through the existing catheter line was beneficial. The dose was 1:1, 1 mL hyaluronidase (150 U/mL) for every 1 mL of extravasated drug. Warm compresses help disperse vinca alkaloids, which helps minimize vesicant toxicity [13].

Dimethyl sulfoxide (DMSO) is an organosulfur solvent that is topically applied to improve absorption of the extravasated solvent. In cases of anthracyclines extravasation, the combination of DMSO and cooling is most commonly described initial therapy for minor anthracyclines extravasation, especially when dexrazoxane is not available. DMSO has been used with success in human anthracycline extravasation. In humans, topical DMSO was applied immediately after extravasation covering twice the area affected. This treatment was repeated twice daily for 14 days with resolution. It is important to note that concomitant use of DMSO and dexrazoxane is not recommended and has been shown, in mice, to decrease dexrazoxane efficacy. However, in a case report of 4 dogs with doxorubicin extravasation, all dogs received dexrazoxane along with topical 90% DMSO ointment every 8 h for 14 days; only 1 dog required surgical debridement but all survived with medical management. Evidence to support DMSO use for doxorubicin extravasation exists; however, the strength and variability of that data do not support DMSO's use as first-line treatment of doxorubicin extravasation [14–18].

Sodium thiosulfate: It is an antidote generally recommended for mechlorethamine (nitrogen mustard) extravasation.

Local injection of corticosteroids has been hypothesized to accelerate wound healing and prevent ulcer formation. Local injection of granulocyte macrophage colony-stimulating factor, which is a glycoprotein growth factor, has been reported to be beneficial to wound healing in cases of doxorubicin extravasation. Local injection of corticosteroids has been hypothesized to accelerate wound healing and prevent ulcer formation. While in vitro animal experimental studies showed no prevention of ulcer formation after corticosteroid injection, it was reported to have clinical benefit on ulcer prevention when used on humans. Variable results have been reported regarding the success of wound healing after the use of local corticosteroids, which depends on the amount of inflammatory cells generated at the site of extravasation. Local injection of granulocyte macrophage colony-stimulating factor, which is a glycoprotein growth factor, has been reported to be beneficial to wound healing in cases of doxorubicin extravasation. The mechanism is believed to be through stimulation of cellular components such as fibroblasts and endothelial cells [19]. Evaluation of blood flow by indocyanine green angiography in the extravasation area predicts the extent of damage and the need of future surgical intervention [20]. ICG angiography was therefore considered a good indicator of local perfusion and a predictor of tissue damage. This method, which can be performed on an outpatient basis, was suitable to identify patients at risk early after extravasation of vesicants.

Indications for surgery in chemotherapy extravasation include full-thickness skin necrosis, chronic ulcer, and persistent pain. It is crucial that all necrotic tissue be removed until bleeding occurs and only healthy tissue left for wound coverage. To ensure complete excision, some surgeons use intraoperative fluorescent dye injection to detect the doxorubicin HCl in the tissue to ensure complete excision. After this, either immediate or delayed surgical reconstruction and skin grafting can be performed [21].

Vacuum-assisted closure (VAC) dressing, this method applies a negative pressure to the wound, aids in aspiration of extravasated vesicant, and improves its environment. There are only few reports in which negative pressure wound healing (NPWH) was used for vesicant extravasation [22].

Hyperbaric oxygen therapy: Hyperbaric oxygen therapy (HBO) is defined by the Undersea and Hyperbaric Medical Society as a therapy consisting of intermittent breathing 100% oxygen in a chamber whose pressure is greater than atmospheric pressure. Its role in chemotherapy extravasation is still unclear, but it is believed that HBO increases production of oxygen free radicals and thus can aid in extravasation wound healing [23, 24].

28.7 Specific Drugs Interactions

Anthracyclines: Although all vesicants can cause tissue damage upon extravasation, anthracyclines, such as daunorubicin, doxorubicin, epirubicin, and idarubicin, have the greatest vesicant potential when compared to other chemotherapeutic agents. While all chemotherapeutic agents cause similar signs upon extravasation, anthracyclines are characterized by causing immediate pain and burning sensation, which can last up to hours and can be severe. Lesions form slowly over weeks and expand over periods of months due to tissue retention of the extravasant vesicant. Weeks after the extravasation episode, surrounding tissue may become red, firm, and tender. The resolution of redness depends on the size of the extravasation area. If the area is small in size, redness will gradually resolve over the following weeks. If extravasation is significant, the center of the redness area becomes necrotic and painful. The accidental leak of anthracyclines can cause severe tissue damage. By cellular uptake and remaining for an extended period of time in tissue, they cause a continuous vicious cycle of tissue damage [25].

Epirubicin is an anthracycline chemotherapy agent used for treatment of several cancers including esophageal, breast, and gastric. Extravasation is a well-recognized and serious complication of any intravenous therapies but especially chemotherapeutic agents. Signs of the injury can be subtle and without prompt recognition and treatment there can be extensive tissue damage and depending on location of injury this can result in significant functional [26].

Vinca alkaloids: Vinca alkaloids, which include vinblastine, vincristine, and vinorelbine, can cause direct cellular damage upon extravasation. Extravasation is known to cause a mostly painful ulceration, local paresthesia, and slow healing. It can cause significant irritation and usually presents with intense pain around intravenous line or port site, erythema, and tenderness. Erythema may be delayed by 1–2 h and even 3 d depending on the dosage of the vinca alkaloid administered. This is followed by blister formation, swelling, and induration and can be complicated by sloughing, ulceration, and tissue necrosis. Vinorelbine, which is a moderate vesicant, also causes common irritation and burning sensations which are prevented by proper dilution, short infusion time, and use of an adequately large vein [27].

Taxanes: Taxanes, including docetaxel and paclitaxel, are most often classified by literature as vesicants although there is no clear delineation. Most reactions following extravasation of taxanes consist of erythema, tenderness, and swelling. There are case reports of patients who had necrosis and skin exfoliation. It is rare that taxane extravasation requires surgical debridement [28].

Oxaliplatin: Platinum compounds have been classified as irritants. Oxaliplatin has been recently reported to have vesicant properties. Extravasation usually begins with a palpable swelling and discomfort upon palpation. Lesion usually progresses to erythematous painful lesions and resemble erysipelas. Long-term outcome is usually healing and necrosis and surgical debridement are rarely needed. The harm caused by oxaliplatin extravasation is not comparable to that of anthracyclines and vinca alkaloids [29].

Mitomycin C (MMC) is a DNA-alkylating chemotherapeutic agent mostly used in the treatment of adenocarcinomas of the gastrointestinal tract. Due to its toxicity, inadvertent extravasation of this medication can cause local skin and soft tissue injury. Acute symptoms are mild with erythema, swelling, and pain. Weeks later, indolent ulcerations can appear with severe local necrosis, resembling doxorubicin extravasation [24, 30–33].

28.8 Conclusion

Safe administration of chemotherapy and prevention of extravasation is a shared responsibility among medical team members. Education of patients about risks and manifestations is essential. Prevention of chemotherapy extravasation is an important quality indicator for certification of chemotherapy infusion centers. While only some healthcare institutions devise their own policies and guidelines regarding extravasation prevention and management, there is a need to have local institution education, training, and guidelines. All institutions that administer intravenous chemotherapy should have known antidotes available. In spite of all efforts to prevent, accidental extravasation still occurs and more research for antidote for many drugs is needed.

References

1. Coyle CE, Griffie J, Czaplewski LM. Eliminating extravasation events: a multidisciplinary approach. J Infus Nurs. 2014;37:157–64.
2. Schrijvers DL. Extravasation: a dreaded complication of chemotherapy. Ann Oncol. 2003;14(Suppl 3):iii26–30. https://doi.org/10.1093/annonc/mdg744. © 2003 European Society for Medical Oncology.
3. Haslik W, Hacker S, Felberbauer FX, Thallinger C, Bartsch R, Kornauth C, et al. Port-a-Cath extravasation of vesicant cytotoxics: surgical options for a rare complication of cancer chemotherapy. Eur J Surg Oncol. 2015;41(3):378–85.
4. Reynolds PM, MacLaren R, Mueller SW, Fish DN, Kiser TH. Management of extravasation injuries: a focused evaluation of noncytotoxic medications. Pharmacotherapy. 2014;34:617–32.
5. Doellman D, Hadaway L, Bowe-Geddes LA, Franklin M, LeDonne J, Papke-O'Donnell L, Pettit J, Schulmeister L, Stranz M. Infiltration and extravasation: update on prevention and management. J Infus Nurs. 2009;32:203–11. https://doi.org/10.1097/NAN.0b013e3181aac042. PMID: 19605999.
6. Cassagnol M, McBride A. Management of chemotherapy extravasations. US Pharm. 2009;34(9):3–11.
7. El-Saghir N, Otrock Z, Mufarrij. U.S. Department of Health and Human Services, National Institutes of Health, National Cancer Institute: Common Terminology Criteria for Adverse Events (CTCAE) (V4.0, May 2009); 2015.
8. Pérez Fidalgo JA, García Fabregat L, Cervantes A, Margulies A, Vidall C, Roila F. Management of chemotherapy extravasation: ESMO—EONS clinical practice guidelines. Eur J Oncol Nurs. 2012;16:528–34. https://doi.org/10.1016/j.ejon.2012.09.004. PMID: 23304728.
9. Schrijvers DL. Extravasation: a dreaded complication of chemotherapy. Ann Oncol. 2003;14 Suppl 3:iii26–30. https://doi.org/10.1093/annonc/mdg744. PMID: 12821535.
10. Mader I, Furst-Weger P, Mader RM, Nogler-Semenitz E, Wassertheurer S. Extravasation of cytotoxic agents. 2nd ed. Wien: Springer; 2010.
11. Mouridsen HT, Langer SW, Buter J, et al. Treatment of anthracycline extravasation with savene (dexrazoxane): results from two prospective clinical multicenter studies. Ann Oncol. 2007;18:546–50.
12. Langer SW, Sehested M, Jensen PB. Treatment of anthracycline extravasation with dexrazoxane. Clin Cancer Res. 2000;6:3680–6.
13. Bertelli G, Dini D, Forno GB, et al. Hyaluronidase as an antidote to extravasation of vinca alkaloids: clinical results. J Cancer Res Clin Oncol. 1994;120:505–6.
14. Fidalgo JA, Pérez L, García Fabregat A, et al. Management of chemotherapy extravasation: ESMO-EONS clinical practice guidelines. Ann Oncol. 2012;23(Suppl 7):vii167–73. Oxford University Press.
15. Venable RO, Saba CF, Endicott MM, et al. Dexrazoxane treatment of doxorubicin extravasation injury in four dogs. J Am Vet Med Assoc. 2012;240(3):304–7.
16. Langer SW. Extravasation of chemotherapy. Curr Oncol Rep. 2010;12(4):242–6. https://doi.org/10.1007/s11912-010-0110-7.
17. Langer SW, Thougaard AV, Sehested M, Jensen PB. Treatment of anthracycline extravasation in mice with dexrazoxane with or without DMSO and hydrocortisone. Cancer Chemother Pharmacol. 2006;57(1):125–8. https://doi.org/10.1007/s00280-005-0022-7.
18. Bertelli G, Gozza A, Forno GB, et al. Topical dimethylsulfoxide for the prevention of soft tissue injury after extravasation of vesicant cytotoxic drugs: a prospective clinical study. J Clin Oncol. 1995;13:2851–5.
19. Hong WK, Bast RC, Hait WN, Kufe DW, Pollock RE, Weichselbaum RR, Holland JF III, Frei E. Cancer medicine, vol. 8. PMPHUSA Ltd; 2010. http://www.pmph-usa.com/t/medicine/general-medicine/p/CM8.

20. Pluschnig U, Haslik W, Bartsch R, Made RM. Extravasation emergencies: state-of-the-art management and progress in clinical research. Memo. 2016;9(4):226–30. https://doi.org/10.1007/s12254-016-0304-2.
21. Al-Benna S, O'Boyle C, Holley J. Extravasation injuries in adults. ISRN Dermatol. 2013;2013:856541. https://doi.org/10.1155/2013/856541. PMID: 23738141.
22. Lucchina S, Fusetti C. Surgical vacuum-assisted closure for treatment of vinorelbine extravasation. Chin J Traumatol. 2009;12:247–9. PMID: 19635221.
23. Gill AL, Bell CN. Hyperbaric oxygen: its uses, mechanisms of action and outcomes. QJM. 2004;97:385–95. https://doi.org/10.1093/qjmed/hch074. PMID: 15208426.
24. Kreidieh FY, Moukadem HA, El Saghir NS. Overview, prevention and management of chemotherapy extravasation. World J Clin Oncol. 2016;7(1):87–97.
25. Conde-Estévez D, Mateu-de Antonio J. Treatment of anthracycline extravasations using dexrazoxane. Clin Transl Oncol. 2014;16:11–7. https://doi.org/10.1007/s12094-013-1100-7. PMID: 23949792.
26. Hale O, Deutsch PG, Lahiri A. Epirubicin extravasation: consequences of delayed management. BMJ Case Rep. 2017;2017:bcr2016218012. https://doi.org/10.1136/bcr-2016. Published 2017 Jan 6.
27. Heijmen L, Vehof J, van Laarhoven HW. Blistering of the hand in a breast cancer patient. Extravasation. Neth J Med. 2011;69(82):85. PMID: 21411846.
28. El Saghir NS, Otrock ZK. Docetaxel extravasation into the normal breast during breast cancer treatment. Anti-Cancer Drugs. 2004;15:401–4. https://doi.org/10.1097/00001813-200404000-00013. PMID: 15057145.
29. Ener RA, Meglathery SB, Styler M. Extravasation of systemic hemato-oncological therapies. Ann Oncol. 2004;15:858–62. https://doi.org/10.1093/annonc/mdh214. PMID: 15151940.
30. Mieczkowska K, Deutsch A, Amin B, et al. Mitomycin extravasation injury: a case series. JAAD Case Rep. 2021;15:69–72. https://doi.org/10.1016/j.jdcr.2021.06.029. Published 2021 Jul 13.
31. Pattison J. Managing cytotoxic extravasation. Nurs Times. 2002;98:32–3.
32. Khanna AK, Khanna A, Asthana AK, Misra MK. Mitomycin C extravasation ulcers. J Surg Oncol. 1985;28(2):108–10. https://doi.org/10.1002/jso.2930280207. PMID: 3918215.
33. Gault DT. Extravasation injuries. Br J Plast Surg. 1993;46(2):91–6.

29 Diathermy Burn Ulcers

Seema Khanna

Electrosurgical units, also called as surgical diathermy are an integral part of any surgical operation theater. They are an indispensable tool for general surgery, all surgical super-specialties, gynecology, orthopedics, ophthalmology, otorhinolaryngology, dermatology, dentistry. Recent advancements in energy devices have led to the introduction of newer modalities such as ultrasound based scalpel device, feedback dependent auto shutdown devices, hybrid devices, radiofrequency ablators, and laser energy devices. However, electrosurgical units (ESU) remain the primary workhorse of the operating surgeon. The advent of laparoscopic surgery has led to further refinements of ESU equipment as well as appearance of newer aspects of safety issues and complications.

Surgical diathermy was invented by Bovie and its first use is credited to Cushing (1927) who used it for the removal of intra-cranial tumors [1]. Although they are extremely safe and the newer versions come with enhanced safety features yet complications to the patient and to the operating room personnel have been reported off and on. The true incidence of diathermy complications is probably more than what is generally believed in the absence of reliable reporting. In USA 500–600 cases of surgical fires are estimated to occur every year [2]. Besides causing harm and occasional death in the patient, destruction of operation room infrastructure, ESU related complications are an important cause of malpractice suits.

S. Khanna (✉)
Department of Surgery, Institute of Medical Sciences, Banaras Hindu University, Varanasi, India

A. K. Khanna, S. K. Tiwary (eds.), *Uncommon Ulcers of the Extremities*,
https://doi.org/10.1007/978-981-99-1782-2_29

29.1 Principles of Surgical Diathermy

Surgical diathermy involves the use of high frequency AC electric current either to cauterize small blood vessels or as a cutting modality. The ESU receives alternating current from the electrical supply at 50–60 Hz and converts it into electromagnetic current in excess of 200 KHz. Depending on the wavelength, diathermy can be used to cut, coagulate, desiccate, or fulgurate tissues.

There are two main modes of electrode configuration used in surgical diathermy [3]:

1. Monopolar mode: Where current flows from an active electrode placed near or in contact with the tissue to be treated to a passive or indifferent or dispersive electrode in contact with the patient's skin elsewhere in the body. The passive electrode is usually in a wide area of contact with the skin of the buttocks or legs.
2. Bipolar mode: Where both the active and passive electrodes are mounted on a pen like device or forceps. The tissue under treatment is grasped between the two electrodes and the current flows only through this tissue and does not spread to other parts of the body. Thus, bipolar mode is a much safer mode compared to monopolar mode.

In patients with cardiac pacemakers only the bipolar diathermy can be used. Use of monopolar diathermy is contraindicated because dispersal of current through the body can interfere with the rhythm and setting of the pacemaker. For the same reason burn injuries are a more frequent occurrence with use of monopolar compared to bipolar diathermy.

29.2 Safety Precautions During Use of ESUs

Besides technical failure, improper or careless use of ESUs can result in burn injuries at the local or distal site, lead to smoke inhalation by OR personnel, and is also a fire hazard. Some simple safety precautions are mandatory when using an ESU especially of the monopolar variety.

1. Ensure good electrical contact between a large area of the skin of patient's back and the dispersive or patient plate which contains the indifferent electrode in monopolar diathermy. Ideally the entire buttock or back of thigh should be in contact. The size of the dispersive electrode pad should be at least 70 cm^2 in area to carry sufficient current back to the ESU and avoid thermal injury at the site.
2. Ensure that patient is not in unintended contact with a metal object which can cause capacitive leakage of current to earth or ground. This can lead to burn at the site of contact (Fig. 29.1).
3. Check that sufficient electrolyte gel is present on the dispersive electrode pad and its wires are in good condition. Disruption of the electrical circuit at the pad can lead to shocks and burns.

Fig. 29.1 Diathermy burns at calf region due to inadequate adhesive jelly on dispersive electrode

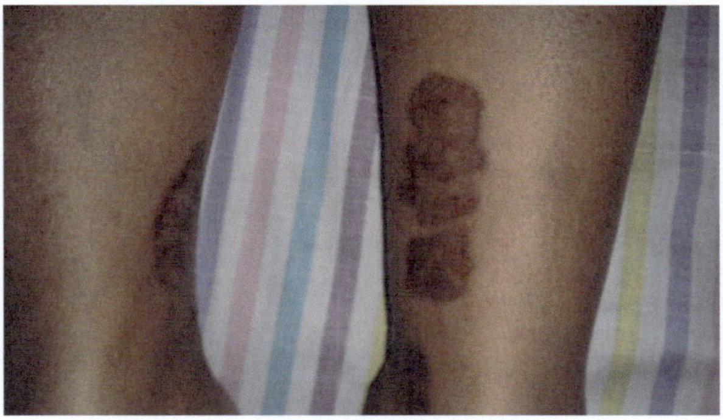

4. Place the dispersive electrode pad on the same side as the surgical procedure and as close as possible to the active electrode.
5. If the patient has a metallic implant, e.g.: a hip implant, the dispersive electrode pad should be placed in such a position that the metallic object does not lie in the path of the returning current.
6. If alcohol based disinfectant has been used for the skin prep it should be allowed to dry before using the active electrode. OR personnel should check that spirit and alcohol based disinfectant have not pooled below the patient on the operation table.
7. Operation theater should ideally have a gas scavenging system to evacuate the diathermy generated smoke. Failing which a pedestal fan should run behind the surgeon to disperse the smoke and vapors generated.
8. Surgeon should check his gloves for any minute perforation or internal hydration due to sweating or fluid seepage which can cause burn to the surgeon's fingertips.

29.3 ESU Related Injuries

Intraoperative injuries secondary to use of ESU are broadly categorized as

(a) Thermal injuries
(b) Diathermy smoke related injuries
(c) ESU related fires
(d) ESU related explosion
(e) Malfunction of electromagnetic devices implanted in patient

29.3.1 Thermal Injuries Due to ESU Use

These injuries can be direct or indirect. Direct injuries are the result of accidental application of the active electrode at an unintended site on the patient. Indirect thermal injury is a consequence of accidental contact of the active electrode to a metal instrument such as a forceps which is in contact to a tissue not intended for diathermy. Another mode of indirect injury is due to spread of current from the shaft of active electrode to tissue in contact.

29.3.2 Mechanisms of Thermal Injury During Diathermy Use

29.3.2.1 Injuries Caused by Active Electrode

1. Inadvertent contact of active electrode with neighboring tissue
2. Inadvertent activation of active electrode due to accidental compression of foot pedal
3. Damage to insulation sleeve of active electrode
4. Inappropriate placement of a hot electrode on patient's skin
5. Channeling of current along vascular pedicles, nerves, or adhesions
6. Perforated gloves or throughout hydrated gloves of operating surgeons

29.3.2.2 Injuries Caused by Dispersive Electrode Pads

1. Poor contact of electrode with patient's skin: either due to small area of contact or drying of the conductive jelly
2. Dispersive electrode placed over bony prominence
3. Dispersive electrode close to ECG leads

29.3.2.3 Injuries Caused by Diversion of Current

Capacitive coupling: This is the induction of stray current to a surrounding conductor through the intact insulation of an active electrode. This is a problem in laparoscopic surgery where active electrode is separated from a metal trocar only by its insulation sheath. The metal trocar gets electrified and the current gets harmlessly dispersed through the abdominal wall. However, if the electrified trocar is separated from the abdominal wall by insulation, then inadvertent contact of trocar with viscera can cause serious injury.

29.3.3 Clinical Profile of Diathermy Induced Skin Burns

The incidence of thermal cutaneous burns due to diathermy was estimated to be 1–2 patients per thousand operation 25 years ago [4]. With the improvement in ESU devices and enhanced safety features the incidence of such burns is negligible now. Most ESU machines now have auto-sensors which prevent activation of the active electrode until the complete electrical circuits including the dispersive electrode are properly positioned and in sound working condition. However technical failures and ignorance of proper usage of the ESU may still lead to an occasional thermal injury.

Diathermy burns are usually detected after the operation. On the evening of surgery the patient may complain of pain or burning sensation at the site where the dispersive electrode was placed or any other site where inadvertent earthing of current took place. The erythema at the site may initially be mistaken for allergic reaction to the disinfectant solution because it is a much more common occurrence than

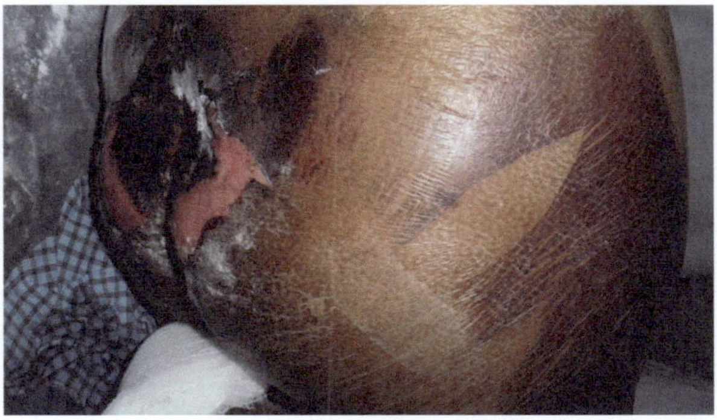

Fig. 29.2 Accidental deep burns at site other than dispersive electrode due to fluid accumulation

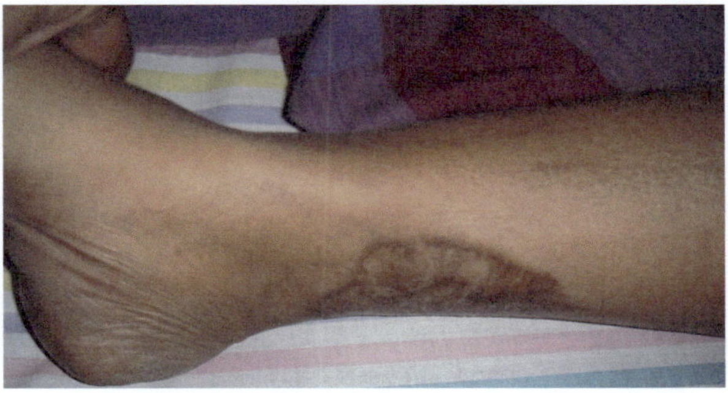

Fig. 29.3 Superficial burn at inactive electrode site

diathermy burns. Burns over the sacrum or heel are likely to be mistaken for pressure sores. Superficial burns may cause only skin erythema which resolves over few days. Deeper burns may start ulcerating after 2–3 days of injury (Fig. 29.2).

When a diathermy burn ulcerates it will take a longer time to heal. This is due to the thrombosis of superficial blood vessels in surrounding skin. The floor of the ulcer will require debridement to remove slough and necrotic tissues. Almost all such ulcers will undergo primary healing over next 2–3 weeks. However there are reports of larger ulcers needing closure with skin graft or flap. Such type of diathermy burns is most commonly located over the gluteal or sacral areas where disinfectant fluid, blood, or leaking urine is most likely to accumulate.

Several reports have pointed out that the commonest cause of electro-surgery burns is use of monopolar diathermy with improperly placed grounding electrode [5]. A loose grounding pad will cause local heat generation and sparking at the contact site. A minimum of 70 cm^2 of firm, hair free skin to grounding pad contact should be ensured. Preferably it should be secured with an adhesive bandage. If the patient's position is changed during surgery, the positioning of the dispersive pad should be checked and adjusted as required. Pads with adhesive properties should be preferred. Most ESUs come with an alarm system which will prevent activation of the electrode if the dispersive pad is not in secure position. Use of bipolar diathermy will eliminate possibility of such type of burn injuries (Fig. 29.3).

29.3.4 Association Between Type of Surgical Procedure and Diathermy Burns

Certain procedures such as tumor ablation and laparoscopic and orthopedic surgery require longer periods of electrocautery use sometimes at higher current settings. Such procedures have a higher risk of diathermy injuries. Also at higher risk are procedures where an intraoperative change of position is required as displacement of dispersive pad may occur. It is recommended that the ESU should be set at short duration duty cycles with auto cutoff after a certain time of 10–15 s.

The causes leading to diathermy associated burn injuries can be categorized into three main groups:

(a) Equipment failure related
(b) OR personnel oversight related
(c) Operative draping and disinfection fluid related

29.3.4.1 Equipment Failure Related

Electrosurgical units with capacity to monitor patient grounding pad contact impedance only should be used. Such machines will automatically switch off if the contact is inadequate or the grounding wire has come loose from the pad. Disposable neutral electrode pads with conductive gel coating although a little expensive should be preferred. Such electrodes are pliant and can be wrapped around the calf or thigh to ensure a good large area contact. These pads adhere firmly even if there is excessive sweating or fluid collection. Also they negate the issue of surface contour irregularity, scars, and creases which can impede a satisfactory contact with a rigid plate electrode.

29.3.4.2 OR Personnel Oversight Related

The surgeon needs to take overall responsibility for all OR events barring those which are under the control of the anesthesiologist. All nursing and technical staff should be familiar with diathermy machine, its potential hazards and the fine tuning required as per the demands of the surgical procedure. This becomes even more relevant when a new machine is procured or there is shifting of OR staff from one OR to another.

29.3.4.3 Operative Draping and Disinfectant Fluid Related

While scrubbing the patient with disinfectant fluid, the surgeon should ensure that the fluid does not seep under the patient or gets pooled up under other potential sites of earthing such as the blood pressure cuff. If cotton drapes are placed before the alcoholic disinfectant has entirely dried up, the linen may act as a wick to draw the solution up to the operative site. Further alcohol vapors trapped under the drapes may be channeled to the operative site and get ignited when a diathermy electrode is activated [6].

When alcohol based disinfectants are used, the surgeon must wait for the solution to evaporate before starting surgery. The hairs must be shaved to prevent pooling of the disinfectant. A safer option is to use povidone iodine or chlorhexidine instead.

29.3.5 Capacitive Coupling Burn

These are also called as alternate site burns because they occur at unusual sites which are not in the surgical field. An interesting case of forehead burn in a patient with titanium plates in her skull illustrates this variety of diathermy burn injuries. The titanium plates had been implanted earlier during a surgery for skull anomalies. The patient was placed prone on the operation table with the grounding pad on the lateral side of thigh. This resulted in capacitive coupling between the active electrode and the alternate grounding source which was the titanium skull plate [7, 8].

Capacitive coupling occurs when an aberrant intraoperative current is created by metallic objects in contact with the body of patient. Such injuries occur when the site comes in contact with metallic IV drip stand, uninsulated area of operation table, ECG leads, temperature probes, or sites of leads of monitoring devices.

29.3.6 Supplemented Oxygen Induced Fire

Patients undergoing surgical procedures of the face and neck region are at risk of fire injury if electrocautery is used in presence of inhalational oxygen. A safe method is to employ endotracheal intubation for delivering of oxygen. However, if a mask or nasal prong is used, then oxygen enriched atmosphere is a fire hazard when electrocautery is used [8].

29.4 Diathermy Injuries and Malpractice Suits

Although electrocautery associated injuries are extremely rare yet when they do occur they may become the reason for malpractice litigation. The important question that arises is whether the injury is secondary to equipment failure or personnel negligence. When injury has occurred, patient should be suitably compensated and receive prompt and best possible treatment to pre-empt a malpractice suit. Further the injury should be reported to create awareness and avoid such injuries in future.

References

1. Cushing H. Meningiomas arising from the olfactory groove and their removal by the aid of electrosurgery. Lancet. 1927;1:1329–39.
2. Choudhry AJ, Haddad NN, Khaswneh MA, Cullinan DC, Zielinski MD. Surgical fires and operative burns: lessons learnt from a 33 years review of medical litigation. Am J Surg. 2017;213(03):558–64.

3. Siddaiah-Subramanya M, Tiang KW, Nyandower M. Complications, implications and prevention of electrosurgical injuries: cornerstone of diathermy use for junior surgical trainees. Surg J. 2017;3:e148–53.
4. Aigner N, Fialka C, Fritz A, Wrahs O, Zoch G. Complications in the use of diathermy. Burns. 1997;23(3):256–64.
5. Saaiq M, Zaib S, Ahmad S. Electrocautery burns: experience with three cases and review of literature. Ann Burns Fire Disasters. 2012;25(4):203–6.
6. Patel R, Chavda KD, Hukkari S. Surgical field fire and skin burns caused by alcohol based skin preparation. J Emerg Trauma Shock. 2010;3:305.
7. Mundinger GS, Rozen SM, Carson B, et al. Full thickness forehead burns over indwelling titanium hardware resulting from an aberrant intraoperative electrocautery circuit. Eplasty. 2007;8:1–7.
8. Engel SJ, Patel NK, Morrison CM, et al. Operating room fires part II. Optimizing safety. Plast Reconstr Surg. 2012;130:681.

Functional Wound Healing 30

Kanhaiya Singh, Shomita S. Mathew-Steiner, and Chandan K. Sen

30.1 Introduction

The fundamental characteristics of a living being is the ability to heal damaged tissue. This includes every kind of traumatic event ranging from a simple paper cut to complex myocardial infraction. Such tissue repair system encompasses two separate processes: replacement and regeneration [1]. During regeneration, a brand-new growth fully restores the morphology and functionality of damaged tissue to its previous normal state. Replacement on the contrary repairs the injured tissue by laying down of connective tissue, a process known as scarring [1]. In humans, the means of recovery following a tissue damage event consists of replacement rather than regeneration [1]. Although this process of tissue repair by replacement may restore few original structures of the damaged tissue; however, it is often associated with structural abnormalities that impair the organ function. One of the classical examples of such impairment is the formation of scar after myocardial infarction [1]. A complete investigation of the size, location, composition, structure and mechanical properties of such scar is critical to determine the functionality of the recovering heart [2]. Similarly, in liver pathology, it is important to access liver synthetic function like serum albumin and prothrombin time in addition to injury markers like serum transaminases and bilirubin levels [3, 4]. However, there is no such standard guidelines to assess the reconstitution of skin functionality after physical insults like wounds. Such determination of skin functionality is critical as any damage in skin integrity can allow dermal absorption of harmful chemicals that can travel into body and cause potential health issues [5]. For example, higher

K. Singh (✉) · S. S. Mathew-Steiner · C. K. Sen
McGowan Institute for Regenerative Medicine, Department of Surgery, University of Pittsburgh School of Medicine, Pittsburgh, PA, USA
e-mail: singhk@pitt.edu

A. K. Khanna, S. K. Tiwary (eds.), *Uncommon Ulcers of the Extremities*,
https://doi.org/10.1007/978-981-99-1782-2_30

penetration of allergens could be correlated to onset of food allergies, allergic rhinitis and asthma, a condition described as "atopic march" seen in atopic dermatitis [6, 7]. Immunological studies have started to provide some insight into the link between skin barrier defects and impact on distant internal organs. Specifically, induction of a systemic T helper 2 inflammatory response and a thymic stromal lymphopoietin-mediated pathway initiated at the defective skin negatively impacts the intestinal and respiratory tract [8]. This chapter addresses the variables that can affect the extent and the quality of healing of skin tissue post-injury [9].

30.2 Human Chronic Wound and Its Burden

Wounds that do not follow normal process of healing and are open for more than a month are classified as chronic wounds [10]. If left untreated these chronic wounds can result in significant medical issues like limb amputation, infection, sepsis, and even death [10]. Chronic wounds are often complicated by comorbidities [10]. Vast majority of subjects suffering from wound healing impairment have other genetic, epigenetic, or metabolic predispositions [11–26]. Chronic wounds impact about 8.2 million Medicare beneficiaries with cost projection ranged from \$28.1 to \$96.8 billion [10, 27]. The global advanced wound care market is projected to reach \$18.7 billion by 2027 [27]. In addition to the direct expenditure toward these non-healing wounds, there is also indirect expenditure that possibly contributes to loss of productivity, family costs, family status, and loss of quality of life.

Diabetic foot ulcers (DFU) are one of the most common reasons for hospitalization of diabetic patients and frequently result in amputation of lower limbs [10, 28]. The rate of amputation in patients with DFU is 38.4% [29]. Infection is a common complication of DFU [10, 28, 30, 31]. In the current standard of care (SoC), wound closure is defined (FDA) by wound area coverage without drainage [32]. Published preclinical large animal works have demonstrated that wounds with a history of biofilm infection may meet above criteria but the repaired wound-site skin is deficient in barrier function [33–35]. This has led to the concept of functional wound closure wherein the current clinical definition of wound closure is supplemented with a functional parameter—restoration of the skin barrier function.

30.3 Skin Barrier System

The skin serves as the largest human organ. It has three layers: the epidermis, the dermis, and the hypodermis. The epidermis is the outer layer of skin which generates protective and defensive functions (Table 30.1) [36]. Presence of epithelial barrier structures in skin is required to isolate our body from the external environment and to maintain homeostasis [37]. The skin's barrier function is predominantly composed of three key elements: (1) the stratum corneum (air–liquid barrier; outermost layer of the skin), (2) tight junctions (liquid–liquid barrier), and the (3) Langerhans cell network (immunological barrier) [37, 38]. The stratum corneum is the

Table 30.1 Multiple protective functions of the outer epidermis

Function	Principal compartment	Structural basis	Biochemical basis	Regulatory signals (receptors)
Permeability[a,b]	Extracellular matrix of SC	Lamellar bilayers	Ceramides, cholesterol, nonessential fatty acids in proper ratio	IL-1α, Ca^{++}, pH, liposensors, serine proteases via PAR2, TPRV1, and 4
Antimicrobial[a,b]	Extracellular matrix of SC	Lamellar bilayers	Antimicrobial peptides, FFA, sphingosine	1,25 (OH)2D3; IL-1α
Antioxidant[b]	Extracellular matrix of SC	Lamellar bilayers	Cholesterol, FFA, secreted vitamin E, redox gradient	?
Cohesion (integrity) → desquamation[a,b]	Extracellular matrix of SC	Corneodesmosomes	Intercellular DSG1/ DSC1 homodimers	pH, Ca^{++}, (TPRV)
Mechanical or rheological[b]	Corneocyte	Cornified envelope; keratin filaments	γ-glutamyl isopeptide bonds	Ca^{++}, CholSO4, liposensors
Chemical (antigen exclusion)[a,b]	Extracellular matrix of SC	Extracellular lacunae	Hydrophilic products of corneodesmosomes	Same as for permeability barrier
Psychosensory interface[b]	Extracellular matrix of SC	Lamellar bilayers	Barrier lipids	Glucocorticoids, heat (TPRV3)
Neurosensory	Stratum granulosum	Neuroreceptors + transmitters	Ion channels, neurotransmitters	Divalent cations; K^+; others?
Hydration[b]	Corneocyte	Cytosolic pool of precursors	Filaggrin proteolytic products; glycerol	Osmotic changes (TPRV1 and 4), aquaporin 3
Ultraviolet light	Corneocyte	Cytosol	Trans-urocanic acid (histidase activity)	
Initiation of inflammation (first-degree cytokine activity)[a,b]	Corneocyte	Cytosol	Proteolytic activation of pro-IL-1α/β	pH, serine protease activation

Reproduced with permission from Springer Nature. The following original report is credited: Peter M Elias [36]

FFA free fatty acids, *IL* interleukin, *PAR2* plasminogen activator type 2 receptor, *SC* stratum corneum

[a] Regulated by SC pH

[b] Abnormal in atopic dermatitis

outermost layer of skin which serves as air–liquid interface barrier, thereby protecting the living layers from desiccation [37, 38]. Each corneocyte in the stratum corneum is sealed together by tight junctions. Claudins proteins are important components of the tight junctions between corneocytes that help to prevent moisture loss through this layer of the skin as well as block access through the skin of external environmental allergens. Another class of proteins called desmogleins mediate cell-to-cell tight junction adhesion in the stratum corneum. Any significant disruption of these epithelial barrier systems increases vulnerability to infection and allergens and results in the onset of skin diseases [37, 38]. Compromised skin barrier function is often associated with different skin diseases like atopic dermatitis, psoriasis, and contact dermatitis [37–39]. One of the striking examples of the importance of these barrier systems is that the transgenic mice with abnormal desmoglein expression die due to water loss and dehydration mediated by lack of corneocyte adhesion [40, 41]. Hence it is important to functionally characterize the significance of barrier function following skin injury. The following section describes the parameters that are important in characterizing the barrier function functionality following skin tissue injury.

30.3.1 Transepidermal Water Loss (TEWL)

Among the defensive functions of skin, the most critical is the permeability barrier, which is determined by TEWL [9, 35, 36]. The first of its kind measurement of TEWL was described in 1911 and today it serves as a standard procedure in a wide variety of dermatological and skin related research activities [42–45]. TEWL represents the diffusion of condensed water through the stratum corneum [43, 46]. An elevated TEWL values represents a compromised skin barrier function and has been associated with a number of skin diseases like atopic dermatitis and psoriasis. Lowered TEWL on indicates recovered skin barrier [43]. Such reduced TEWL is often associated with larger surface corneocytes and an increased number of corneocyte layers [47]. In addition, the elevated levels of TEWL is frequently correlated with low hydration levels of TEWL measurement can also screen treatments having a beneficial effect on the barrier function and aids in monitoring the effect of topical treatment in an objective and non-invasive way in human skin [44].

TEWL represents a flux density, i.e., a quantity of water per unit area per unit time (elaborated by Imhof et al. [46]). The commonly used methods of measurement of TEWL are indirect and measure the flux density of water evaporating from the skin surface (Imhof et al. [46]). The practical unit for TEWL measurement is $g\ m^{-2}\ h^{-1}$.

$$\text{Flux density} = \frac{\text{Mass of Water}}{\text{Area} \times \text{Time}}$$

Based on the application different types of TEWL devices can be used. Some of the examples are (1) open-chamber TEWL device, (2) unventilated-chamber TEWL device, and (3) condenser-chamber TEWL device [47] (Fig. 30.1). The disadvantages of this method are that it can be easily disturbed by the perspiration of the volunteers and by topically applied substances, for instance, application of hydrophobic wound healing creams [48]. It should be recognized that different anatomical sites within an individual have different inherent TEWL levels. For example, TEWL levels are generally high at the palm and soles because of the presence of low sebaceous lipid content at these sites [49]. Other regional differences in the TEWL measurement can be attributed to skin temperature, microvascular

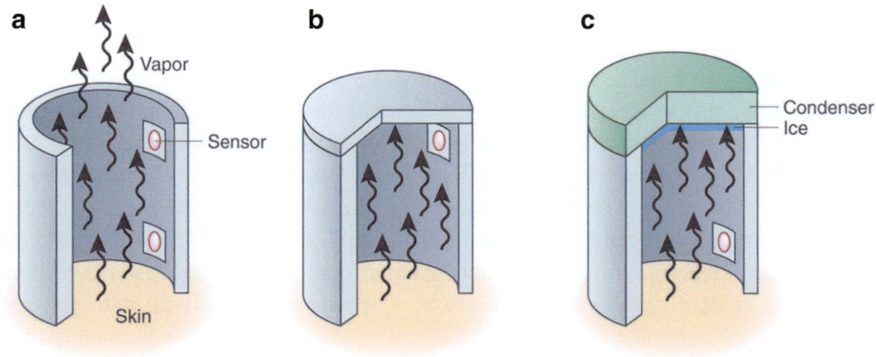

Fig. 30.1 TEWL devices. (**a**) Open-chamber TEWL device. A hollow cylinder is placed in contact with the skin, and water vapor diffuses through the open chamber. Spatially separated temperature and relative humidity sensors detect the humidity gradient. (**b**) Unventilated-chamber TEWL device. The upper end of the chamber is closed, resulting in water vapor collecting in the chamber. The temperature and relative humidity sensors detect the rate of increase of relative humidity. (**c**) Condenser-chamber TEWL device. The upper end of the chamber is closed by a condenser that removes water vapor from the chamber, enabling continuous TEWL measurements to be recorded. Water vapor density is measured by sensors in the chamber and condenser. *TEWL* transepidermal water loss. (Reproduced under the terms of Elsevier. The following original report is credited: Alexander et al. [47])

abundance, and occlusion [49]. Hence it is important to adhere to the set guidelines that address the external factors affecting TEWL in research studies and achieve consistency and accuracy [44, 45]. A room temperature of 18–21 °C, relative humidity of 40–60%, no exposure to direct light, no recent (<12 h) application are some of the external factors that are employed while collecting TEWL measurement [47]. Importantly, proper calibration of the TEWL equipment and its components should be done before taking the TEWL measurements.

30.3.2 Molecular Determinants of Skin Barrier Function

During initial phase of wound healing, epithelial cells dismantle cell–cell adhesion and tight junctions to acquire a mesenchymal phenotype by a process known as epithelial-to-mesenchymal transition (EMT) [9, 14]. This process stimulates and mobilizes stationary keratinocytes in the skin toward the wound bed, enabling re-epithelialization [50]. Many well-defined regulators like extracellular growth factors, transcription factors (e.g., Twist and Zeb1), microRNAs (e.g., miR-200b, miR-200c, miR-9), and other microenvironmental cues govern the process of EMT [14, 16, 51, 52]. Any defect in such injury induced EMT process leads to impairment of wound healing [14]. However, following successful re-epithelialization, epithelial cells give up their migratory behavior, reconstitute apico-basal polarization, and re-establish junctional complexes by the process of mesenchymal-to-epithelial transition (MET) [53]. This process of MET reconstitutes apical junctional complexes encompassing tight junctions and adherens junctions and restores the barrier function of repaired skin. Although the essentials of such EMT↔MET have not been well characterized yet, the mechanisms may reasonably be hypothesized to be an iterative process. Such coordinated inherent reversible plasticity of skin cells is crucial for proper wound repair (Fig. 30.2) [9]. Given the fact that this tissue EMT↔MET is responsive to individual's glycemic status renders extraordinary significance to this process in the context of diabetic wounds [14, 54]. For example, work by our group recently identified ZEB1, an EMT regulator, as a significant mechanistic hub across different cellular compartments in wounds. ZEB1 is responsive to the glycemic status of the injury microenvironment in both epithelial and endothelial cell compartments. In epithelial cells, sustained hyperglycemia impaired the ZEB1-EMT pathway toward wound epithelialization. Future studies unveiling the molecular underpinnings of cutaneous wound epithelial plasticity will reveal regulatory hubs orchestrating wound re-epithelialization.

30.3.3 Metabolic Determinants of Skin Barrier Function

Biochemically, one of the major contributors of the epithelial barrier is lipids produced in the lamellar bodies of the stratum granulosum [55]. These lipids increase the adhesion between corneocytes and create an multilamellar epidermal barrier [55]. Composition wise ceramides constitute 50% of lipids forming the multilamellar barrier of skin followed by cholesterol (25%) and fatty acids (FAs) (15%) [55–57]. Chemically, ceramides are composed of a sphingoid base, which is a long-chain amino alcohol, and a FA joined by an amide bond [55]. The sphingoid base may consist of dihydrosphingosine (dS), sphingosine (S), phytosphingosine (P), or 6-hydroxy sphingosine (H) [55, 58]. The FA may be a non-hydroxyl FA (N), an α-hydroxyl FA (A), or an esterified ω-hydroxyl FA (EO) [55, 58]. In addition to providing extracellular barrier function, ceramides act as a secondary messenger intracellularly. Intracellular ceramides play important role in signal transduction during various processes like cell growth, senescence, diabetes, insulin resistance, and inflammation [55, 59–61]. Biosynthesis of ceramide directly regulates the cutaneous barrier function and prevents TEWL [60, 62]. It has been reported that 9 out of 11 ceramide classes found in human stratum corneum has significant correlations with TEWL [63]. Any significant changes in the skin ceramide content are associated with a number of diseases such as atopic dermatitis, psoriasis, and impaired wound healing [62]. Additionally, inhibition of cholesterol or fatty acid also impairs barrier function by adversely affecting lamellar body formation [64].

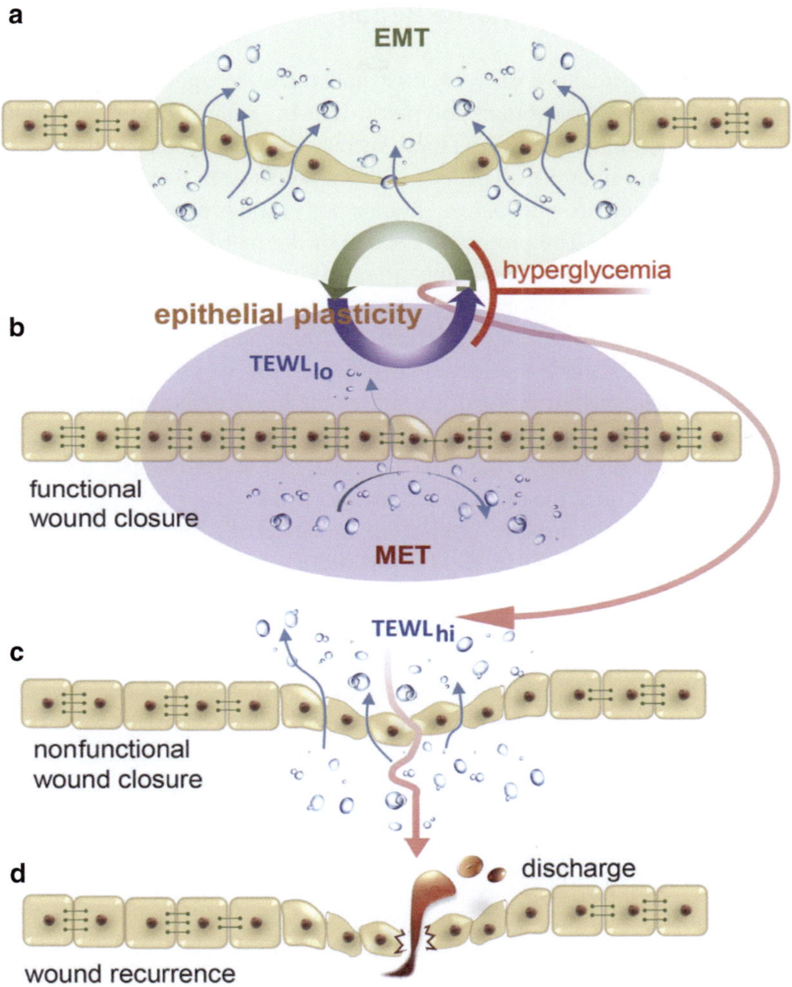

Fig. 30.2 Hyperglycemia restrains cutaneous epithelial plasticity necessary for functional wound closure. A hypothetical paradigm depicts (**a**) and (**b**) in which EMT↔MET is central for re-epithelialization and restoration of the barrier function of the repaired skin. During EMT, epithelial cells dismantle cell adhesion and tight junction structures in an effort to acquire a mesenchymal phenotype favoring re-epithelialization. MET helps to reconstitute the AJCs restoring the barrier function of the repaired skin. (**c**) Hyperglycemia is a barrier to such plasticity and as such hinders re-epithelialization, restoration of barrier function, or both. The result is wound chronicity or non-functional wound closure. (**d**) Closure of wound without the restoration of skin barrier function predisposes the closed wound to recidivism as evident in preclinical porcine studies. The incidence of wound recurrence is high in patients with diabetes. TEWL is a measure of skin barrier function. TEWLhi represents TEWL-deficient skin barrier function. TEWLlo represents TEWL-restored skin barrier function indicative of functional wound closure. Horizontal rivets between cells represent functional AJC. These are low or absent in mesenchymal cells compromising barrier function. *AJC* apical junctional complex, *EMT* epithelial-to-mesenchymal transition, *MET* mesenchymal-to-epithelial transition, *TEWL* transepidermal water loss. (Reproduced under the terms of Elsevier. The following original report is credited: Sen and Roy [9])

30.4 Biofilm and Skin Tissue Repair

Microbes have the innate ability to exist and thrive in aggregates/communities sheathed within an extracellular polymeric matrix, called the biofilm mode of growth. The communities could be single species or multi-species including bacteria, fungi, and other microbes. This is a survival mechanism that enables microbial adaptation to harsh environments (e.g., human body) and is perceived as an invisible threat to human health. The protective cocoon of the matrix is impervious to standard antimicrobials [65–80], including silver [35] and the host's immune system. Within the matrix, the microbial cells can communicate with each other using chemical (quorum sensing) and electrical (ion channels) signaling, share genes (e.g., antibiotic resistance) that promote efficient use of resources and activate pathogenic mechanisms. Additionally, a subpopulation of cells within the biofilm is responsive to physiological and microenvironment changes and exhibits a persistent phenotype. These can survive the direct exposure to antimicrobials and result in recurrent infections once the therapy has been stopped.

Biofilm infection is directly implicated in numerous human soft tissue and device-related infections [67, 71, 81–119]. Biofilm infection in an open wound is a significant threat to wound healing [120–122]. Current standard clinical microbiology tests do not detect a biofilm as this form of infection is not reliably culturable [69, 109, 115] and cannot be reliably eliminated even by aggressive debridement [35]. In fact, debridement may inadvertently move some of the infectious elements into deeper tissue [35] potentially causing complications. The vast majority of the current biofilm literature represents in vitro studies [68, 69, 80, 87, 123–131]. The clinical relevance of such approach is arguable because the struggle between biofilm infection and host defense defines a clinically relevant biofilm [71, 78, 81, 97–101, 105, 106, 108, 115, 119, 128, 132–136]. Clinically, consistent with the CDC and NIH estimates [137], there is a rapidly growing evidence demonstrating that the presence of biofilm clearly threatens human health. In the context of medical devices and food safety, the FDA recognized this threat and sought to avoid biofilm infection [138–140]. However, clinically relevant systematic mechanism-directed studies are scanty due to the ethics of experimentally generating biofilms in humans. To understand the cascade of events that lead to pathological impact of biofilm infection, relevant preclinical wound infection studies are needed. Such understanding requires controlled experimental preclinical studies. Pig being the most reliable preclinical model for wounds [141], we developed the first [128] burn biofilm model in pigs [35]. The progressive interaction between bacteria and the host is an iterative process that helps evolve an acute-phase infection to a pathogenic biofilm. Thus, long-term (weeks) wound infection studies are needed to understand the crosstalk between host and bacteria [128]. This model led to the observation that biofilm-infected burn wounds may close, but the repaired skin lacking barrier function leaves the wound site functionally compromised [35].

30.4.1 Biofilm and Skin Barrier Function

The breaching of the skin following wounding leaves the body vulnerable to external threats. The physiological response to this breach is the onset of the wound healing cascade culminating on re-epithelialization and closure of the breach. As mentioned earlier, wound re-epithelialization relies on EMT. This promotes increased motility of keratinocytes caused by cytoskeletal reorganization until the wound is closed. Gap closure engages a return to epithelial phenotype with the restoration of intercellular junctional proteins and formation of a tight skin barrier that protects the body from external assaults. Published studies identified that while biofilm infection does not compromise visual closure of wounds, the "repaired" skin has significant barrier function defects. Specifically, biofilm infection silences several junctional proteins including E-cadherin, ZO-1 and ZO-2 through a microRNA (miRNA) dependent process. Although bacterial infection [142, 143] is known to perturb tight junctions and miRNA [144–146] and is known to regulate epithelial barrier function, these studies were the first to highlight a role for biofilm-induced miRNA in compromising skin barrier function.

30.4.2 Biofilm and Wound Recurrence

Recurrence in chronic wounds is a known phenomenon whereby a wound that appears to heal visually per FDA guidance [32] reopens weeks, months, or years after initial closure. One study estimated that ~40% of patients had diabetic foot ulcer recurrence within a year of healing and 65% do so within 5 years [147]. Once scenario in the context of biofilm infection is related to faulty barrier formation, as described above, whereby the entry of pathogens could establish infection and thereby reopen the wound or the persistent biofilm within the closed wound could seed a new round of infection to reopen the wound. Biofilm forming bacteria come armed with virulence factors that target various host proteins. For example, a study using in vivo graded *Staphylococcus aureus* biofilm infection established a cause-and-effect relationship with skin collagen levels via a miRNA-matrix metalloproteinase (MMP) axis. Only biofilm forming *S. aureus* strains were able to markedly inhibit collagen I by inducing MMP-2 through depletion of miR-143. Such activation of MMP-2 inhibited collagen I, a major structural protein of the skin extracellular matrix, culminating in poor wound tensile strength of the repaired skin. Loss of structural collagen [148] markedly changes the biomechanical properties of the skin such that they are vulnerable to external trauma and could reopen.

30.4.3 The Theft Biofilm Concept

During the process of host–microbe interaction, mechanistic underpinnings of biofilm infection are contextual and depend on the host tissue microenvironment [39]. Recently, the theft biofilm concept has been proposed which demonstrates that

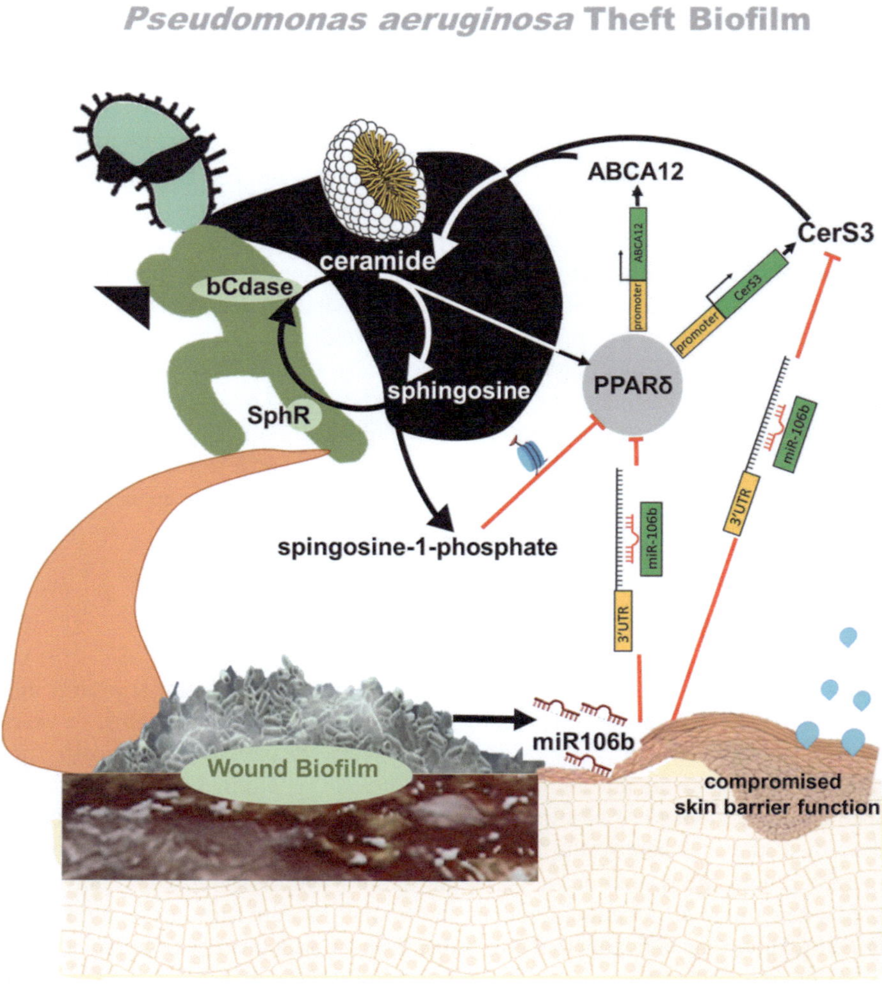

Fig. 30.3 The theft biofilm concept. In cutaneous wounds, *Pseudomonas aeruginosa* forms pathogenic theft biofilm. Such biofilm severity relies on the theft of host lipids (ceramides) causing potent induction of bacterial ceramidase (*bcdase*). Skin lipid homeostasis is disrupted such that the site of wound repair is deficient in barrier function exacerbating host pathology. (Reproduced under the terms of Wolters Kluwer Health, Inc. The following original report is credited: Sinha et al. [39])

microbial biofilm involves larceny of host factors toward bolstering pathogenicity and promotes host vulnerability [39] (Fig. 30.3). Bacterial pathogens such as *Pseudomonas aeruginosa* are armed with virulence factors that target host proteins, lipids, carbohydrates, and other molecules. The host microenvironment presents offenses and defenses that trigger pathogen responses. *P. aeruginosa* exploits host lipids to enable immune evasion [149, 150] and establish biofilm [151]. In the skin, *P. aeruginosa* infection responds to cues from host skin and robustly induced bacterial ceramidases. Ceramidases target essential skin lipids, i.e., ceramides, that are the first line of the skin barrier defense. Pathogenic *P. aeruginosa* biofilm, thereby, responds iteratively to host factors. The presence of ceramides in the breached and infected skin activated bacterial ceramidases to metabolize host ceramides producing sphingosine (Sph) and sphingosine-1-phosphate (S1P). Sph and S1P further induced bacterial ceramidase and inhibited proliferator activated receptor (PPAR)δ, respectively. *P. aeruginosa* biofilm silences (PPAR)δ via miR-106b. Decreased (PPAR)δ inhibited ABCA12 expression, thereby disrupting skin lipid homeostasis and compromising barrier function [39].

30.5 TEWL as a Reliable Measurement of Skin Barrier Function in Biofilm Infected Wounds

Biofilm-infected wounds may achieve closure without restoring the barrier function of the repaired skin. Such barrier function-deficient skin exhibits compromised biomechanical properties of closed wounds and favors wound recurrence. Hence the concept of "functional wound closure" states that wound closure is only complete when defects caused by injury are covered by skin with a restored barrier function. Thus, measurement of barrier function restoration is an important element characterizing biofilm-infected wound closure [33–35]. TEWL, as described above, is the most widely used objective measurement that characterizes skin barrier function. $TEWL_{hi}$ represents deficient skin barrier function and $TEWL_{lo}$ represents restored/close to normal skin barrier function indicative of functional closure. The skin barrier is disturbed in pathological conditions (e.g., atopic dermatitis [36, 152–154], psoriasis [155, 156], and biofilm infection [34, 35]) and physiological conditions (e.g., aging and menopause) [54] and are objectively assessed as $TEWL_{hi}$. This measure has been validated in humans and animal models by different groups [35, 157, 158]. For example, in atopic dermatitis, increased TEWL, reflecting skin barrier dysfunction, is a major pathological feature that can be robustly correlated with severity of disease and response to treatment not only in adults but also neonates [36, 152–154].

Several preclinical porcine studies [35, 128, 159, 160], using polymicrobial biofilm infection caused by clinically isolated bacteria demonstrated that a history of biofilm infection compromises barrier function of the repaired skin as manifested by high TEWL [35, 128, 159, 160]. Pilot clinical studies in DFU suggested a strong correlation between $TEWL_{hi}$ and increased risk for recurrence of DFU. These studies laid the foundation for the first NIH Diabetic Foot Consortium (DFC) clinical trial (NCT04558775) to assess the value of TEWL as a biomarker predicting DFU recurrence. The scope of this study is to find the right type of treatment or measurement that will predict wound recurrence. TEWL will be measured on the closed wound site and a location similar to the wound site (reference site). Enrollment of the participants will be done within 2 weeks after closure of their DFU. Participants will be followed weekly for 16 weeks by phone until the earliest time of DFU wound recurrence or 16 weeks. Participants who experience a DFU wound recurrence and a subset of participants who do not experience a DFU wound recurrence by week 16 will be asked to attend one final visit. Successful completion of this study may identify TEWL as an essential biomarker for the assessment of DFU healing progress and prognosis.

30.6 Conclusion

The current standard of care that informs the clinical decision-making process in wound care is for a physician to visually assess the wound for closure. The validity of that clinical decision-making process is questionable in the light of the emergent concept of functional wound closure. Wounds infected by bacteria in biofilm configuration may close, as appreciated visually, but functionally remains open because the repaired skin lacks barrier function. Such defective repair of wounds lends itself to a higher rate of recurrence or post-closure complication in patients. The notion that continued care, until functional wound closure is achieved, is necessary to minimize recurrence and amputation would be of transformative value in the delivery of DFU care. In this context TEWL is being most widely used objective measurement for assessing the barrier function of skin in healthy individuals but also patients with skin diseases that are associated with skin barrier dysfunction, such as aging, atopic dermatitis, and chronic wounds. Finally, this chapter explains the premise of measurement of skin barrier function being investigated by NIH Diabetic Foot Consortium as the new biomarker that may predict DFU wound recurrence.

Acknowledgment This work was supported in part by National Institute of Diabetes and Digestive and Kidney Diseases grants DK128845, DK119099, DK135447, and DK125835 to CKS and DK136814 to KS. This work was also supported in part by U.S. Department of Defense grants W81XWH-22-1-0146 to KS and W81XWH-21-1-0033 to CKS. Research programs led by CKS were supported by the Lilly Endowment Indiana Collaborative Initiative for Talent Enrichment (INCITE) program and John Templeton Foundation grant 61742.

References

1. Krafts KP. Tissue repair: the hidden drama. Organogenesis. 2010;6:225–33.
2. Richardson WJ, Clarke SA, Quinn TA, Holmes JW. Physiological implications of myocardial scar structure. Compr Physiol. 2015;5:1877–909.
3. Agrawal S, Dhiman RK, Limdi JK. Evaluation of abnormal liver function tests. Postgrad Med J. 2016;92:223–34.
4. Limdi JK, Hyde GM. Evaluation of abnormal liver function tests. Postgrad Med J. 2003;79:307–12.
5. Hudson TJ. Skin barrier function and allergic risk. Nat Genet. 2006;38:399–400.
6. Campbell DE. Role of food allergy in childhood atopic dermatitis. J Paediatr Child Health. 2012;48:1058–64.
7. Smith AR, Knaysi G, Wilson JM, Wisniewski JA. The skin as a route of allergen exposure: part I. Immune components and mechanisms. Curr Allergy Asthma Rep. 2017;17:6.
8. Zhu TH, Zhu TR, Tran KA, Sivamani RK, Shi VY. Epithelial barrier dysfunctions in atopic dermatitis: a skin-gut-lung model linking microbiome alteration and immune dysregulation. Br J Dermatol. 2018;179:570–81.

9. Sen CK, Roy S. The hyperglycemia stranglehold stifles cutaneous epithelial mesenchymal plasticity and functional wound closure. J Invest Dermatol. 2021;141:1382–5.
10. Sen CK. Human wound and its burden: updated 2020 compendium of estimates. Adv Wound Care (New Rochelle). 2021;10:281–92.
11. Rustagi Y, Abouhashem AS, Verma P, Verma SS, Hernandez E, Liu S, Kumar M, Guda PR, Srivastava R, Mohanty SK, Kacar S, Mahajan S, Wanczyk KE, Khanna S, Murphy MP, Gordillo GM, Roy S, Wan J, Sen CK, Singh K. Endothelial phospholipase Cgamma2 improves outcomes of diabetic ischemic limb rescue following VEGF therapy. Diabetes. 2022;71:1149.
12. Bhamidipati T, Sinha M, Sen CK, Singh K. Laser capture microdissection in the spatial analysis of epigenetic modifications in skin: a comprehensive review. Oxidative Med Cell Longev. 2022;2022:4127238.
13. Zhou X, Brown BA, Siegel AP, El Masry MS, Zeng X, Song W, Das A, Khandelwal P, Clark A, Singh K, Guda PR, Gorain M, Timsina L, Xuan Y, Jacobson SC, Novotny MV, Roy S, Agarwal M, Lee RJ, Sen CK, Clemmer DE, Ghatak S. Exosome-mediated crosstalk between keratinocytes and macrophages in cutaneous wound healing. ACS Nano. 2020;14:12732–48.
14. Singh K, Sinha M, Pal D, Tabasum S, Gnyawali SC, Khona D, Sarkar S, Mohanty SK, Soto-Gonzalez F, Khanna S, Roy S, Sen CK. Cutaneous epithelial to mesenchymal transition activator ZEB1 regulates wound angiogenesis and closure in a glycemic status-dependent manner. Diabetes. 2019;68:2175–90.
15. Sinha M, Sen CK, Singh K, Das A, Ghatak S, Rhea B, Blackstone B, Powell HM, Khanna S, Roy S. Direct conversion of injury-site myeloid cells to fibroblast-like cells of granulation tissue. Nat Commun. 2018;9:936.
16. Singh K, Pal D, Sinha M, Ghatak S, Gnyawali SC, Khanna S, Roy S, Sen CK. Epigenetic modification of microRNA-200b contributes to diabetic vasculopathy. Mol Ther. 2017;25:2689–704.
17. Singh K, Agrawal NK, Gupta SK, Sinha P, Singh K. Increased expression of TLR9 associated with pro-inflammatory S100A8 and IL-8 in diabetic wounds could lead to unresolved inflammation in type 2 diabetes mellitus (T2DM) cases with impaired wound healing. J Diabetes Complicat. 2016;30:99–108.
18. Singh K, Agrawal NK, Gupta SK, Mohan G, Chaturvedi S, Singh K. Decreased expression of heat shock proteins may lead to compromised wound healing in type 2 diabetes mellitus patients. J Diabetes Complicat. 2015;29:578–88.
19. Singh K, Agrawal NK, Gupta SK, Mohan G, Chaturvedi S, Singh K. Increased expression of endosomal members of toll-like receptor family abrogates wound healing in patients with type 2 diabetes mellitus. Int Wound J. 2016;13:927–35.
20. Singh K, Singh K. Carcinogenesis and diabetic wound healing: evidences of parallelism. Curr Diabetes Rev. 2015;11:32–45.
21. Singh K, Agrawal NK, Gupta SK, Mohan G, Chaturvedi S, Singh K. Genetic and epigenetic alterations in Toll like receptor 2 and wound healing impairment in type 2 diabetes patients. J Diabetes Complicat. 2015;29:222–9.
22. Singh K, Agrawal NK, Gupta SK, Mohan G, Chaturvedi S, Singh K. Differential expression of matrix metalloproteinase-9 gene in wounds of type 2 diabetes mellitus cases with susceptible -1562C>T genotypes and wound severity. Int J Low Extrem Wounds. 2014;13:94–102.
23. Singh K, Singh VK, Agrawal NK, Gupta SK, Singh K. Genetic alterations in toll-like receptor 4 signaling pathway and impairment of wound healing in patients with type 2 diabetes. Int J Low Extrem Wounds. 2014;13:162–3.
24. Singh K, Agrawal NK, Gupta SK, Singh K. Association of variant rs7903146 (C/T) single nucleotide polymorphism of TCF7L2 gene with impairment in wound healing among north Indian type 2 diabetes population: a case-control study. Int J Low Extrem Wounds. 2013;12:310–5.
25. Singh K, Agrawal NK, Gupta SK, Singh K. A functional single nucleotide polymorphism -1562C>T in the matrix metalloproteinase-9 promoter is associated with type 2 diabetes and diabetic foot ulcers. Int J Low Extrem Wounds. 2013;12:199–204.

26. Singh K, Singh VK, Agrawal NK, Gupta SK, Singh K. Association of Toll-like receptor 4 polymorphisms with diabetic foot ulcers and application of artificial neural network in DFU risk assessment in type 2 diabetes patients. Biomed Res Int. 2013;2013:318686.
27. Nussbaum SR, Carter MJ, Fife CE, DaVanzo J, Haught R, Nusgart M, Cartwright D. An economic evaluation of the impact, cost, and Medicare policy implications of chronic nonhealing wounds. Value Health. 2018;21:27–32.
28. Falanga V. Wound healing and its impairment in the diabetic foot. Lancet. 2005;366:1736–43.
29. Kim SY, Kim TH, Choi JY, Kwon YJ, Choi DH, Kim KC, Kim MJ, Hwang HK, Lee KB. Predictors for amputation in patients with diabetic foot wound. Vasc Specialist Int. 2018;34:109–16.
30. Bjarnsholt T, Kirketerp-Moller K, Jensen PO, Madsen KG, Phipps R, Krogfelt K, Hoiby N, Givskov M. Why chronic wounds will not heal: a novel hypothesis. Wound Repair Regen. 2008;16:2–10.
31. Davis SC, Martinez L, Kirsner R. The diabetic foot: the importance of biofilms and wound bed preparation. Curr Diab Rep. 2006;6:439–45.
32. US Department of Health and Human Services F. Guidance for industry: chronic cutaneous ulcer and burn wounds-developing products for treatment. 2006;2014.
33. Roy S, Santra S, Das A, Dixith S, Sinha M, Ghatak S, Ghosh N, Banerjee P, Khanna S, Mathew-Steiner S, Ghatak PD, Blackstone BN, Powell HM, Bergdall VK, Wozniak DJ, Sen CK. Staphylococcus aureus biofilm infection compromises wound healing by causing deficiencies in granulation tissue collagen. Ann Surg. 2020;271:1174–85.
34. Barki KG, Das A, Dixith S, Ghatak PD, Mathew-Steiner S, Schwab E, Khanna S, Wozniak DJ, Roy S, Sen CK. Electric field based dressing disrupts mixed-species bacterial biofilm infection and restores functional wound healing. Ann Surg. 2019;269:756–66.
35. Roy S, Elgharably H, Sinha M, Ganesh K, Chaney S, Mann E, Miller C, Khanna S, Bergdall VK, Powell HM, Cook CH, Gordillo GM, Wozniak DJ, Sen CK. Mixed-species biofilm compromises wound healing by disrupting epidermal barrier function. J Pathol. 2014;233:331–43.
36. Elias PM. Skin barrier function. Curr Allergy Asthma Rep. 2008;8:299–305.
37. Kubo A, Nagao K, Amagai M. Epidermal barrier dysfunction and cutaneous sensitization in atopic diseases. J Clin Invest. 2012;122:440–7.
38. Bouwstra JA, Ponec M. The skin barrier in healthy and diseased state. Biochim Biophys Acta. 2006;1758:2080–95.
39. Sinha M, Ghosh N, Wijesinghe DS, Mathew-Steiner SS, Das A, Singh K, Masry ME, Khanna S, Inoue H, Yamazaki K, Kawada M, Gordillo GM, Roy S, Sen CK. Pseudomonas aeruginosa theft biofilm require host lipids of cutaneous wound. Ann Surg. 2021;277:e634.
40. Hogan MB, Peele K, Wilson NW. Skin barrier function and its importance at the start of the atopic march. J Allergy (Cairo). 2012;2012:901940.
41. Elias PM, Matsuyoshi N, Wu H, Lin C, Wang ZH, Brown BE, Stanley JR. Desmoglein isoform distribution affects stratum corneum structure and function. J Cell Biol. 2001;153:243–9.
42. Akdeniz M, Gabriel S, Lichterfeld-Kottner A, Blume-Peytavi U, Kottner J. Transepidermal water loss in healthy adults: a systematic review and meta-analysis update. Br J Dermatol. 2018;179:1049–55.
43. du Plessis J, Stefaniak A, Eloff F, John S, Agner T, Chou TC, Nixon R, Steiner M, Franken A, Kudla I, Holness L. International guidelines for the in vivo assessment of skin properties in non-clinical settings: part 2. Transepidermal water loss and skin hydration. Skin Res Technol. 2013;19:265–78.
44. Rogiers V, Group E. EEMCO guidance for the assessment of transepidermal water loss in cosmetic sciences. Skin Pharmacol Appl Ski Physiol. 2001;14:117–28.
45. Pinnagoda J, Tupker RA, Agner T, Serup J. Guidelines for transepidermal water loss (TEWL) measurement. A report from the Standardization Group of the European Society of Contact Dermatitis. Contact Dermatitis. 1990;22:164–78.
46. Imhof RE, De Jesus ME, Xiao P, Ciortea LI, Berg EP. Closed-chamber transepidermal water loss measurement: microclimate, calibration and performance. Int J Cosmet Sci. 2009;31:97–118.

47. Alexander H, Brown S, Danby S, Flohr C. Research techniques made simple: transepidermal water loss measurement as a research tool. J Invest Dermatol. 2018;138:2295–300.e1.
48. Alborova A, Lademann J, Kramer A, Richter H, Patzelt A, Sterry W, Koch S. In vivo analysis of wound healing by optical methods. GMS Krankenhhyg Interdiszip. 2008;3:Doc10.
49. Brancaleon L, Bamberg MP, Sakamaki T, Kollias N. Attenuated total reflection-Fourier transform infrared spectroscopy as a possible method to investigate biophysical parameters of stratum corneum in vivo. J Invest Dermatol. 2001;116:380–6.
50. Yan C, Grimm WA, Garner WL, Qin L, Travis T, Tan N, Han YP. Epithelial to mesenchymal transition in human skin wound healing is induced by tumor necrosis factor-alpha through bone morphogenic protein-2. Am J Pathol. 2010;176:2247–58.
51. Lamouille S, Xu J, Derynck R. Molecular mechanisms of epithelial-mesenchymal transition. Nat Rev Mol Cell Biol. 2014;15:178–96.
52. De Craene B, Berx G. Regulatory networks defining EMT during cancer initiation and progression. Nat Rev Cancer. 2013;13:97–110.
53. Thiery JP, Acloque H, Huang RY, Nieto MA. Epithelial-mesenchymal transitions in development and disease. Cell. 2009;139:871–90.
54. Miller T. Chapter 14—Clinical testing to uphold an anti-aging claim. In: Dayan N, editor. Skin aging handbook. Norwich, NY: William Andrew Publishing; 2009. p. 363–89.
55. Cha HJ, He C, Zhao H, Dong Y, An IS, An S. Intercellular and intracellular functions of ceramides and their metabolites in skin (review). Int J Mol Med. 2016;38:16–22.
56. Candi E, Schmidt R, Melino G. The cornified envelope: a model of cell death in the skin. Nat Rev Mol Cell Biol. 2005;6:328–40.
57. Coderch L, Lopez O, de la Maza A, Parra JL. Ceramides and skin function. Am J Clin Dermatol. 2003;4:107–29.
58. Robson KJ, Stewart ME, Michelsen S, Lazo ND, Downing DT. 6-Hydroxy-4-sphingenine in human epidermal ceramides. J Lipid Res. 1994;35:2060–8.
59. Ruvolo PP. Intracellular signal transduction pathways activated by ceramide and its metabolites. Pharmacol Res. 2003;47:383–92.
60. Geilen CC, Wieder T, Orfanos CE. Ceramide signalling: regulatory role in cell proliferation, differentiation and apoptosis in human epidermis. Arch Dermatol Res. 1997;289:559–66.
61. Hannun YA. Functions of ceramide in coordinating cellular responses to stress. Science. 1996;274:1855–9.
62. Meckfessel MH, Brandt S. The structure, function, and importance of ceramides in skin and their use as therapeutic agents in skin-care products. J Am Acad Dermatol. 2014;71:177–84.
63. Ishikawa J, Narita H, Kondo N, Hotta M, Takagi Y, Masukawa Y, Kitahara T, Takema Y, Koyano S, Yamazaki S, Hatamochi A. Changes in the ceramide profile of atopic dermatitis patients. J Invest Dermatol. 2010;130:2511–4.
64. Feingold KR. Thematic review series: skin lipids. The role of epidermal lipids in cutaneous permeability barrier homeostasis. J Lipid Res. 2007;48:2531–46.
65. Andersson DI. Persistence of antibiotic resistant bacteria. Curr Opin Microbiol. 2003;6:452–6.
66. Anwar H, Dasgupta M, Lam K, Costerton JW. Tobramycin resistance of mucoid Pseudomonas aeruginosa biofilm grown under iron limitation. J Antimicrob Chemother. 1989;24:647–55.
67. Cooper RA, Bjarnsholt T, Alhede M. Biofilms in wounds: a review of present knowledge. J Wound Care. 2014;23:570, 572–4, 576–80 passim.
68. Costerton JW. Introduction to biofilm. Int J Antimicrob Agents. 1999;11:217–21; discussion 237–9.
69. Fux CA, Costerton JW, Stewart PS, Stoodley P. Survival strategies of infectious biofilms. Trends Microbiol. 2005;13:34–40.
70. Hoiby N, Bjarnsholt T, Givskov M, Molin S, Ciofu O. Antibiotic resistance of bacterial biofilms. Int J Antimicrob Agents. 2010;35:322–32.
71. Hoiby N, Ciofu O, Johansen HK, Song ZJ, Moser C, Jensen PO, Molin S, Givskov M, Tolker-Nielsen T, Bjarnsholt T. The clinical impact of bacterial biofilms. Int J Oral Sci. 2011;3:55–65.
72. Hoyle BD, Jass J, Costerton JW. The biofilm glycocalyx as a resistance factor. J Antimicrob Chemother. 1990;26:1–5.

73. Lewis K. Multidrug tolerance of biofilms and persister cells. Curr Top Microbiol Immunol. 2008;322:107–31.
74. Patel R. Biofilms and antimicrobial resistance. Clin Orthop Relat Res. 2005:41–7.
75. Perez F, Hujer AM, Hujer KM, Decker BK, Rather PN, Bonomo RA. Global challenge of multidrug-resistant Acinetobacter baumannii. Antimicrob Agents Chemother. 2007;51:3471–84.
76. Rodriguez-Bano J, Marti S, Soto S, Fernandez-Cuenca F, Cisneros JM, Pachon J, Pascual A, Martinez-Martinez L, McQueary C, Actis LA, Vila J, Spanish Group for the Study of Nosocomial I. Biofilm formation in Acinetobacter baumannii: associated features and clinical implications. Clin Microbiol Infect. 2008;14:276–8.
77. Romling U, Balsalobre C. Biofilm infections, their resilience to therapy and innovative treatment strategies. J Intern Med. 2012;272:541–61.
78. Rybtke MT, Jensen PO, Hoiby N, Givskov M, Tolker-Nielsen T, Bjarnsholt T. The implication of Pseudomonas aeruginosa biofilms in infections. Inflamm Allergy Drug Targets. 2011;10:141–57.
79. Schweizer HP. Efflux as a mechanism of resistance to antimicrobials in Pseudomonas aeruginosa and related bacteria: unanswered questions. Genet Mol Res. 2003;2:48–62.
80. Stewart PS, Costerton JW. Antibiotic resistance of bacteria in biofilms. Lancet. 2001;358:135–8.
81. Nistico L, Kreft R, Gieseke A, Coticchia JM, Burrows A, Khampang P, Liu Y, Kerschner JE, Post JC, Lonergan S, Sampath R, Hu FZ, Ehrlich GD, Stoodley P, Hall-Stoodley L. Adenoid reservoir for pathogenic biofilm bacteria. J Clin Microbiol. 2011;49:1411–20.
82. Costerton JW. Anaerobic biofilm infections in cystic fibrosis. Mol Cell. 2002;10:699–700.
83. Dunne WM Jr. Bacterial adhesion: seen any good biofilms lately? Clin Microbiol Rev. 2002;15:155–66.
84. Marrie TJ, Sung JY, Costerton JW. Bacterial biofilm formation on nasogastric tubes. J Gastroenterol Hepatol. 1990;5:503–6.
85. Nickel JC, Heaton J, Morales A, Costerton JW. Bacterial biofilm in persistent penile prosthesis-associated infection. J Urol. 1986;135:586–8.
86. Sung JY, Leung JW, Shaffer EA, Lam K, Costerton JW. Bacterial biofilm, brown pigment stone and blockage of biliary stents. J Gastroenterol Hepatol. 1993;8:28–34.
87. Parsek MR, Singh PK. Bacterial biofilms: an emerging link to disease pathogenesis. Annu Rev Microbiol. 2003;57:677–701.
88. Matsukawa M, Kunishima Y, Takahashi S, Takeyama K, Tsukamoto T. Bacterial colonization on intraluminal surface of urethral catheter. Urology. 2005;65:440–4.
89. Costerton JW, Montanaro L, Arciola CR. Bacterial communications in implant infections: a target for an intelligence war. Int J Artif Organs. 2007;30:757–63.
90. Speer AG, Cotton PB, Rode J, Seddon AM, Neal CR, Holton J, Costerton JW. Biliary stent blockage with bacterial biofilm. A light and electron microscopy study. Ann Intern Med. 1988;108:546–53.
91. Dasgupta MK, Kowalewaska-Grochowska K, Costerton JW. Biofilm and peritonitis in peritoneal dialysis. Perit Dial Int. 1993;13(Suppl 2):S322–5.
92. Holland SP, Pulido JS, Miller D, Ellis B, Alfonso E, Scott M, Costerton JW. Biofilm and scleral buckle-associated infections. A mechanism for persistence. Ophthalmology. 1991;98:933–8.
93. Arciola CR, Campoccia D, Speziale P, Montanaro L, Costerton JW. Biofilm formation in staphylococcus implant infections. A review of molecular mechanisms and implications for biofilm-resistant materials. Biomaterials. 2012;33:5967–82.
94. Costerton JW, Montanaro L, Arciola CR. Biofilm in implant infections: its production and regulation. Int J Artif Organs. 2005;28:1062–8.
95. Davis LE, Cook G, Costerton JW. Biofilm on ventriculo-peritoneal shunt tubing as a cause of treatment failure in coccidioidal meningitis. Emerg Infect Dis. 2002;8:376–9.
96. Costerton JW. Biofilm theory can guide the treatment of device-related orthopaedic infections. Clin Orthop Relat Res. 2005:7–11.

97. Yousif A, Jamal MA, Raad I. Biofilm-based central line-associated bloodstream infections. Adv Exp Med Biol. 2015;830:157–79.
98. Wolcott RD, Ehrlich GD. Biofilms and chronic infections. JAMA. 2008;299:2682–4.
99. Wolcott RD, Rhoads DD, Dowd SE. Biofilms and chronic wound inflammation. J Wound Care. 2008;17:333–41.
100. James GA, Swogger E, Wolcott R, Pulcini E, Secor P, Sestrich J, Costerton JW, Stewart PS. Biofilms in chronic wounds. Wound Repair Regen. 2008;16:37–44.
101. Kennedy P, Brammah S, Wills E. Burns, biofilm and a new appraisal of burn wound sepsis. Burns. 2010;36:49–56.
102. Stoodley P, Conti SF, DeMeo PJ, Nistico L, Melton-Kreft R, Johnson S, Darabi A, Ehrlich GD, Costerton JW, Kathju S. Characterization of a mixed MRSA/MRSE biofilm in an explanted total ankle arthroplasty. FEMS Immunol Med Microbiol. 2011;62:66–74.
103. Qvist T, Eickhardt S, Kragh KN, Andersen CB, Iversen M, Hoiby N, Bjarnsholt T. Chronic pulmonary disease with Mycobacterium abscessus complex is a biofilm infection. Eur Respir J. 2015;46:1823–6.
104. Clinton A, Carter T. Chronic wound biofilms: pathogenesis and potential therapies. Lab Med. 2015;46:277–84.
105. Wolcott RD, Rhoads DD, Bennett ME, Wolcott BM, Gogokhia L, Costerton JW, Dowd SE. Chronic wounds and the medical biofilm paradigm. J Wound Care. 2010;19:45–6, 48–50, 52–3.
106. Romero R, Schaudinn C, Kusanovic JP, Gorur A, Gotsch F, Webster P, Nhan-Chang CL, Erez O, Kim CJ, Espinoza J, Goncalves LF, Vaisbuch E, Mazaki-Tovi S, Hassan SS, Costerton JW. Detection of a microbial biofilm in intraamniotic infection. Am J Obstet Gynecol. 2008;198(135):e1–5.
107. Bjarnsholt T, Tolker-Nielsen T, Givskov M, Janssen M, Christensen LH. Detection of bacteria by fluorescence in situ hybridization in culture-negative soft tissue filler lesions. Dermatol Surg. 2009;35(Suppl 2):1620–4.
108. Vyas KS, Wong LK. Detection of biofilm in wounds as an early indicator for risk for tissue infection and wound chronicity. Ann Plast Surg. 2016;76:127–31.
109. Hall-Stoodley L, Hu FZ, Gieseke A, Nistico L, Nguyen D, Hayes J, Forbes M, Greenberg DP, Dice B, Burrows A, Wackym PA, Stoodley P, Post JC, Ehrlich GD, Kerschner JE. Direct detection of bacterial biofilms on the middle-ear mucosa of children with chronic otitis media. JAMA. 2006;296:202–11.
110. Elgharably H, Mann E, Awad H, Ganesh K, Ghatak PD, Gordillo G, Sai-Sudhakar CB, Roy S, Wozniak DJ, Sen CK. First evidence of sternal wound biofilm following cardiac surgery. PLoS One. 2013;8:e70360.
111. Xiang J, Sun Z, Song F, Han LZ, Huan JN. [Formation of bacterial biofilm on deep vein catheters in burn patients and its significance]. Zhonghua Shao Shang Za Zhi. 2010;26:95–9.
112. Kowalewska-Grochowska K, Richards R, Moysa GL, Lam K, Costerton JW, King EG. Guidewire catheter change in central venous catheter biofilm formation in a burn population. Chest. 1991;100:1090–5.
113. Dallo SF, Weitao T. Insights into acinetobacter war-wound infections, biofilms, and control. Adv Skin Wound Care. 2010;23:169–74.
114. Homoe P, Bjarnsholt T, Wessman M, Sorensen HC, Johansen HK. Morphological evidence of biofilm formation in Greenlanders with chronic suppurative otitis media. Eur Arch Otorhinolaryngol. 2009;266:1533–8.
115. Stoodley P, Ehrlich GD, Sedghizadeh PP, Hall-Stoodley L, Baratz ME, Altman DT, Sotereanos NG, Costerton JW, Demeo P. Orthopaedic biofilm infections. Curr Orthop Pract. 2011;22:558–63.
116. Schaudinn C, Gorur A, Keller D, Sedghizadeh PP, Costerton JW. Periodontitis: an archetypical biofilm disease. J Am Dent Assoc. 2009;140:978–86.
117. Bjarnsholt T, Jensen PO, Fiandaca MJ, Pedersen J, Hansen CR, Andersen CB, Pressler T, Givskov M, Hoiby N. Pseudomonas aeruginosa biofilms in the respiratory tract of cystic fibrosis patients. Pediatr Pulmonol. 2009;44:547–58.

118. Singh PK, Schaefer AL, Parsek MR, Moninger TO, Welsh MJ, Greenberg EP. Quorum-sensing signals indicate that cystic fibrosis lungs are infected with bacterial biofilms. Nature. 2000;407:762–4.
119. Percival SL, Hill KE, Williams DW, Hooper SJ, Thomas DW, Costerton JW. A review of the scientific evidence for biofilms in wounds. Wound Repair Regen. 2012;20:647–57.
120. Schultz G, Bjarnsholt T, James GA, Leaper DJ, McBain AJ, Malone M, Stoodley P, Swanson T, Tachi M, Wolcott RD. Consensus guidelines for the identification and treatment of biofilms in chronic nonhealing wounds. Wound Repair Regen. 2017;25:744–57.
121. Malone M, Bjarnsholt T, McBain AJ, James GA, Stoodley P, Leaper D, Tachi M, Schultz G, Swanson T, Wolcott RD. The prevalence of biofilms in chronic wounds: a systematic review and meta-analysis of published data. J Wound Care. 2017;26:20–5.
122. Gajula B, Munnamgi S, Basu S. How bacterial biofilms affect chronic wound healing: a narrative review. IJS Glob Health. 2020;3.
123. Alhede M, Bjarnsholt T, Givskov M, Alhede M. Pseudomonas aeruginosa biofilms: mechanisms of immune evasion. Adv Appl Microbiol. 2014;86:1–40.
124. Anwar H, Strap JL, Costerton JW. Growth characteristics and expression of iron-regulated outer-membrane proteins of chemostat-grown biofilm cells of Pseudomonas aeruginosa. Can J Microbiol. 1991;37:737–43.
125. Anwar H, van Biesen T, Dasgupta M, Lam K, Costerton JW. Interaction of biofilm bacteria with antibiotics in a novel in vitro chemostat system. Antimicrob Agents Chemother. 1989;33:1824–6.
126. Davies DG, Parsek MR, Pearson JP, Iglewski BH, Costerton JW, Greenberg EP. The involvement of cell-to-cell signals in the development of a bacterial biofilm. Science. 1998;280:295–8.
127. Drenkard E, Ausubel FM. Pseudomonas biofilm formation and antibiotic resistance are linked to phenotypic variation. Nature. 2002;416:740–3.
128. Ganesh K, Sinha M, Mathew-Steiner SS, Das A, Roy S, Sen CK. Chronic wound biofilm model. Adv Wound Care (New Rochelle). 2015;4:382–8.
129. Liu YJ, Xie J, Zhao LJ, Qian YF, Zhao Y, Liu X. Biofilm formation characteristics of Pseudomonas lundensis isolated from meat. J Food Sci. 2015;80:M2904.
130. Remis JP, Costerton JW, Auer M. Biofilms: structures that may facilitate cell-cell interactions. ISME J. 2010;4:1085–7.
131. Wellman N, Fortun SM, McLeod BR. Bacterial biofilms and the bioelectric effect. Antimicrob Agents Chemother. 1996;40:2012–4.
132. Keller D, Costerton JW. Oral biofilm: entry and immune system response. Compend Contin Educ Dent. 2009;30:24–32; quiz 34, 36.
133. Rhoads DD, Wolcott RD, Percival SL. Biofilms in wounds: management strategies. J Wound Care. 2008;17:502–8.
134. Starkey M, Hickman JH, Ma L, Zhang N, De Long S, Hinz A, Palacios S, Manoil C, Kirisits MJ, Starner TD, Wozniak DJ, Harwood CS, Parsek MR. Pseudomonas aeruginosa rugose small-colony variants have adaptations that likely promote persistence in the cystic fibrosis lung. J Bacteriol. 2009;191:3492–503.
135. Wanger G, Gorby Y, El-Naggar MY, Yuzvinsky TD, Schaudinn C, Gorur A, Sedghizadeh PP. Electrically conductive bacterial nanowires in bisphosphonate-related osteonecrosis of the jaw biofilms. Oral Surg Oral Med Oral Pathol Oral Radiol. 2013;115:71–8.
136. Wolcott R, Costerton JW, Raoult D, Cutler SJ. The polymicrobial nature of biofilm infection. Clin Microbiol Infect. 2013;19:107–12.
137. Wolcott R, Dowd S. The role of biofilms: are we hitting the right target? Plast Reconstr Surg. 2011;127(Suppl 1):28S–35S.
138. FDA. Public workshop-biofilms, medical devices and anti-biofilm technology-challenges and opportunities; 2014.
139. FDA. Draft guidance for industry and FDA Staff-Premarket notification (510(k)) submissions for medical devices that include antimicrobial agents; 2007.
140. FDA. GMPs—Section two: literature review of common food safety problems and applicable controls; 2004.

141. Sullivan TP, Eaglstein WH, Davis SC, Mertz P. The pig as a model for human wound healing. Wound Repair Regen. 2001;9:66–76.
142. Ireton K. Molecular mechanisms of cell-cell spread of intracellular bacterial pathogens. Open Biol. 2013;3:130079.
143. Clark CA, Thomas LK, Azghani AO. Inhibition of protein kinase C attenuates Pseudomonas aeruginosa elastase-induced epithelial barrier disruption. Am J Respir Cell Mol Biol. 2011;45:1263–71.
144. Yang Y, Ma Y, Shi C, Chen H, Zhang H, Chen N, Zhang P, Wang F, Yang J, Yang J, Zhu Q, Liang Y, Wu W, Gao R, Yang Z, Zou Y, Qin H. Overexpression of miR-21 in patients with ulcerative colitis impairs intestinal epithelial barrier function through targeting the Rho GTPase RhoB. Biochem Biophys Res Commun. 2013;434:746–52.
145. Ye D, Guo S, Al-Sadi R, Ma TY. MicroRNA regulation of intestinal epithelial tight junction permeability. Gastroenterology. 2011;141:1323–33.
146. Yi R, O'Carroll D, Pasolli HA, Zhang Z, Dietrich FS, Tarakhovsky A, Fuchs E. Morphogenesis in skin is governed by discrete sets of differentially expressed microRNAs. Nat Genet. 2006;38:356–62.
147. Armstrong DG, Boulton AJM, Bus SA. Diabetic foot ulcers and their recurrence. N Engl J Med. 2017;376:2367–75.
148. Bellini MH, Caldini ET, Scapinelli MP, Simoes MJ, Machado DB, Nurmberg R. Increased elastic microfibrils and thickening of fibroblastic nuclear lamina in canine cutaneous asthenia. Vet Dermatol. 2009;20:139–43.
149. Toledo A, Benach JL. Hijacking and use of host lipids by intracellular pathogens. Microbiol Spectr. 2015;3.
150. Grassme H, Jendrossek V, Riehle A, von Kurthy G, Berger J, Schwarz H, Weller M, Kolesnick R, Gulbins E. Host defense against Pseudomonas aeruginosa requires ceramide-rich membrane rafts. Nat Med. 2003;9:322–30.
151. Dar HH, Tyurina YY, Mikulska-Ruminska K, Shrivastava I, Ting HC, Tyurin VA, Krieger J, St Croix CM, Watkins S, Bayir E, Mao G, Armbruster CR, Kapralov A, Wang H, Parsek MR, Anthonymuthu TS, Ogunsola AF, Flitter BA, Freedman CJ, Gaston JR, Holman TR, Pilewski JM, Greenberger JS, Mallampalli RK, Doi Y, Lee JS, Bahar I, Bomberger JM, Bayir H, Kagan VE. Pseudomonas aeruginosa utilizes host polyunsaturated phosphatidylethanolamines to trigger theft-ferroptosis in bronchial epithelium. J Clin Invest. 2018;128:4639–53.
152. Flohr C, England K, Radulovic S, McLean WH, Campbel LE, Barker J, Perkin M, Lack G. Filaggrin loss-of-function mutations are associated with early-onset eczema, eczema severity and transepidermal water loss at 3 months of age. Br J Dermatol. 2010;163:1333–6.
153. Chamlin SL, Kao J, Frieden IJ, Sheu MY, Fowler AJ, Fluhr JW, Williams ML, Elias PM. Ceramide-dominant barrier repair lipids alleviate childhood atopic dermatitis: changes in barrier function provide a sensitive indicator of disease activity. J Am Acad Dermatol. 2002;47:198–208.
154. Sugarman JL, Fluhr JW, Fowler AJ, Bruckner T, Diepgen TL, Williams ML. The objective severity assessment of atopic dermatitis score: an objective measure using permeability barrier function and stratum corneum hydration with computer-assisted estimates for extent of disease. Arch Dermatol. 2003;139:1417–22.
155. Nikam VN, Monteiro RC, Dandakeri S, Bhat RM. Transepidermal water loss in psoriasis: a case-control study. Indian Dermatol Online J. 2019;10:267–71.
156. Montero-Vilchez T, Segura-Fernández-Nogueras M-V, Pérez-Rodríguez I, Soler-Gongora M, Martinez-Lopez A, Fernández-González A, Molina-Leyva A, Arias-Santiago S. Skin barrier function in psoriasis and atopic dermatitis: transepidermal water loss and temperature as useful tools to assess disease severity. J Clin Med. 2021;10:359.
157. Fluhr JW, Feingold KR, Elias PM. Transepidermal water loss reflects permeability barrier status: validation in human and rodent in vivo and ex vivo models. Exp Dermatol. 2006;15:483–92.
158. Damien F, Boncheva M. The extent of orthorhombic lipid phases in the stratum corneum determines the barrier efficiency of human skin in vivo. J Invest Dermatol. 2010;130:611–4.

159. Ganesh K, Das A, Dixith S, Ghatak PD, Mathew-Steiner S, Schwab E, Khanna S, Wozniak D, Roy S, Sen CK. Electric field based dressing disrupts mixed-species bacterial biofilm infection and restores functional wound healing. Ann Surg. 2019;269(4):756–66.
160. Roy SSS, Das A, Dixith S, Sinha M, Ghatak S, Ghosh N, Banerjee P, Khanna S, Mathew-Steiner S, Das Ghatak P, Blackstone B, Powell HM, Bergdall VK, Wozniak DJ, Sen CK. Staphylococcus aureus biofilm infection compromises wound healing by causing deficiencies in granulation tissue collagen. Ann Surg. 2018;271:1174.

MIX
Papier aus verantwortungsvollen Quellen
Paper from responsible sources
FSC® C105338
www.fsc.org

If you have any concerns about our products,
you can contact us on
ProductSafety@springernature.com

In case Publisher is established outside the EU,
the EU authorized representative is:
Springer Nature Customer Service Center GmbH
Europaplatz 3, 69115 Heidelberg, Germany

Printed by Libri Plureos GmbH
in Hamburg, Germany